Health Care Science Technology

Career Foundations

Kathryn A. Booth, R.N., M.S.

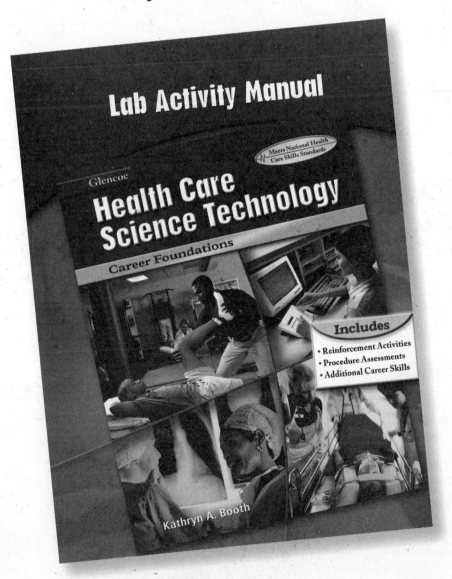

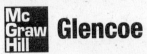

Glencoe

New York, New York   Columbus, Ohio   Chicago, Illinois   Woodland Hills, California

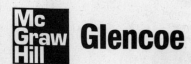

Glencoe

The *McGraw·Hill* Companies

Send all inquiries to:
Glencoe/McGraw-Hill
21600 Oxnard Street, Suite 500
Woodland Hills, CA 91367

ISBN: 0-07-829737-0 *Student Edition*

Printed in the United States of America
6 7 8 9 10 047 08

Safety Notice

The reader is expressly advised to consider and use all safety precautions described in this textbook or that might also be indicated by undertaking the activities described herein. In addition, common sense should be exercised to help avoid all potential hazards and, in particular, to take relevant safety precautions concerning any known or likely hazards involved in health care, or in use of the procedures described in *Health Care Science Technology: Career Foundations,* such as the risk of infection.

Publisher and Author assume no responsibility for the activities of the reader or for the subject matter experts who prepared this book. Publisher and Author make no representation or warranties of any kind, including but not limited to, the warranties of fitness for particular purpose or merchantability, nor for any implied warranties related thereto, or otherwise. Publisher and Author will not be liable for damages of any type, including any consequential, special or exemplary damages resulting, in whole or in part, from reader's use or reliance upon the information, instructions, warnings or other matter contained in this textbook.

Brand Disclaimer

Publisher does not necessarily recommend or endorse any particular company or brand name product that may be discussed or pictured in this textbook. Brand name products are used because they are readily available, likely to be known to the reader, and their use may aid in the understanding of the text. Publisher recognizes that other brand names or generic products may be substituted and work as well or better than those featured in the textbook.

Contents

Preface for the Student

Using the Lab Activity Manual

This Lab Activity Manual has three Parts: Part A, Part B, and Part C. To understand how to use each Part, take a few minutes to read the following.

Part A presents Reinforcement Activities for all chapters and Procedure Assessments for all procedures in the textbook. The Reinforcement Activities consist of several types of questions, including matching, true-false, multiple choice, short answer, and fill-in-the-blank. These questions cover the main points of each chapter. Once you have read the chapter, answer these questions to check your understanding of the information. Ask your teacher to grade your work. Be sure to include your name and the date at the top of each page. Review your graded questions. Then review the information you need to answer correctly the questions you missed.

CHAPTER 4   Name _____   Date _____

First Aid and CPR   Reinforcement Activities

True/False

Write "T" in the blank provided if the statement is true. Write "F" if the statement is false.

_____ 1. Providing first aid correctly can mean the difference between life and death.

_____ 2. First aid providers must assume that all blood and body fluids are infectious.

Your performance of each Procedure in the textbook can be measured through completion of the Procedure Assessment. These follow the Reinforcement Activities. Each Procedure Assessment includes the step-by-step procedure. Each Assessment includes a suggested point value for the correct completion of each step. The following method can help you become proficient in performing the procedures. As you read this, refer to the Procedure Assessment sample on page ix.

1. *Self-practice.* Review the steps for each procedure. Then complete the procedure. Ensure your accuracy by referring to the textbook if necessary. Evaluate your performance in the Self Practice column.

2. *Peer practice.* Complete the procedure with a partner or in a group if a make-believe client is required. During this practice, a student acting as the evaluator can prompt you and alert you to mistakes. If you make a mistake, your evaluator should review the step with you. You should then complete the procedural step correctly. You should then continue the practice. The evaluator should evaluate your performance in the Peer Practice column. Repeat your practice of the procedure until you have correctly completed all of the steps.

3. *Peer testing.* Complete the procedure with a different student evaluator. Complete each step of the procedure. The evaluator should not prompt you or alert you to errors. The evaluator should evaluate your performance in the Peer Testing column. If you miss more than three steps, review the missed steps with the evaluator and complete the procedure again.

4. *Final testing.* Complete the procedure with your teacher or a teacher-designated individual as the evaluator. The evaluator should evaluate your performance in the Final Testing column. The final evaluator will provide the score you will receive on the procedure in the Total Earned column. A Comments section is for the evaluator's comments regarding your performance during practice or testing. The evaluator should include here any suggestions related to steps you performed incorrectly or did not perform. A Signature line and a Date line are provided for the evaluator.

Name _____   Date _____

First Aid and CPR

PROCEDURE 4A2:
Using a Face Shield—No Trauma

PROCEDURE ASSESSMENT

Procedure Steps	Suggested Points	Self Practice	Peer Practice	Peer Testing	Final Testing	Total Earned
PREPROCEDURE						
1. Gather equipment and unwrap face shield.	17					
PROCEDURE						
2. Place face shield over client's mouth.	17					
• Insert shield's extension tube into mouth.	16					
3. Open client's airway, using head tilt-chin lift method.	16					
4. Pinch client's nose and blow into shield's extension tube.	17					

Part B introduces additional career skills relating to many of the textbook chapters. The procedure for each skill contains background information and is presented in a step-by-step format just as in the textbook. If you enjoy or excel in a particular area of health care and would like to learn more, you will find this material useful. Read and review these procedures directly from Part B of this Lab Activity Manual. They may be handy references for you during your job shadowing experience or clinical rotation.

Part C provides a Procedure Assessment for each procedure introduced in Part B. If required by your teacher or facility, you may use these Procedure Assessments for practice and evaluation of any of the procedures.

PART A

Reinforcement Activities and Procedure Assessment

Health Care Career Clusters

Reinforcement Activities

Matching

Write the letter of the phrase that best matches each numbered item in the blank provided. (Answers may be used more than once.)

_____ 1. Administrative medical assistant	**a.** Therapeutic Service Careers.
_____ 2. Medical technologist	**b.** Diagnostic Service Careers.
_____ 3. Advanced practice nurse	**c.** Health Informatics Service Careers.
_____ 4. Geneticist	**d.** Support Services Careers.
_____ 5. Psychologist	**e.** Biotechnology Research and Development Careers.
_____ 6. Biomedical engineer	
_____ 7. Pharmacist	
_____ 8. Chiropractor	
_____ 9. Central supply technician	
_____ 10. Clinical laboratory scientist	
_____ 11. Home health aide	
_____ 12. Toxicologist	

Multiple Choice

Circle the letter that best answers the question or completes the statement.

13. A program of study from a technical school, community college, or state college resulting in an Associate of Applied Science degree is a
    a. one-year program of study.
    b. two-year program of study.
    c. four-year program of study.
    d. six-year program of study.

14. Health informatics service personnel perform
    a. client diagnostic testing.
    b. client recordkeeping.
    c. client safety training.
    d. client meal menu plans.

15. *Robert's Rules of Order, Newly Revised* is meant to serve as
    a. a guideline for proper classroom behavior.
    b. a guideline for conducting meetings.
    c. a guideline for proper job conduct.
    d. a guideline for government employees.

16. The belief that health care workers should understand how their role fits into their department, organization, and the health care environment, falls under which National Health Care Skill Standard?
 a. systems
 b. legal responsibilities
 c. communication
 d. teamwork

17. Health care workers should know the various ways of giving and obtaining information. This statement is part of which National Health Care Skill Standard?
 a. systems
 b. legal responsibilities
 c. communication
 d. teamwork

18. A person who organizes and manages his or her own business is called a/an
 a. professional.
 b. technician.
 c. technologist.
 d. entrepreneur.

19. The first level of the nursing health care career pathway is the profession
 a. nurse practitioner.
 b. nursing assistant.
 c. registered nurse.
 d. licensed vocational nurse.

20. The certified dietary manager career belongs to which career cluster?
 a. Therapeutic Service
 b. Diagnostic Service
 c. Health Informatics Service
 d. Support Services

21. Health care workers should apply knowledge and demonstrate technical skills required within their profession. This is part of which National Health Care Skill Standard?
 a. technical skills
 b. information technology skills
 c. legal responsibilities
 d. systems

22. The career field of bioinformatics was formed by the merging of
 a. biology and health informatics.
 b. health informatics and computer science.
 c. biology and computer science.
 d. computer science and microbiology.

Fill in the Blank

Write the word (or words) that best completes the sentence in the blank provided.

23. A _____ is a chosen profession or occupation.

24. Any career dealing with the administration of treatment falls within the _____ Service Career Pathway.

25. A set of rules to conduct a meeting in an efficient manner is known as

_____.

26. Voting on a _____ can occur by voice, roll call, general consent, division, or ballot.

27. Have a _____ for your meeting, create an _____, and do not allow everyone to _____ at once.

True/False

Write "T" in the blank provided if the statement is true. Write "F" if the statement is false.

_____ **28.** Emergency Medical Services include careers that are categorized in the Therapeutic Service Careers.

_____ **29.** A Diagnostic Service Career worker would identify a particular disease or characteristic of a disease.

_____ **30.** Upon completion of an associate's degree, students may go on and work on their master's degree.

_____ **31.** Continuing education is not necessary for those in the health care industry.

_____ **32.** The degree above a master's degree is a doctorate.

Health Care Systems

Reinforcement Activities

Matching

Write the letter of the phrase that best matches each numbered item in the blank provided.

_____ **1.** HMO

_____ **2.** CDC

_____ **3.** WHO

_____ **4.** Medicare

_____ **5.** Medicaid

a. The national agency responsible for monitoring and prevention of disease.

b. A type of health insurance focusing on wellness and disease prevention.

c. Provides health insurance to people over age 65 as well as those who are disabled or have kidney failure.

d. An international health agency whose goal is to improve all people's level of health.

e. Provides health insurance to certain low-income pregnant women, children, and the aged, blind, and disabled.

Multiple Choice

Circle the letter that best answers the question or completes the statement.

6. Health care organizations that receive financial support primarily by contributions and fundraising events are
   a. health maintenance organizations.
   b. long-term care facilities.
   c. volunteer and nonprofit agencies.
   d. government hospitals.

7. A type of hospital that has shareholders who expect a profit is a
   a. military hospital.
   b. specialty hospital.
   c. religious hospital.
   d. private hospital.

8. Ethical codes still followed by physicians were first practiced by
   a. Rhazes.
   b. Hippocrates.
   c. Galen.
   d. Lister.

9. Facilities that perform tests on blood and other body fluids are
   a. laboratories.
   b. practitioner's offices.
   c. clinics.
   d. out-patient care.

10. If a person does not have health insurance and cannot afford to pay for care, a hospital may
   a. treat the person and reduce fees for all patients.
   b. allow the person to work in trade for services provided.
   c. treat the person and increase fees for all patients.
   d. refer the person to a specialist.

Fill in the Blank

Write the word (or words) that best completes the sentence in the blank provided.

11. An important concern for health care workers and society in general is the demand for health services by the _____ generation.

12. The invention of the _____ in the Renaissance period allowed publication of manuscripts and illustrations of medical discoveries.

13. The amount of money an insured person must pay for services before an insurance company will contribute to the cost of services provided is a _____.

14. _____ includes procedures used by health care workers to prevent the spread of infection.

15. Many surgeries that once required several days' hospitalization are now done in _____.

16. Volunteer health organizations conduct _____, provide _____, and _____ for specific diseases.

True/False

Write "T" in the blank provided if the statement is true. Write "F" if the statement is false.

_____ 17. Home care is often more expensive than care provided in a nursing home or hospital.

_____ 18. The Department of Health and Human Services deals with health issues in the United States.

_____ 19. Some type of health insurance covers every person in the United States.

_____ 20. Prevention of illness is more cost-effective than treating disease.

Matching

Write the letter of the phrase that best matches each numbered item in the blank provided.

_____ 21. Hospital

_____ 22. Long-term care facility

_____ 23. Practitioner's office

_____ 24. Clinics

_____ 25. Laboratories

_____ 26. Emergency medical services

_____ 27. Home health care

_____ 28. Rehabilitation services

_____ 29. Hospices

a. Provide care to ill and injured as quickly as possible.

b. Care for clients who are terminally ill.

c. Includes private, nonprofit, government, and specialized.

d. Clients found here require regular health care services.

e. Tests on blood and other body fluids are performed here.

f. Provides care for acute, sudden, and chronic illness.

g. Helps clients to regain physical and mental abilities.

h. Care is provided in the home.

i. More than one practitioner is usually found here.

Safety and Infection Control Practices

Reinforcement Activities

Matching

Write the letter of the phrase that best matches each numbered item in the blank provided.

_____ **1.** CDC

_____ **2.** Type D fire extinguisher

_____ **3.** Type A fire extinguisher

_____ **4.** OSHA

_____ **5.** Type B fire extinguisher

_____ **6.** Staphylococci

_____ **7.** Streptococci

_____ **8.** Virus

_____ **9.** Fungi

_____ **10.** Spirilla

_____ **11.** Bacilli

a. Fire extinguisher used on paper, cloth, or wood.

b. Fire extinguisher containing carbon dioxide.

c. Fire extinguisher used only on burning metals.

d. Governing agency that oversees disease activity in the United States.

e. Governing agency that oversees the health and welfare of the United States workforce.

f. Corkscrew shaped bacteria

g. Causes ringworm

h. Appears in clusters

i. Appears in chains

j. Smallest microorganism

k. Rod shaped

True/False

Write "T" in the blank provided if the statement is true. Write "F" if the statement is false.

_____ **12.** When moving a heavy object, try to push or pull instead of lifting the item.

_____ **13.** Do not bend your knees when picking up an object off the floor.

_____ **14.** Class B fire extinguishers are to be used on paper fires.

_____ **15.** The proper way to operate a fire extinguisher is to aim at the top of the flame and spray in an up and down motion.

_____ **16.** To gain knowledge about a chemical you are using, you would refer to the MSDS supplied by the chemical's manufacturer.

_____ **17.** RACE is an acronym standing for **R**un away from the fire, **A**ctivate the alarm, **C**onfine personnel, and **E**xtinguish the fire.

_____ **18.** Class D fire extinguishers extinguish combustible metals.

_____ **19.** Disinfection methods kill all microorganisms.

_____ **20.** An electron microscope is needed to view viruses.

_____ **21.** The Brightfield microscope is most commonly used in laboratories.

_____ **22.** The shortest objective is the highest power of magnification on the microscope.

_____ **23.** Rickettsiae are parasites.

_____ **24.** Tuberculosis is caused by a virus.

Multiple Choice

Circle the letter that best answers the question or completes the statement.

25. MSDS is an acronym for
    a. Material Satisfaction Data Sheet.
    b. Multipurpose System Data Sheet.
    c. Material Safety Data Sheet.
    d. Material Safety Development System.

26. The best way to confine a fire is to
    a. fan the fire, pushing the flames in the opposite direction.
    b. close all windows and doors.
    c. open the windows to allow the smoke to escape.
    d. none of the above.

27. The three elements needed to start a fire are
    a. air, oxygen, and fuel.
    b. fuel, heat, and carbon dioxide.
    c. fuel, heat, and oxygen.
    d. oxygen, carbon dioxide, and nitrogen.

28. If you are in serious danger because of a large fire, you should
    a. use the acronym PASS with the fire extinguisher.
    b. evacuate the area quickly.
    c. open all windows to let out the smoke.
    d. leave quickly; everyone else will know there is fire soon enough.

29. When working with a client in a hospital bed, it is best to have the bed at
    a. a safe level for the client.
    b. a good working height for your back.
    c. the lowest possible level.
    d. none of the above.

30. OSHA is a
    a. state agency governing safety in the workplace.
    b. federal agency governing safety in the workplace.
    c. hospital organization agency governing safety in the workplace.
    d. private agency governed by insurance companies.

31. The A in the acronym PASS means
    a. aim at the base of the fire.
    b. activate fire alarm.
    c. announce that you are about to use a fire extinguisher.
    d. always stand 3 feet from a fire when using an extinguisher.

32. Which of the following is most effective in destroying all microorganisms and their spores?
   a. disinfection.
   b. sterilization.
   c. antiseptics.
   d. sanitization.

33. Light in a microscope is controlled by which of the following?
   a. objectives.
   b. mechanical stage.
   c. fine adjustment.
   d. iris diaphragm.

34. Which of the following techniques used by healthcare workers *best* prevents the spread of microorganisms?
   a. sterilization.
   b. handwashing.
   c. disinfection.
   d. isolation.

35. Identify the example listed below of a fomite
   a. staphylococci.
   b. streptococci.
   c. bed linen.
   d. autoclave.

36. A client is admitted to the hospital for eye surgery. The client then acquires a respiratory infection and is said to have which of the following conditions?
   a. tuberculosis.
   b. nosocomial infection.
   c. varicella.
   d. airborne precautions.

37. Which of the following is an example of a systemic response to infection?
   a. fever.
   b. swelling.
   c. redness.
   d. tenderness.

Fill in the Blank
Write the word (or words) that best completes the sentence in the blank provided.

38. A(n) _____ is an instrument used to kill all microorganisms and their spores.

39. Resistant microorganisms that are hard to kill are called _____.

40. Infections capable of being spread to others are called _____.

41. A _____ host is one who is capable of becoming infected.

Name _____ Date _____

42. Medications that are used to kill bacteria are called _____.

43. _____ are guidelines established by the CDC to prevent the spread of infectious diseases.

Labeling

In the space provided, write the word(s) that identifies the corresponding part on the diagram.

44. Label the parts of the microscope in the figure below.

(a.) _____   (g.) _____

(b.) _____   (h.) _____

(c.) _____   (i.) _____

(d.) _____   (j.) _____

(e.) _____   (k.) _____

(f.) _____   (l.) _____

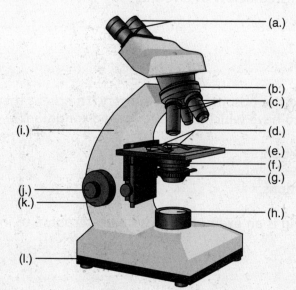

Safety and Infection Control Practices

PROCEDURE 3A:
Using a Fire Extinguisher

········· **PROCEDURE ASSESSMENT** ·········

Procedure Steps	Suggested Points	Self Practice	Peer Practice	Peer Testing	Final Testing	Total Earned
PREPROCEDURE						
1. Gather equipment.	9					
2. Ensure extinguisher can be used on a paper fire.	11					
3. Check charge on extinguisher.	11					
PROCEDURE						
4. Start the PASS procedure.						
• Pull extinguisher's pin and grasp its handle.	11					
• Aim extinguisher at simulated fire's base.	11					
• Squeeze extinguisher's handle.	11					
• Sweep nozzle from side to side.	11					
POSTPROCEDURE						
5. Store extinguisher.	7					
6. Clean area.	7					
7. Recharge extinguisher.	11					
TOTAL POSSIBLE POINTS	100					

Comments:

_____

_____

_____

_____

_____

_____

_____

_____

_____

Signatures: **Date:**

SCORING   *See Preface for scoring instructions.*

Safety and Infection Control Practices

PROCEDURE 3B:
Practicing Proper Body Mechanics

PROCEDURE ASSESSMENT

Procedure Steps	Suggested Points	Self Practice	Peer Practice	Peer Testing	Final Testing	Total Earned
PREPROCEDURE						
1. Gather equipment	3					
2. Place equipment in lab or classroom	3					
PROCEDURE						
3. Begin with good posture						
• Place feet 6 to 10 inches apart	5					
• Keep back straight and head up	5					
• Keep shoulders back and knees flexed	5					
4. Practice lifting object						
• Place object on floor or low table	3					
• Bend from hips and knees	5					
• Keep feet apart and back straight	4					
• Lift object and bring it close to your body	5					
• Set object down	5					
5. Practice moving a heavy object						
• Place object on floor in front of you and place table to your right or left	2					
• Lift object, using back muscles and keeping object close to body	5					
• Pivot and place object on table	5					
• Pick up object from table	5					
• Pivot and place object on floor to your side	4					
• Keep back straight and use hips and knees to lower object	5					
6. Push and pull a heavy object						
• Check and unlock wheels on wheelchair or bed	3					
• Stand behind object	2					
• Keep arms slightly bent and feet apart	5					
• Lean into object and push it 5 feet	5					
• Stop object and lock and unlock wheels	3					
• Pull object back to original location	5					

PROCEDURE 3B: Practicing Proper Body Mechanics *(continued)*

Procedure Steps POSTPROCEDURE	Suggested Points	Self Practice	Peer Practice	Peer Testing	Final Testing	Total Earned
7. Store equipment and clean area	3					
8. Use correct body mechanics	5					
TOTAL POSSIBLE POINTS	100					

Comments:

_____

_____

_____

_____

_____

_____

_____

_____

Signatures: _____ Date: _____

SCORING   *See Preface for scoring instructions.*

Safety and Infection Control Practices

PROCEDURE 3C:
Operating a Microscope

PROCEDURE ASSESSMENT

Procedure Steps	Suggested Points	Self Practice	Peer Practice	Peer Testing	Final Testing	Total Earned
PREPROCEDURE						
1. Gather supplies and equipment	6					
2. Wash hands and put on gloves and face shield	8					
3. Label slides with client's name	5					
4. Plug in microscope and turn on light switch	6					
PROCEDURE						
5. Place specimen slide on stage, frosted end up	5					
6. Carefully raise substage so it doesn't touch slide	6					
7. Turn revolving nosepiece to 10X and focus coarse-adjustment dial	5					
8. Turn fine-adjustment dial	6					
9. Adjust substage diaphragm level or mirror for correct lighting	6					
10. Turn nosepiece to intermediate-power objective and adjust fine-focus dial	5					
11. Use oil sparingly when using oil-immersion lens objective or high-power field	6					
12. After identifying specimen, properly dispose of biohazardous material	7					
POSTPROCEDURE						
13. Clean ocular lens	5					
14. Turn off microscope light and store equipment	5					
15. Disinfect work area	7					
16. Remove gloves and face shield and wash hands	7					
17. Record test results	5					
TOTAL POSSIBLE POINTS	**100**					

Comments: _____

_____

_____

_____

Signatures: _____ Date: _____

SCORING *See Preface for scoring instructions.*

Safety and Infection Control Practices

PROCEDURE 3D:
Hand Washing

PROCEDURE ASSESSMENT

Procedure Steps	Suggested Points	Self Practice	Peer Practice	Peer Testing	Final Testing	Total Earned
PREPROCEDURE						
1. Remove rings and other jewelry	7					
2. Gather supplies and equipment	7					
3. Turn on water and adjust temperature	6					
PROCEDURE						
4. Wet hands thoroughly	8					
5. Lather up with soap	8					
6. Rub hands together	7					
7. Rinse with fingers pointed downward	7					
8. Lather up with soap again	8					
9. Clean fingernails with orange stick or nail brush	7					
10. Rinse with fingers pointed downward	7					
11. Use paper towel to turn off faucet	8					
12. Dry hands with paper towels, then discard towels	7					
POSTPROCEDURE						
13. Clean area without recontaminating hands	7					
14. Apply lotion, if desired	6					
TOTAL POSSIBLE POINTS	100					

Comments: _____

_____

_____

_____

_____

_____

_____

_____

Signatures: _____   **Date:** _____

SCORING   *See Preface for scoring instructions.*

Safety and Infection Control Practices

PROCEDURE 3E:
Donning and Removing Personal Protective Equipment

PROCEDURE ASSESSMENT

Procedure Steps	Suggested Points	Self Practice	Peer Practice	Peer Testing	Final Testing	Total Earned
PREPROCEDURE						
1. Gather supplies	3					
2. Remove jewelry and watch	2					
3. Wash hands	5					
PROCEDURE						
4. Put on a facemask and goggles or mask with face shield						
• Cover mouth and nose with mask and place bendable strip over nose	4					
• Tie upper strings at back of head or pull elastic band around head	3					
• Tie lower strings at neck, ensuring mask covers chin	3					
• Pinch bendable metal strip over nose	4					
5. Put on gown						
• Unfold gown and pull sleeves up arms, with opening in back	4					
• Tie gown at neck	3					
• Overlap gown at back to close it	4					
• Tie gown at waist	3					
6. Put on gloves	4					
7. Pull glove cuffs up over sleeves	2					
8. Provide client care as required	2					
POSTPROCEDURE						
9. Remove gloves						
• Remove first glove by grasping it below cuff	4					
• Pull glove down over hand so it is inside out	4					
• Hold removed glove with other gloved hand	2					
• Reach inside other glove with first two fingers of ungloved hand	2					
• Pull glove down, inside out, over other glove	3					
• Place gloves in biohazardous waste container	4					

PROCEDURE 3E: Donning and Removing Personal Protective Equipment (continued)

Procedure Steps	Suggested Points	Self Practice	Peer Practice	Peer Testing	Final Testing	Total Earned
POSTPROCEDURE						
10. Wash hands	5					
11. Remove gown						
• Untie gown at neck	3					
• Reach inside gown to opposite shoulder and remove gown	2					
• Reach other arm inside sleeve and pull it down	3					
• Hold gown away from you as you fold it inside out	2					
• Place gown in biohazardous waste container	4					
12. Wash hands	5					
13. Remove mask						
• Touch only strings	3					
• Place mask in biohazardous waste container	3					
14. Wash hands	5					
TOTAL POSSIBLE POINTS	100					

Comments: _____

_____

_____

_____

_____

_____

_____

_____

_____

Signatures: _____ **Date:** _____

SCORING *See Preface for scoring instructions.*

First Aid and CPR

Reinforcement Activities

True/False

Write "T" in the blank provided if the statement is true. Write "F" if the statement is false.

_____ 1. Providing first aid correctly can mean the difference between life and death.

_____ 2. First aid providers must assume that all blood and body fluids are infectious.

_____ 3. The purpose of the initial assessment is to identify and provide first aid for life-threatening conditions.

_____ 4. When performing a physical exam, you generally start at the feet and work your way up the body.

_____ 5. Tapping the client's shoulder is one way to help determine the client's level of responsiveness.

_____ 6. For adult one person and two people CPR, give 5 compressions followed by 1 ventilation.

_____ 7. Direct pressure and a tourniquet are the best methods of controlling bleeding.

_____ 8. Anaphylaxis presents with severe chest pain radiating down the right arm.

_____ 9. When washing chemicals off the body, flush with water for 10 minutes.

_____ 10. If you suspect an electrical injury, be sure to turn off the power before touching the client.

_____ 11. Always check the scene of an accident or illness and make sure it is safe to approach before offering your assistance.

_____ 12. Never move a client involved in an accident, unless there is a danger of further injury.

_____ 13. To provide rescue breaths to an infant, cover the infant's nose and mouth with your mouth.

_____ 14. A second-degree burn involves an injury to the outer layer of skin only.

_____ 15. First aid for a minor first or second-degree burn is to cool the area with water.

_____ 16. During a grand mal epileptic seizure, the client may soil their clothes.

_____ 17. The most severe bleeding usually comes from veins.

_____ 18. If possible, one of the treatments to stop severe bleeding is elevation of the wound.

_____ 19. A third-degree burn is less serious than a first-degree burn.

_____ 20. The purpose of rescue breathing is to relieve the obstructed windpipe or airway of an unconscious person.

_____ 21. The purpose of cardiopulmonary resuscitation (CPR) is to restore blood circulation as well as airflow into the lungs.

_____ 22. The client's blood is bright red and gushing forth in spurts synchronized with the client's pulse. This bleeding must be from a vein.

_____ 23. For an adult client requiring CPR, provide chest compressions at a rate of 100 per minute.

_____ 24. Pack an amputated finger directly in ice and call EMS.

_____ 25. If a client is in shock, you should elevate the feet 6 to 8 inches.

_____ 26. Chemical splashes to the skin or eyes require 10 minutes of flushing with water.

Matching

Write the letter of the phrase that best matches each numbered item in the blank provided.

_____ 27. Anaphylaxis

_____ 28. Heart attack

_____ 29. Heat cramps

_____ 30. Barrier devices

_____ 31. Stroke

_____ 32. Cardiac arrest

_____ 33. Symptom

_____ 34. Shock

_____ 35. Burn

_____ 36. Sign

a. Disruption of the blood supply to the brain which causes neurological impairment.

b. Devices used in rescue breathing.

c. Evidence for a disease or injury that is physically observed, felt or heard.

d. Severe life threatening allergic reaction affecting all body systems.

e. An injury to the skin and underlying tissues caused by heat.

f. A state of poor tissue perfusion.

g. Caused by blockage of a coronary artery.

h. A sudden and unexpected stopping of the heart.

i. Evidence for a disease or injury that is relayed to the rescuer by the client.

j. Painful muscle contractions resulting from exposure to heat.

Multiple Choice

Circle the letter that best answers the question or completes the statement.

37. The first action you take in an emergency is
    a. open the airway.
    b. assess the scene for dangers.
    c. determine unresponsiveness.
    d. determine what is wrong with the client.

38. Which of the following signs or symptoms best describes a heart attack?
    a. shortness of breath.
    b. a headache that does not get better.
    c. sharp stabbing chest pains that last only a few seconds.
    d. squeezing or crushing discomfort behind the breastbone that lasts more than a few minutes.

39. Which of the following signs or symptoms best describes a client having a stroke?
    a. chest pain, fatigue, nausea, and vomiting.
    b. no response, chest pain, and shortness of breath.
    c. facial droop, arm weakness, and slurred speech.
    d. sharp, stabbing chest pains with nausea and vomiting.

40. What is the best sign that your rescue breaths are providing air to the client's lungs?
    a. you can feel a pulse.
    b. the client's color changes.
    c. it is not possible to tell this.
    d. the client's chest rises with each breath.

41. What is the ratio of chest compressions to breaths when two people are providing CPR on an adult?
    a. 5:1
    b. 5:2
    c. 15:1
    d. 30:2

42. Signs of internal injuries include all of the following, except
    a. bright red blood spurting from an extremity.
    b. vomiting a coffee ground-like substance.
    c. bleeding from rectum.
    d. dark, tarry stools.

43. The best way to control a bleeding wound is to
    a. apply a tourniquet.
    b. apply direct pressure.
    c. cover the wound with a loose dressing then apply an ice pack.
    d. cover the wound with a bandage and apply a loose dressing.

44. The signs and symptoms of shock include which of the following?
  a. altered mental status.
  b. pink, cool, clammy skin.
  c. normal breathing.
  d. slow heart rate.

45. Other care for clients in shock includes all of the following except
  a. loosening tight clothing.
  b. maintaining an open airway.
  c. giving the client water if the client is thirsty to prevent dehydration.
  d. covering the client to keep the client warm if in a cold environment.

46. The first step a first-aid provider should take in making the initial assessment is
  a. assess the client's airway.
  b. assess the client's breathing.
  c. assess the client's signs of circulation.
  d. assess the client's level of responsiveness.

47. When in the process of assessing your client you encounter a life-threatening major bleed, you should
  a. stop your assessment and call EMS immediately.
  b. continue your assessment and treat life-threatening injuries after the assessment is complete.
  c. stop your assessment and treat the major bleed as soon as you discover it.
  d. stop your assessment of the client and ask about past medical problems.

48. Anaphylactic shock is caused by
  a. burns.
  b. severe infection.
  c. allergic reactions.
  d. severe blood loss.

49. The type of injury when toes, hands, feet, or other limbs are completely cut through or torn off is known as
  a. avulsion.
  b. puncture.
  c. amputation.
  d. laceration.

50. The first step a first-aid provider should take in treating a bleeding wound is to
  a. clean the wound with soap and water.
  b. control bleeding with direct pressure.
  c. further expose the wound.
  d. treat for shock.

51. Burns involving the skin are classified as
  a. superficial.
  b. full-thickness burns.
  c. partial-thickness burns.
  d. all of the above.

52. All of the following are ways of caring for a burn victim except
   a. *do not* remove rings or jewelry.
   b. wrap burned area with sterile dressing.
   c. check the ABC's and treat for shock.
   d. cool burning area with water, then remove clothing.

53. Using the rule of nines, what percentage of the body would be burned if the entire back, and one leg and both arms were involved?
   a. 18 percent
   b. 36 percent
   c. 54 percent
   d. 72 percent

54. When treating burns the first aider should *not*
   a. apply ointments, sprays, or butter.
   b. cool the burn with water.
   c. leave any blisters unbroken.
   d. remove any rings or jewelry.

55. The primary first aid procedure for chemical burns is to wash away the chemical with flowing water for a period of
   a. 5 minutes.
   b. 10 minutes.
   c. 15 minutes.
   d. 20 minutes.

56. The American Heart Association has summarized the most important factors that affect survival of cardiac arrest in its "Chain of Survival" concept. Which of the following are parts of that concept?
   a. early access and CPR.
   b. early defibrillation.
   c. early advanced care.
   d. all of the above.

57. One of the first steps in treating a client who is suffering from an inhaled poison is to
   a. remove contaminated clothing.
   b. remove the person from the source.
   c. perform a head to toe examination.
   d. open the airway and perform rescue breathing.

58. Signs and symptoms of carbon monoxide poisoning include
   a. pale skin.
   b. dizziness.
   c. slow heart beat.
   d. chest pain radiating down the left arm.

59. Signs and symptoms of a musculoskeletal injury include all of the following, except
   a. pain at the site of injury
   b. swelling
   c. deformity
   d. nausea

60. Signs and symptoms of hypothermia include all of the following except
    a. shivering.
    b. cool abdomen.
    c. joint/muscle stiffness.
    d. alterations in mental status.

61. Which of the following is a true emergency and requires rapid cooling and immediate transport to the hospital?
    a. heat stroke.
    b. heat cramps.
    c. heat exhaustion.
    d. first-degree burn.

62. The signs and symptoms of heat stroke include
    a. lack of sweating with red skin.
    b. cool moist skin.
    c. nausea and vomiting.
    d. severe cramps in the legs.

63. When assessing a client's ABCs the "B" stands for
    a. breather.
    b. breathing.
    c. bleeding.
    d. basic.

64. When checking for breathing, the first-aid provider should move the client onto the
    a. left side.
    b. right side.
    c. stomach with face down.
    d. back with face up.

65. When determining adequate or inadequate breathing, the first-aid provider should look for chest rise and fall and listen and feel for air exchange at the
    a. nose only.
    b. chest.
    c. mouth only.
    d. nose and mouth.

66. The very first step to aid a client who is not breathing is to
    a. establish responsiveness.
    b. open the airway.
    c. check for breathing.
    d. check for signs of circulation.

67. The recommended maneuver for opening the airway of a client with possible head, neck or back injury is the
    a. head-tilt.
    b. jaw-thrust.
    c. head-tilt, neck lift.
    d. head-tilt, chin-lift.

68. Finger sweeps are used in infants and children
    a. after opening the airway.
    b. after administering back blows.
    c. after administering chest thrusts.
    d. at no time unless you can actually see the obstruction.

69. Which of the following is the correct order in clearing the airway of an unconscious infant?
    a. 5 chest thrusts, 5 back blows, look for and remove any visible objects, attempt to ventilation.
    b. look for and remove any visible objects, attempt to ventilate, 5 chest thrusts, 5 back blows.
    c. 5 back blows, 5 chest thrusts, look for and remove any visible objects, attempt to ventilate.
    d. look for and remove any visible objects, 5 chest thrusts, attempt to ventilate, 5 back blows.

70. If vinyl or latex gloves are not available when performing first aid, what should you do?
    a. if first aid is being given, gloves are not needed.
    b. find a substitute such as plastic bags or thick towels.
    c. wait for emergency assistance to arrive to start first aid.
    d. call EMS immediately.

71. You know that you have successfully cleared the airway when
    a. the chest rises and falls.
    b. the client regains consciousness.
    c. the tongue is no longer obstructing the airway.
    d. the foreign object is expelled from the mouth.

72. During CPR what should you do after determining that the adult client is not breathing?
    a. start chest compressions.
    b. check for signs of circulation.
    c. give 2 breaths, taking one second per breath.
    d. give 2 breaths, taking 3-5 seconds per breath.

73. In the ABC method of cardiopulmonary resuscitation, the C stands for
    a. open the airway.
    b. check for breathing.
    c. check for signs of circulation.
    d. provide chest compressions.

74. The compression rate for 1-rescuer adult CPR is
    a. 80 to 100 per minute.
    b. 60-100 per minute.
    c. 60-80 per minute.
    d. 100 per minute.

75. The ratio of ventilations to compressions during 1-rescuer adult CPR is
    a. 2 every 30 compressions.
    b. 2 every 5 compressions.
    c. 1 every 15 compressions.
    d. 1 every 5 compressions.

76. What is the ratio of ventilations to compressions on an infant in one-rescuer CPR?
    a. 1 ventilation to 3 compressions.
    b. 1 ventilation to 5 compressions.
    c. 2 ventilations to 30 compressions.
    d. 1 ventilations to 15 compressions.

77. On an adult client, the CPR compression site is
    a. the center of the chest, between the nipples.
    b. centered on the upper half of the sternum.
    c. centered in the middle of the sternum.
    d. centered one finger below the nipples.

78. Once CPR has been started it should be continued until any of the following except
    a. there is a return of circulation.
    b. you are too exhausted to continue.
    c. the family of the client tells you to stop.
    d. you turn care over to another trained rescuer of equal or a higher level of training.

79. Give sugar to a client if which of the following criteria are true?
    a. the client is alert enough to swallow.
    b. the client's mental status is altered.
    c. the client has a history of diabetes.
    d. all the above.

80. In caring for a seizing client remember
    a. protect the client from embarrassment.
    b. place a padded tongue depressor or similar object in the mouth to prevent the client from biting his or her tongue.
    c. hold the client still so that he does not injure himself.
    d. never place anything in his mouth.

First Aid and CPR

PROCEDURE 4A1:
Using a Face Mask—No Trauma

P R O C E D U R E   A S S E S S M E N T

Procedure Steps	Suggested Points	Self Practice	Peer Practice	Peer Testing	Final Testing	Total Earned
PREPROCEDURE						
1. Obtain the correct size of face mask.	6					
2. Stand by client's head and open the airway.	7					
PROCEDURE						
3. If you are a lone rescuer, use the side technique:	5					
• Put mask on client's face so top is over bridge of nose and base is between lower lip and chin.	4					
• Position yourself so you can perform rescue breaths and CPR.	4					
• Seal mask's upper edge with one hand.	4					
• Hold down mask's lower edge with thumb of other hand, then use fingers to execute chin lift.	4					
• Compress mask to create seal.	4					
4. If there are two rescuers, use the head technique:	5					
• Put mask on client's face so apex is over bridge of nose and base is between lower lip and chin.	4					
• Position yourself at client's head.	4					
• Hold down mask's lower edge with both thumbs.	4					
• Use fingers to lift jaw and tilt head back.	4					
• Squeeze mask against client's face.	4					
• Squeeze firmly to make airtight seal.	4					
5. Take a deep breath and blow into mask's valve.	6					
6. Deliver rescue breaths:	7					
• 1 second/breath for an adult						
• 1 second/breath for a child or infant						
7. Watch for client's chest to rise.	6					
8. Take mouth from valve and allow air to escape.	7					

PROCEDURE 4A1: Using a Face Mask—No Trauma *(continued)*

Procedure Steps POSTPROCEDURE	Suggested Points	Self Practice	Peer Practice	Peer Testing	Final Testing	Total Earned
9. Deliver rescue breaths until client recovers or help arrives.	7					
TOTAL POSSIBLE POINTS	100					

Comments: _____

_____

_____

_____

_____

_____

_____

_____

_____

Signatures: _____ **Date:** _____

SCORING *See Preface for scoring instructions.*

First Aid and CPR

PROCEDURE 4A2:
Using a Face Shield—No Trauma

PROCEDURE ASSESSMENT

Procedure Steps	Suggested Points	Self Practice	Peer Practice	Peer Testing	Final Testing	Total Earned
PREPROCEDURE						
1. Gather equipment and unwrap face shield.	17					
PROCEDURE						
2. Place face shield over client's mouth.	17					
• Insert shield's extension tube into mouth.	16					
3. Open client's airway, using chin lift method.	16					
4. Pinch client's nose and blow into shield's extension tube.	17					
POSTPROCEDURE						
5. Continue rescue breaths until client recovers or help arrives.	17					
TOTAL POSSIBLE POINTS	100					

Comments: _____

_____

_____

_____

_____

_____

_____

_____

_____

_____

Signatures: _____   **Date:** _____

SCORING   *See Preface for scoring instructions.*

Name _____   Date _____

First Aid and CPR

PROCEDURE 4A3:
Using a Two-Rescuer Bag-Valve Mask—No Trauma

P R O C E D U R E   A S S E S S M E N T

Procedure Steps	Suggested Points	Self Practice	Peer Practice	Peer Testing	Final Testing	Total Earned
PREPROCEDURE						
1. Gather equipment.	8					
2. Position yourself at top of client's head.	7					
3. Open client's airway using chin lift method.	8					
PROCEDURE						
4. Place your thumbs over top of mask and index and middle fingers over bottom of mask.	7					
5. Place top of mask over bridge of client's nose.	10					
• Lower mask over mouth and lower chin.	8					
6. Use your ring and pinky fingers to pull client's jaw toward you.	9					
7. Operate bag-valve mask:	10					
• First rescuer: Maintain mask seal and head tilt.	8					
• Second rescuer: Connect bag to mask and squeeze bag until chest rises. Squeeze every 5-6 seconds for adult and every 3-5 seconds for infant or child.	8					
8. Second rescuer: Release pressure on bag, allowing it to refill with air.	8					
POSTPROCEDURE						
9. Provide rescue breaths until client recovers or help arrives.	9					
TOTAL POSSIBLE POINTS	100					

Comments: _____

_____

_____

_____

_____

_____

_____

Signatures: _____   Date: _____

SCORING   See Preface for scoring instructions.

First Aid and CPR

PROCEDURE 4A4:
Using a One-Rescuer Bag-Valve Mask—No Trauma

························· PROCEDURE ASSESSMENT ·························

Procedure Steps	Suggested Points	Self Practice	Peer Practice	Peer Testing	Final Testing	Total Earned
PREPROCEDURE						
1. Gather equipment.	9					
2. Position yourself at top of client's head.	9					
3. Open client's airway using head tilt-chin lift method.	10					
PROCEDURE						
4. Place top of mask over bridge of client's nose.	12					
• Lower mask over mouth and upper chin.	10					
5. Use thumb and index finger to form a "C" around ventilation port of mask.	12					
• Use other fingers to hold client's jaw to mask; these fingers should form an "E" on the jaw.	10					
6. Use other hand to squeeze bag:	9					
• Every 5-6 seconds for adult.						
• Every 3-5 seconds for infant or child.						
7. Release pressure on bag; allow bag to refill with air.	10					
POSTPROCEDURE						
8. Provide rescue breaths until client recovers or help arrives.	9					
TOTAL POSSIBLE POINTS	100					

Comments: _____
_____
_____
_____
_____
_____
_____
_____
_____
_____

Signatures: _____   **Date:** _____

SCORING   *See Preface for scoring instructions.*

First Aid and CPR

PROCEDURE 4B1:
One-Rescuer Cardiopulmonary Resuscitation—Adult

PROCEDURE ASSESSMENT

Procedure Steps	Suggested Points	Self Practice	Peer Practice	Peer Testing	Final Testing	Total Earned
PREPROCEDURE						
1. Check client's responsiveness:	3					
• Tap client's shoulder.	2					
• Shout, "Are you OK?"	2					
2. If client is unresponsive, shout for help or call 911.	3					
PROCEDURE						
3. Open client's airway:	3					
• Tilt head back using chin lift method.	2					
a. If you think client has neck or back injury, use jaw thrust method.						
• Remove obstructions from client's mouth.	2					
4. Check for breathing:	3					
• Put your ear next to client's mouth and watch chest.	2					
• Look for chest movement, listen for breaths, and feel for air movement.	2					
• If client is breathing, put him in recovery position:	3					
a. Kneel beside client and place nearest arm straight out from body.	2					
b. Position other arm with back of hand against client's cheek.	2					
c. Grab and bend client's knee opposite you.	2					
d. Protect client's head and pull opposite knee over and to ground.	2					
e. Position top leg to balance client on his side.	2					
f. Tilt head up, make sure hand is under cheek and cover client with blanket.	2					
• If client isn't breathing/is breathing weakly, give 2 rescue breaths, 1 second per breath, using one of these methods:	3					
a. Mouth-to-mouth or mouth-to-nose.	2					
b. Mouth-to-mask device.	2					
c. Bag-valve mask ventilation.	2					

Procedure Steps	Suggested Points	Self Practice	Peer Practice	Peer Testing	Final Testing	Total Earned
PROCEDURE						
• Make sure client's chest is rising/falling. If not, reposition airway. If chest still does not rise, client may have airway obstruction.	2					
5. Check for signs of circulation:	3					
• Check for breathing, coughing, movement, and normal skin color.	2					
• Check for carotid pulse.	2					
a. Locate client's trachea with your index and middle fingers.	2					
b. Put fingers into groove between trachea and side of neck.	2					
c. Feel for pulse for 5 to 10 seconds.	2					
• If client isn't breathing, but you see signs of circulation, give rescue breaths every 5-6 seconds.	2					
• If you can't find pulse/circulation, start CPR and prepare to use AED, if available.	2					
6. Perform chest compressions:	3					
• Unless you suspect neck or back injury, move the client to a firm surface such as the ground or floor.	2					
• Place the heel of one hand on the center of the chest between the nipples.	2					
• Place the other hand on top of the first.	3					
• Lean forward so your shoulders are over client; keep arms straight.	2					
• Keep heel of hand on chest, but don't touch chest with fingers.	2					
• Give 30 chest compressions at rate of 100 per minute, then 2 rescue breaths.	2					
• With each compression, push down on breast bone 1½ to 2 inches.	2					
• Let chest return to normal state between compressions.	2					
• Do 5 cycles (2 minutes) of 30 compressions/2 breaths.	2					

Procedure Steps	Suggested Points	Self Practice	Peer Practice	Peer Testing	Final Testing	Total Earned
POSTPROCEDURE						
7. After you perform CPR, recheck circulation:	3					
• After 5 cycles of 30 to 2, recheck for signs of circulation.	2					
• If still no breathing/circulation, resume CPR, starting with compressions.	2					
• If you see signs of circulation but no breathing, give rescue breaths every 5-6 seconds.	2					
• Recheck for signs of circulation every few minutes.	2					
TOTAL POSSIBLE POINTS	100					

Comments:

_____

_____

_____

_____

_____

_____

_____

_____

_____

_____

Signatures: _____ **Date:** _____

SCORING   *See Preface for scoring instructions.*

Name _____   Date _____

First Aid and CPR

PROCEDURE 4B2:
Two-Rescuer Cardiopulmonary Resuscitation—Adult

-------- **PROCEDURE ASSESSMENT** --------

Procedure Steps	Suggested Points	Self Practice	Peer Practice	Peer Testing	Final Testing	Total Earned
PREPROCEDURE						
1. Check client's responsiveness.	4					
2. Call EMS.	4					
PROCEDURE (Rescuer 1)						
3. Open airway and check for breathing.	5					
4. If client isn't breathing/is breathing weakly, give 2 rescue breaths, 1 second per breath.	4					
a. If chest doesn't rise/fall, reposition airway.	4					
5. Check for signs of circulation:	5					
a. Check for breathing, coughing, movement, and normal skin color.	4					
b. Check for carotid pulse for 5 to 10 seconds.	4					
c. If client isn't breathing, but you see signs of circulation, give rescue breaths every 5-6 seconds.	4					
d. If you can't find pulse/circulation, start CPR and prepare to use AED, if available.	4					
PROCEDURE (Rescuer 2)						
6. Perform CPR:	5					
a. Unless you suspect neck or back injury, move the client to a firm surface such as the ground or floor.						
b. Place the heel of one hand on the center of the chest between the nipples.	4					
c. Put the other hand over the first.	4					
d. Lean forward so your shoulders are over client; keep arms straight.	4					
e. Keep heel of hand on chest, but don't touch chest with fingers.	4					
f. Give 30 chest compressions at rate of 100 per minute, then 2 rescue breaths.	4					
g. With each compression, push down on breast bone 1½ to 2 inches.	4					

PROCEDURE 4B2: Two-Rescuer Cardiopulmonary Resuscitation—Adult *(continued)*

Procedure Steps	Suggested Points	Self Practice	Peer Practice	Peer Testing	Final Testing	Total Earned
h. Let chest return to normal state between compressions.	4					
i. Do 5 cycles (2 minutes) of 30 compressions/2 breaths.	4					
POSTPROCEDURE						
7. Recheck circulation:	5					
• After 5 cycles of 30 to 2, recheck for signs of circulation.	4					
• If still no breathing/circulation, resume CPR, starting with compressions.	4					
• If you see signs of circulation but no breathing, give rescue breaths every 5-6 seconds.	4					
• Recheck for signs of circulation every few minutes or until EMS arrives.	4					
TOTAL POSSIBLE POINTS	**100**					

Comments:

_____

_____

_____

_____

_____

_____

_____

_____

_____

Signatures: _____   Date: _____

SCORING   *See Preface for scoring instructions.*

First Aid and CPR

PROCEDURE 4B3:
Cardiopulmonary Resuscitation for Infants and Children

P R O C E D U R E A S S E S S M E N T

Procedure Steps	Suggested Points	Self Practice	Peer Practice	Peer Testing	Final Testing	Total Earned
PREPROCEDURE						
1. Check for responsiveness:	4					
• Tap child on shoulder. Tap infant on soles of feet.	2					
• Shout, "Are you OK?"	2					
• Send someone to call EMS. If you are alone, continue assessment.	2					
2. If client is unresponsive, place client face up on firm surface, like floor.	4					
PROCEDURE						
3. Open airway:	4					
• Tilt head back using head tilt-chin lift method.	2					
• With pinky finger, remove obstructions, if any, from mouth.	2					
a. Don't perform blind finger sweeps.	1					
• If you think client has neck/back injury, use jaw thrust method.	2					
4. Check for breathing:	2					
• Put your ear next to client's mouth and watch chest.	2					
• Look for chest movement, listen for breaths, and feel for air movement.	2					
• If client is breathing and has no back/ neck injury, put him in recovery position.	2					
• If client isn't breathing/is breathing weakly, give 2 gentle rescue breaths, 1 second per breath.	2					
• If a barrier device or bag-valve mask is available, use it. Be sure to follow the recommended procedures for using these devices.	2					
• To give rescue breaths to infant:	3					
a. Cover infant's mouth and nose with your mouth.	1					
b. If your mouth is small, cover infant's mouth with your mouth and pinch the nose closed with your fingers.	1					
c. Deliver rescue breaths.	1					
• To give rescue breaths to child:	3					
a. Cover child's mouth with your mouth.	1					
b. Pinch child's nose closed with your fingers.	1					
c. Deliver rescue breaths.	1					

PROCEDURE 4B3: Cardiopulmonary Resuscitation for Infants and Children (continued)

Procedure Steps	Suggested Points	Self Practice	Peer Practice	Peer Testing	Final Testing	Total Earned
• Watch for chest to rise; allow for exhalation between breaths.	2					
• Use barrier device or bag-valve mask, if available.	2					
5. Check for signs of circulation	4					
• Check for breathing, coughing, movement, and normal skin color.	2					
• Check for pulse. For child, use carotid pulse in neck; for infant, use brachial pulse.	2					
a. To find brachial pulse, feel on inner side of upper arm between elbow and armpit.	1					
b. Feel for pulse for 5 to 10 seconds.	1					
• If client isn't breathing, but you see signs of circulation and heart rate is above 60 beats per minute (in infant):	2					
a. Instead of chest compressions, give gentle rescue breaths every 3-5 seconds.	1					
• If you can't find pulse/circulation or if heart rate is less than 60 beats per minute with poor circulation (in infant), start CPR.	2					
6. Perform CPR:	4					
• For infants, follow these steps:	3					
a. Imagine line drawn from one nipple to other nipple.	1					
b. Put two fingers of one hand midway between nipples and one finger's width below imaginary line.	1					
c. Maintain airway with other hand. Compress breastbone with fingers, about ⅓ to ½ the depth of the chest. Make sure your fingers aren't on very bottom of breastbone.	1					
d. Give 30 compressions, at a rate of 100 per minute, followed by 2 ventilations.	1					
e. After 2 minutes of CPR, check for signs of circulation. If you are alone, activate EMS.	1					
f. If you don't see signs of circulation or if heart rate is less than 60 beats per minute with poor circulation, resume 30 to 2 cycle, starting with compressions.	1					
g. If you see signs of good circulation and heart rate is above 60 beats per minute, but breathing is absent or poor, continue rescue breaths every 3-5 seconds.	1					

PROCEDURE 4B3: Cardiopulmonary Resuscitation for Infants and Children (continued)

Procedure Steps	Suggested Points	Self Practice	Peer Practice	Peer Testing	Final Testing	Total Earned
h. If infant starts breathing and has no head/neck injuries, put him in recovery position.	1					
i. Otherwise, continue CPR, checking every few minutes for signs of circulation.	1					
• For children, follow these steps:	3					
a. Locate middle of breastbone (sternum).	1					
b. Put heel of one or both hands (depending on size of child) on lower half of sternum, between the nipples.	1					
c. Compress sternum $\frac{1}{3}$ to $\frac{1}{2}$ the depth of the chest. Give 30 compressions, at rate of 100 per minute, then give 2 rescue breaths.	1					
d. Release chest to allow it to expand, but don't take hand away.	1					
e. Continue 30 to 2 cycle; after 2 minutes, check for signs of circulation. If you are alone, activate EMS.	1					
f. If you don't see signs of circulation, resume 30 to 2 cycle, starting with compressions.	1					
g. If you see signs of circulation, but breathing is absent or poor, continue rescue breaths every 3-5 seconds.	1					
h. If child starts breathing and has no head/neck injuries, put him in recovery position.	1					
i. Otherwise, continue CPR, checking every few minutes for signs of circulation.	1					
POSTPROCEDURE						
7. Continue CPR and rescue breathing or remain with client until EMS arrives.	4					
TOTAL POSSIBLE POINTS	100					

Comments:

Signatures: Date:

SCORING   *See Preface for scoring instructions.*

First Aid and CPR

PROCEDURE 4C1:
Foreign Body Airway Obstruction in a Responsive Adult or Child

PROCEDURE ASSESSMENT

Procedure Steps	Suggested Points	Self Practice	Peer Practice	Peer Testing	Final Testing	Total Earned
PREPROCEDURE						
1. Ask, "Are you choking?"	6					
If client indicates yes, tell client you can help.						
2. Ask client to stand.	5					
PROCEDURE						
3. Stand behind client. Place your fist against client's abdomen, just above navel.	5					
4. Grasp your fist with other hand and perform quick inward/upward thrusts into client's abdomen.	6					
5. Continue thrusting until object is expelled or client becomes unresponsive.	5					
6. If client becomes unresponsive, call EMS and do the following steps:	5					
7. Put client on his or her back.	5					
8. Tilt client's head back using head tilt-chin lift maneuver.	5					
9. Look into mouth; if you see object, remove it with index finger.	6					
10. Begin CPR.	6					
• Each time the airway is opened during CPR, check the client's mouth. If you see the object, remove it using a finger sweep.	5					
11. Continue CPR until the object is removed or trained medical personnel relieve you.	6					
12. If object is removed, open airway.	5					
13. If client isn't breathing/is breathing poorly, give 2 rescue breaths.	5					

PROCEDURE 4C1: Foreign Body Airway Obstruction in a Responsive Adult or Child *(continued)*

Procedure Steps	Suggested Points	Self Practice	Peer Practice	Peer Testing	Final Testing	Total Earned
14. Check for signs of circulation; if there are none, resume CPR.	5					
• If client has signs of circulation but breathing is absent/poor, give rescue breaths, every 5-6 seconds for adult and every 3-5 seconds for child.	5					
• Continue rescue breaths until help arrives or client starts breathing.	5					
• If client starts breathing, put him in recovery position.	5					
POSTPROCEDURE						
15. Monitor breathing and signs of circulation until help arrives.	5					
TOTAL POSSIBLE POINTS	100					

Comments: _____

_____

_____

_____

_____

_____

_____

_____

_____

_____

_____

Signatures: _____   **Date:** _____

SCORING   *See Preface for scoring instructions.*

Name _____ Date _____

First Aid and CPR

PROCEDURE 4C2:
Foreign Body Airway Obstruction in an Unresponsive Adult or Child

PROCEDURE ASSESSMENT

Procedure Steps	Suggested Points	Self Practice	Peer Practice	Peer Testing	Final Testing	Total Earned
PREPROCEDURE						
1. Tap client's shoulder and shout, "Are you OK?"	8					
2. If client is unresponsive, shout for help or call 911.	6					
PROCEDURE						
3. Open airway and tilt head back using chin lift method.	8					
• Look into mouth and remove obstructions.	8					
• Don't use blind finger sweeps.						
4. Begin CPR.	6					
• Each time the airway is opened during CPR, check the client's mouth.	4					
• If you see the object, remove it using a finger sweep.	4					
5. Continue CPR until the object is removed or trained medical personnel relieve you.	6					
POSTPROCEDURE						
6. If object is removed, open airway.	8					
7. If client isn't breathing/is breathing poorly, give 2 rescue breaths.	8					
8. If you don't see signs of circulation, resume CPR.	8					
• If client has signs of circulation but breathing is absent/poor, perform rescue breaths, every 5-6 seconds for adult and every 3-5 seconds for child.	8					

PROCEDURE 4C2: Foreign Body Airway Obstruction in an Unresponsive Adult or Child (continued)

Procedure Steps	Suggested Points	Self Practice	Peer Practice	Peer Testing	Final Testing	Total Earned
• Continue rescue breaths until help arrives or client starts breathing.	6					
• If client starts breathing, put him or her in recovery position.	6					
9. Monitor breathing/signs of circulation until help arrives.	6					
TOTAL POSSIBLE POINTS	100					

Comments: _____
_____
_____
_____
_____
_____
_____
_____
_____
_____

Signatures: _____ Date: _____

SCORING   *See Preface for scoring instructions.*

First Aid and CPR

PROCEDURE 4C3:
Foreign Body Airway Obstruction in a Responsive Infant

PROCEDURE ASSESSMENT

Procedure Steps	Suggested Points	Self Practice	Peer Practice	Peer Testing	Final Testing	Total Earned
PREPROCEDURE						
Look for signs of airway obstruction:	4					
• Difficulty in breathing.	2					
• Inability to make sounds or cry.	2					
• A high-pitched wheezy sound or no sound while inhaling.	2					
• Weak, ineffective coughs.	2					
• Blue lips or skin.	2					
PROCEDURE						
1. Place the infant in rescue position:	4					
• Sit or kneel and rest your arm on your knee or lap.	2					
• Place infant face down on your arm	2					
• His legs should straddle your forearm.	2					
• Support his jaw and head with your hand.	2					
2. Forcefully strike infant's back up to 5 times between shoulder blades.	4					
3. If object is not expelled:	4					
• Place free hand on infant's back.	2					
• Hold his head with your other hand.	2					
• Support infant between your forearms and turn his body as a unit.	2					
4. Support infant's head with hand of same arm.	4					
• Keep infant's head lower than rest of his body.	2					
5. Give up to 5 chest thrusts:	4					
• Place 2 fingers over sternum in same position used for chest compressions.	2					
• Compress chest upward toward infant's head.	2					
• Stop if object is expelled.	2					
6. Alternate back blows and chest thrusts until object is expelled or infant becomes unresponsive.	4					
7. If infant becomes unresponsive, call EMS.	4					
8. Open infant's mouth and look inside.	4					
• If you see object, remove it with your pinky.	2					
• Don't use blind finger sweeps.						

PROCEDURE 4C3: Foreign Body Airway Obstruction in a Responsive Infant (continued)

Procedure Steps	Suggested Points	Self Practice	Peer Practice	Peer Testing	Final Testing	Total Earned
9. Begin CPR.	4					
• Each time the airway is opened during CPR, check the infant's mouth.	2					
• If you see the object, remove it using a finger sweep.	2					
10. Continue CPR until the object is removed or trained medical personnel relieve you.	3					
POSTPROCEDURE						
11. If object is removed, open infant's airway.	4					
12. If infant isn't breathing/is breathing poorly, give 2 rescue breaths.	4					
13. Continue rescue breaths until infant starts breathing or help arrives.	3					
• If infant starts breathing, continue to monitor the airway.	2					
14. If you see no signs of circulation, resume CPR.	4					
• If infant has signs of circulation, but breathing is absent/poor, give rescue breaths every 3-5 seconds.	2					
TOTAL POSSIBLE POINTS	100					

Comments: _____

_____

_____

_____

_____

_____

_____

_____

_____

_____

Signatures: _____ Date: _____

SCORING See Preface for scoring instructions.

Name _____   Date _____

First Aid and CPR

PROCEDURE 4C4:
Foreign Body Airway Obstruction in an Unresponsive Infant

PROCEDURE ASSESSMENT

Procedure Steps	Suggested Points	Self Practice	Peer Practice	Peer Testing	Final Testing	Total Earned
PREPROCEDURE						
1. Check for responsiveness:	6					
• Tap soles of infant's feet. Shout, "Are you OK?"	3					
• If available, send someone to call EMS. If you're alone, continue assessment.	3					
2. If infant is unresponsive, place him or her on back on firm surface such as floor.	6					
PROCEDURE						
3. Open airway:	6					
• Tilt head back using chin lift method.	4					
• Look in mouth; remove obstructions with pinky. Don't perform blind finger sweeps.	3					
4. Check for breathing:	6					
• Put your ear next to infant's mouth and watch chest.	4					
• Look for rise/fall of chest, listen for breathing, and feel for air movement.	3					
5. If infant isn't breathing, give 2 rescue breaths, 1 second per breath.	6					
• If chest doesn't rise, reposition airway and try again.	4					
6. If attempts to provide rescue breaths are unsuccessful, begin CPR.	6					
• Each time the airway is opened during CPR, check the infant's mouth.	3					
• If you see the object, remove it using a finger sweep.	3					
7. Continue CPR until the object is removed or trained medical personnel relieve you.	6					
8. Repeat steps 5 through 7 until rescue breaths are effective.	6					

PROCEDURE 4C4: Foreign Body Airway Obstruction in an Unresponsive Infant (continued)

Procedure Steps	Suggested Points	Self Practice	Peer Practice	Peer Testing	Final Testing	Total Earned
POSTPROCEDURE						
9. If object is expelled, open infant's airway.	6					
10. If infant isn't breathing/is breathing poorly, give 2 rescue breaths.	6					
11. If you see no signs of circulation, resume CPR.	6					
• If you see signs of circulation but breathing is absent/poor, give rescue breaths every 3-5 seconds.	4					
TOTAL POSSIBLE POINTS	**100**					

Comments:

_____

_____

_____

_____

_____

_____

_____

_____

_____

Signatures: _____ **Date:** _____

SCORING   *See Preface for scoring instructions.*

First Aid and CPR

PROCEDURE 4D:
Heart Attack and Stroke

····· **P R O C E D U R E   A S S E S S M E N T** ·····

Procedure Steps	Suggested Points	Self Practice	Peer Practice	Peer Testing	Final Testing	Total Earned
PREPROCEDURE						
1. Immediately call EMS.	6					
2. Check the ABCs. Provide CPR, if appropriate.	7					
PROCEDURE (Heart Attack)						
• Help client to least painful position.	8					
a. Client shouldn't walk or overexert himself or herself.	7					
• Loosen restrictive clothing (necktie or belt).	7					
• Remain calm and reassure client.	6					
• Ask client about history of cardiac disease and current medications.	6					
• If client has nitroglycerine, the client should take it.	8					
a. Client should sit or lie down, as nitroglycerine lowers blood pressure.	7					
PROCEDURE (Stroke)						
• Help client lie down and elevate head and shoulders.	6					
• Loosen restrictive clothing (necktie or belt).	5					
• Reassure client.	6					
• Place unresponsive but breathing client into recovery position.	6					
• Keep airway open. Don't let client eat or drink anything.	7					
POSTPROCEDURE						
3. If client becomes unresponsive, check ABCs and start CPR, if needed.	8					
TOTAL POSSIBLE POINTS	100					

Comments: _____

_____

_____

_____

Signatures: _____   Date: _____

SCORING   *See Preface for scoring instructions.*

Name _____ Date _____

First Aid and CPR

PROCEDURE 4E:
Minor Wound Care

····················· **PROCEDURE ASSESSMENT** ·····················

Procedure Steps	Suggested Points	Self Practice	Peer Practice	Peer Testing	Final Testing	Total Earned
PREPROCEDURE						
1. Wash your hands.	10					
2. Put on latex or vinyl gloves.	8					
PROCEDURE						
3. If possible, put wound under running water; wash inside it with soap and water.	8					
• Otherwise, pour soapy water over wound and rinse.	7					
4. If bleeding restarts, apply direct pressure with clean gauze.	8					
5. Pat wound dry with sterile gauze/clean cloth.	7					
6. Don't use iodine, hydrogen peroxide, or alcohol to clean wound, unless directed to by a professional.	10					
• Don't use antibiotic ointments on puncture wounds or wounds that require sutures.	8					
7. Apply adhesive strip or appropriate dressing.	7					
POSTPROCEDURE						
8. Remove gloves and wash hands.	10					
9. Tell client to change dressing daily, or more often if it gets wet or dirty.	8					
10. Tell client to check wound for signs of infection and call doctor with questions.	9					
TOTAL POSSIBLE POINTS	**100**					

Comments: _____

_____

_____

_____

_____

_____

Signatures: _____ **Date:** _____

SCORING *See Preface for scoring instructions.*

First Aid and CPR

PROCEDURE 4F:
Controlling External Bleeding

P R O C E D U R E　A S S E S S M E N T

Procedure Steps	Suggested Points	Self Practice	Peer Practice	Peer Testing	Final Testing	Total Earned
PREPROCEDURE						
1. Gather needed equipment.	4					
2. Assess scene for hazards.	5					
3. Move client only if necessary.	3					
4. Check client for ABCs and bleeding.	4					
5. Call EMS, if appropriate.	4					
PROCEDURE						
6. Don't touch wound with bare hands. Put on latex or vinyl gloves, use waterproof material or ask client to apply pressure to wound, if possible.	5					
7. Expose wound by cutting or removing clothing.	4					
8. Put sterile gauze pad or clean cloth over bleeding site.	3					
9. Apply direct pressure to site using fingers and palm.	5					
• Don't apply direct pressure to eye injury, skull fracture or site of impaled object.	4					
10. Keep pressure on site for 5 to 10 minutes.	3					
11. If there are no neck/back injuries or badly broken bones, elevate injured arm or leg above level of heart.	3					
12. Continue direct pressure.	5					
• If bleeding leaks through gauze, put more dressing on top of first layer.	4					
• Replace top dressing with another if bleeding seeps through.	4					
• Don't remove dressing that is directly on wound.	4					
13. Apply roller (pressure) bandage on top of gauze above and below wound.	3					
14. Make pressure bandage secure.	5					
• Check pulse below bandage to ensure bandage isn't too tight.	4					
15. Quickly obtain help for client.	4					
16. Assess client and treat for shock, if necessary.	4					
17. Comfort client.	3					

PROCEDURE 4F: Controlling External Bleeding (continued)

Procedure Steps	Suggested Points	Self Practice	Peer Practice	Peer Testing	Final Testing	Total Earned
18. When you can't apply direct pressure, wrap roller gauze around fingers to form loop and apply "doughnut" to wound.	4					
POSTPROCEDURE						
19. Care for wound.	3					
20. Remove gloves and wash hands.	6					
TOTAL POSSIBLE POINTS	100					

Comments:

Signatures: _____ **Date:** _____

SCORING *See Preface for scoring instructions.*

First Aid and CPR

PROCEDURE 4G:
Internal Bleeding

P R O C E D U R E   A S S E S S M E N T

Procedure Steps	Suggested Points	Self Practice	Peer Practice	Peer Testing	Final Testing	Total Earned
PREPROCEDURE						
1. Gather needed equipment.	7					
2. Ensure scene is safe and put on latex or vinyl gloves.	10					
3. Seek immediate medical attention.	8					
4. Check client's responsiveness and ABCs.	9					
• Supply first aid to restore ABCs, if needed.						
• Control all major external bleeding.	8					
PROCEDURE						
5. If you are certain there is no head/neck/back injury, put client on left side and elevate legs 8 to 12 inches.	7					
6. Cover client with blankets or coats.	8					
7. Don't let client eat or drink anything.	9					
8. Reassure client.	11					
9. Monitor ABCs until help arrives.	11					
POSTPROCEDURE						
10. Remove gloves and wash hands.	12					
TOTAL POSSIBLE POINTS	**100**					

Comments:

_____

_____

_____

_____

_____

_____

_____

_____

Signatures: _____ **Date:** _____

SCORING   *See Preface for scoring instructions.*

First Aid and CPR

PROCEDURE 4H:
Shock

PROCEDURE ASSESSMENT

Procedure Steps	Suggested Points	Self Practice	Peer Practice	Peer Testing	Final Testing	Total Earned
PREPROCEDURE						
1. Gather needed equipment. Ensure scene is safe and put on latex or vinyl gloves.	8					
2. Call EMS immediately.	7					
3. Check client's responsiveness and ABCs.	8					
• Supply first aid to restore ABCs, if needed.						
• Control all major external bleeding.	7					
PROCEDURE						
4. Lay client on back unless he has neck/back injuries. If client is nauseous, place him on left side.	9					
5. Raise client's legs 8 to 12 inches only if there are no neck/back injuries.	9					
6. Loosen constrictive clothing (necktie or belt).	8					
7. Cover client with blankets or coats; put them under client too.	9					
8. Do not give client food or drink.	9					
9. Reassure client.	9					
POSTPROCEDURE						
10. Stay with client until EMS arrives.	7					
11. Remove gloves and wash hands.	10					
TOTAL POSSIBLE POINTS	100					

Comments: _____

_____

_____

_____

_____

_____

_____

_____

Signatures: _____ **Date:** _____

SCORING   *See Preface for scoring instructions.*

Name _____ Date _____

First Aid and CPR

PROCEDURE 4I:
Anaphylaxis

P R O C E D U R E   A S S E S S M E N T

Procedure Steps	Suggested Points	Self Practice	Peer Practice	Peer Testing	Final Testing	Total Earned
PREPROCEDURE						
1. Gather needed equipment.	13					
2. Ensure scene is safe and put on latex or vinyl gloves.	16					
3. Seek immediate medical attention or call EMS.	14					
4. Check client's responsiveness and ABCs.	14					
• Supply first aid to restore ABCs, if necessary.						
PROCEDURE						
5. If client has doctor-prescribed bee sting kit, help him use it immediately.	15					
6. Obtain immediate medical assistance.	14					
POSTPROCEDURE						
7. Remain with client until EMS arrives.	14					
TOTAL POSSIBLE POINTS	100					

Comments: _____

_____

_____

_____

_____

_____

_____

_____

_____

Signatures: _____ **Date:** _____

SCORING *See Preface for scoring instructions.*

Name _____ Date _____

First Aid and CPR

PROCEDURE 4J:
Burns

PROCEDURE ASSESSMENT

Procedure Steps	Suggested Points	Self Practice	Peer Practice	Peer Testing	Final Testing	Total Earned
PREPROCEDURE						
1. Ensure scene is safe.	3					
2. Seek immediate medical attention or call EMS.	3					
3. Stop burning process:	4					
• For electrical burn, turn off power.	3					
• If client is on fire, have him or her drop and roll, smother flames with blanket, or douse client with water.	3					
• For chemical burn, follow steps below.						
4. Check client's responsiveness, airway, breathing and circulation.	3					
• Supply first aid to restore ABCs, if needed.						
PROCEDURE						
5. Estimate depth or degree of burn. Clients can have more than one type.	4					
• First-degree thermal burn (reddened area):	3					
a. Immerse burned area in cool water or apply cool wet cloth.	2					
b. Keep area immersed until site is pain-free.	2					
c. If possible, keep site elevated.	2					
d. Don't apply butter, grease or other coating.	2					
• Second-degree thermal burn (reddened area with blisters):	3					
a. Immerse burned area in cool water or apply cool wet cloth.	2					
b. Keep area immersed until site is pain-free.	2					
c. Cover burn with dry, non-adhesive sterile dressing. Don't break blisters.	2					
d. Keep burn dry.	2					
e. Assess burn area for signs of infection.	2					
• Third-degree thermal burn (waxy or leathery look):	3					
a. Cover burn with dry, non-adhesive sterile dressing.	2					
b. Treat client for shock. Elevate his legs and cover him with clean sheet.	2					
c. Reassure client.	2					

PROCEDURE 4J: Burns (continued)

Procedure Steps	Suggested Points	Self Practice	Peer Practice	Peer Testing	Final Testing	Total Earned
• Chemical burn:	3					
a. Remove chemicals by flushing site with water. Use shower or hose if available. If chemical is dry powder, first brush off, then flush.	2					
b. Remove contaminated clothing and jewelry.	2					
c. Flush site, including eyes, with water for 20 minutes.	2					
d. Cover site with sterile dressing/clean cloth.	2					
• Electrical burn:	3					
a. Unplug or disconnect electrical device, or turn off power at circuit breaker panel.	2					
b. Seek immediate medical attention or call EMS.	2					
c. If you suspect spinal injury or if client has violent muscle contractions, don't move client. Open airway using jaw thrust method.	2					
d. Treat client for shock.	2					
6. Estimate surface area of body burned:	3					
• Use rule of nines to calculate percentage.	2					
7. Identify body areas that are burned.	3					
• Burns to face, hands, feet, and genitals are most serious.						
8. Determine severity of burn:	3					
• Minor burns can be treated at home.						
• Moderate to critical burns must be treated at a hospital.						
9. Perform first aid procedures as described previously.	3					
POSTPROCEDURE						
10. Stay with client until help arrives.	3					
11. Wash your hands.	5					
TOTAL POSSIBLE POINTS	**100**					

Comments:

_____

_____

_____

_____

_____

Signatures: _____ Date: _____

SCORING   *See Preface for scoring instructions.*

First Aid and CPR

PROCEDURE 4K:
Injuries to Bones, Joints, and Muscles

PROCEDURE ASSESSMENT

Procedure Steps	Suggested Points	Self Practice	Peer Practice	Peer Testing	Final Testing	Total Earned
PREPROCEDURE						
1. Gather needed equipment.	4					
2. Put on latex or vinyl gloves.	6					
3. Ensure scene is safe.	5					
4. Check client's responsiveness and ABCs.	5					
• Supply first aid to restore ABCs, if needed.						
• Control all major external bleeding.						
PROCEDURE						
5. If possible, remove clothing over area and assess injury.	6					
• Ask client to explain how injury occurred.	4					
6. Look/feel for deformity, bruises, open wounds, depressions, tenderness and swelling, or exposed bone ends.	6					
• Cover open wounds with sterile dressing.	4					
• Check for movement/sensation, if possible.	4					
• Have client wiggle fingers or toes, touch a finger or toe, and identify site touched.	4					
7. Don't move injured part.	6					
8. Consider splinting injured site:	6					
• Extend splints above and below joints of injured site.	5					
• Pad splints at bony areas and injury sites with clothes or towels.	5					
• Support injured site and apply splints.	5					
• Use strips of cloth, roller gauze, etc. to tie splints in place.	5					
• Ensure splints are snug but don't impair circulation. Leave fingers and toes exposed.	5					
9. Apply ice pack only if client has pulse at site of injury.	5					
10. Have client rest and elevate injured area.	5					
POSTPROCEDURE						
11. Call EMS or take client to hospital.	5					
TOTAL POSSIBLE POINTS	**100**					

PROCEDURE 4K: Injuries to Bones, Joints, and Muscles *(continued)*

Comments:

_____
_____
_____
_____
_____
_____
_____
_____
_____

Signatures: _____ Date: _____

SCORING   *See Preface for scoring instructions.*

Name _____   Date _____

First Aid and CPR

PROCEDURE 4L:
Diabetic Emergencies

PROCEDURE ASSESSMENT

Procedure Steps	Suggested Points	Self Practice	Peer Practice	Peer Testing	Final Testing	Total Earned
PREPROCEDURE						
1. Ensure scene is safe.	13					
2. Check client's responsiveness and ABCs. Supply first aid to restore ABCs, if necessary.	12					
PROCEDURE						
3. Recognize signs of hypoglycemia or hyperglycemia.	13					
4. For hypoglycemia, give some form of sugar (soda, etc.) if these conditions are present:	13					
• The client is a known diabetic.	12					
• The client is alert enough to swallow.	12					
5. If you aren't sure whether client has high or low blood sugar, give client sugar.	13					
POSTPROCEDURE						
6. If symptoms don't reverse after 15 to 20 minutes, seek medical attention.	12					
TOTAL POSSIBLE POINTS	100					

Comments: _____
_____
_____
_____
_____
_____
_____
_____
_____
_____

Signatures: _____   Date: _____

SCORING   *See Preface for scoring instructions.*

Name _____ Date _____

First Aid and CPR

PROCEDURE 4M:
Seizures

· · · · · · · · · · · · · · · · P R O C E D U R E   A S S E S S M E N T · · · · · · · · · · · · · · · ·

Procedure Steps	Suggested Points	Self Practice	Peer Practice	Peer Testing	Final Testing	Total Earned
PREPROCEDURE						
Ensure scene is safe.						
PROCEDURE						
1. If client is standing or sitting, lower client to floor.	8					
2. Cushion client's head with pillow.	7					
3. Loosen restrictive clothing.	8					
4. Clear area of furniture or equipment so client doesn't strike it.	9					
5. Turn client on left side.	8					
6. Look for appropriate medical identification.	9					
7. Don't hold client down or restrict movements.	8					
8. Time the seizure, if possible.	7					
9. Don't put any object in client's mouth.	8					
10. Stay with client until seizure ends.	9					
POSTPROCEDURE						
11. Obtain medical assistance as necessary.	9					
12. Wash your hands.	10					
TOTAL POSSIBLE POINTS	**100**					

Comments:

_____

_____

_____

_____

_____

_____

_____

_____

_____

Signatures: _____   **Date:** _____

SCORING   *See Preface for scoring instructions.*

First Aid and CPR

PROCEDURE 4N:
Heat Emergencies

PROCEDURE ASSESSMENT

Procedure Steps	Suggested Points	Self Practice	Peer Practice	Peer Testing	Final Testing	Total Earned
PREPROCEDURE						
1. Gather needed equipment.	3					
2. Stop client's activity and move him or her to cool location.	3					
3. If you suspect heat stroke, call EMS immediately.	3					
PROCEDURE						
• Heat cramps:	6					
a. Give client a sport drink diluted to ½ strength.	5					
b. Don't let client return to activity for a few hours after cramp subsides.	5					
c. Stretch cramping muscle.	5					
• Heat exhaustion:	6					
a. Loosen or remove clothing.	5					
b. Place client in supine position with legs elevated 8 to 12 inches.	5					
c. Sponge client with cool water.	5					
d. If client is responsive and not nauseated, give client water to drink.	5					
e. If condition doesn't improve after 15 to 20 minutes, seek medical assistance.	5					
• Heat stroke:	6					
a. Remove all non-cotton clothing.	5					
b. Soak client with water, especially neck and head.	5					
c. Fan client to increase rate of evaporation.	5					
d. Use ice packs on neck, armpits, and groin. Don't let client shiver.	5					
e. Keep client lying down with feet elevated.	5					
f. Massage extremities.	5					
POSTPROCEDURE						
4. Stay with client until condition subsides or EMS arrives.	3					
TOTAL POSSIBLE POINTS	**100**					

PROCEDURE 4N: Heat Emergencies *(continued)*

Comments: _____
_____
_____
_____
_____
_____
_____
_____
_____
_____

Signatures: _____ Date: _____

SCORING   *See Preface for scoring instructions.*

First Aid and CPR

PROCEDURE 40:
Cold-Related Emergencies

PROCEDURE ASSESSMENT

Procedure Steps	Suggested Points	Self Practice	Peer Practice	Peer Testing	Final Testing	Total Earned
PREPROCEDURE						
1. Gather needed equipment.	3					
2. Check client's responsiveness and ABCs. Supply first aid to restore ABCs, if necessary. It may take a full minute to check for breathing and pulse if client has hypothermia.	4					
3. Quickly move client out of the cold.	4					
PROCEDURE						
• Hypothermia:						
a. Handle client with extreme care.	5					
• Put blankets, towels, etc., above and below client.	4					
• Remove wet clothing and replace with dry clothing/covering.	4					
• Keep client flat.	4					
• Don't allow client to move or exercise.	4					
b. Call EMS.	4					
c. Cover body, including head.	3					
• Frost nip:						
a. If you can't bring client out of cold, place the fingers in his or her armpits and cover cheeks, ears, and nose with a gloved hand.	2					
b. Remove all wet clothing.	2					
c. Immerse chilled body parts in warm (not hot) water until all sensation returns.	3					
• Frostbite:						
a. Remove wet clothing and replace with dry clothing/covering.	2					
b. Call EMS or take client to hospital.	3					
c. If feet are affected, carry client.	2					
d. If affected part is partly thawed or if client is more than 1 hour from a hospital, immerse frozen part in warm water (102 degrees F). Add more warm water as needed.	3					

PROCEDURE 4O: Cold-Related Emergencies (continued)

Procedure Steps	Suggested Points	Self Practice	Peer Practice	Peer Testing	Final Testing	Total Earned
e. Do not:	4					
• Use direct heat (fire or heating pad).	2					
• Thaw area if it might refreeze.	2					
• Rub frostbitten skin or rub snow on area.	3					
• Allow client to smoke.	2					
• Break any blisters.	3					
• Let client drink alcohol.	2					
f. Rewarming takes up to 40 minutes and is accompanied by a burning sensation.						
• Skin may blister, swell, and turn red, blue, or purple.						
• Thawed skin is pink and no longer numb.						
g. Apply sterile dressing to thawed area.	5					
• Don't disturb blisters.	4					
• Put dressing between fingers and toes if they were affected.	4					
h. Wrap rewarmed areas to prevent refreezing.	4					
• Ask client to keep thawed areas motionless.	4					
i. Seek emergency care quickly.						
4. Stay with client until help arrives.	5					
TOTAL POSSIBLE POINTS	**100**					

Comments:

_____

_____

_____

_____

_____

_____

_____

_____

_____

Signatures: _____ Date: _____

SCORING *See Preface for scoring instructions.*

Name _____ Date _____

First Aid and CPR

PROCEDURE 4P:
Poisons

PROCEDURE ASSESSMENT

Procedure Steps	Suggested Points	Self Practice	Peer Practice	Peer Testing	Final Testing	Total Earned
PREPROCEDURE						
1. Ensure scene is safe.	5					
2. Check client's responsiveness and ABCs.	4					
• Supply first aid to restore ABCs.	3					
• Place unresponsive client on his left side.	3					
PROCEDURE						
• Ingested poisons:						
a. Call poison control center immediately.	5					
b. If client is unresponsive or acting strangely, call EMS and poison control.	4					
c. When you call poison control, tell them:	4					
Age and weight if client is a child. Name of the substance involved. Amount of substance that was swallowed. Amount of time elapsed since substance was swallowed.						
d. Follow poison control's directions:	5					
• Dilute poison with milk or water only if told to do so.	4					
• For a child, give 8 to 16 ounces of milk or water.	4					
e. Induce vomiting only if told to do so.	4					
f. Save all containers and vomit to aid in poison identification.	5					
• Carbon monoxide and inhaled poisoning:						
a. Get client out of poisonous environment only if it's safe to do so.	4					
b. Call 911 or local EMS number.	4					
c. Put client on his left side if he is nauseated or unresponsive.	4					
• Absorbed poisons:						
a. If contact is with poisonous plant:	4					
• Wash skin with soap and water or alcohol.	3					
b. If contact is with insecticide, pesticide, or another chemical:	4					
• Wash site with lots of water for 20 minutes.	3					
• Don't contaminate yourself with poison.	3					

PROCEDURE 4P: Poisons *(continued)*

Procedure Steps	Suggested Points	Self Practice	Peer Practice	Peer Testing	Final Testing	Total Earned
c. If client isn't breathing and you think poison is on client's face or in mouth:	5					
• Rinse area and attempt ventilation with barrier device.	4					
• If barrier device isn't available, close client's mouth and do rescue breathing through nose.	4					
• If necessary, use cloth to cover nose to avoid direct contact.	4					
POSTPROCEDURE						
3. Stay with client until EMS arrives.	4					
TOTAL POSSIBLE POINTS	100					

Comments:

Signatures: Date:

SCORING   *See Preface for scoring instructions.*

Medical Terminology   Reinforcement Activities

Fill in the Blank

Write the word (or words) that best completes the sentence in the blank provided.

1. _____ are found at the beginning of the word and describe, modify, or limit the term.

2. When the vowel *O* is placed after a word root, it becomes a _____.

3. The _____ provides the basic meaning of the word.

4. Placed at the end of the word, the _____ changes the word's meaning.

5. The singular form of bacteria is _____.

6. The posterior part of the brain is called the _____.

7. The bones of the body also function as a storage area for excess _____.

8. _____ is a decrease in the size of an organ or tissue.

9. Two word roots used for kidneys are _____ and _____.

10. A disease-causing agent would be called a _____.

11. BMR is the abbreviation for _____.

12. IM is the abbreviation for _____.

13. _____ is the study of skin and its diseases.

14. If you suffered from cervicodynia, the pain would be in your _____.

Matching

Write the letter of the phrase that best matches each numbered item in the blank provided.

_____ 15. Neur		**a.** A word root meaning nerve.
_____ 16. Tachy		**b.** Combining form meaning nerve.
_____ 17. Pathy		**c.** Suffix meaning excision or removal.
_____ 18. Leuk/o		**d.** Out of bed.
_____ 19. Neur/o		**e.** Suffix meaning disease condition.
_____ 20. Dia		**f.** Do not resuscitate.
_____ 21. Contra		**g.** Prefix meaning across or through.
_____ 22. OOB		**h.** Prefix meaning against.
_____ 23. Ectomy		**i.** Repeat as needed.

_____ 24. PRN, prn   j. Descriptive term meaning fast.

_____ 25. DNR   k. Prefix meaning through, complete.

_____ 26. Trans   l. Word part for the color white.

Multiple Choice

Circle the answer that best answers the question or completes the statement.

27. *-ectomy* is a frequently used
    a. word root.
    b. prefix.
    c. suffix.
    d. combining form.

28. The word root *cardi* refers to the
    a. neck.
    b. head.
    c. heart.
    d. liver.

29. The prefix *hyper-* refers to
    a. above.
    b. below.
    c. within.
    d. before.

30. The commonly used directional term *hemi* means
    a. away from.
    b. toward.
    c. around.
    d. half.

31. The word root *rhin* refers to the
    a. chin.
    b. spine.
    c. mind.
    d. nose.

Anatomy and Physiology

Reinforcement Activities

Matching

Write the letter of the phrase that best matches each numbered item in the blank provided.

_____ 1. Esophagus

_____ 2. Paraplegia

_____ 3. Cytoplasm

_____ 4. Deglutition

_____ 5. Venules

_____ 6. Interneurons

_____ 7. Hypogastric region

_____ 8. Hydrocephalus

_____ 9. Hemoptysis

_____ 10. Meninges

_____ 11. Thyroid cartilage

_____ 12. Mandible

_____ 13. Glomerulus

_____ 14. Nervous tissue

_____ 15. Gangrene

_____ 16. Orthopnea

_____ 17. Cochlea

_____ 18. Diarthroses

_____ 19. Osteocytes

_____ 20. Pylorus

a. The area just below the umbilical region.

b. This substance performs the work of the cell, such as reproduction and movement.

c. Carries messages to and from the brain and spinal cord from all parts of the body.

d. The passageway for food.

e. Difficulty in breathing, especially while lying down.

f. Spitting of blood from the lungs or bronchial tubes.

g. Tiny veins that connect to the capillaries.

h. The bone containing the sockets for the lower teeth.

i. Joints that move freely, such as the knee.

j. Carry and process sensory information.

k. Three layers of membranes that cover the brain and spinal cord.

l. Overproduction of cerebrospinal fluid in the brain.

m. Paralysis from the waist down.

n. Snail-shaped structure important to equilibrium.

o. The process of swallowing.

p. On the largynx, also known as the Adam's apple.

q. The first place where urine is formed in the kidney, it filters fluid from the blood.

r. Death of tissue due to loss of blood supply.

s. The cells of bone.

t. The narrowed bottom part of the stomach.

True/False

Write "T" in the blank provided if the statement is true. Write "F" if the statement is false.

_____ 21. The epidermis does not contain blood vessels.

_____ 22. The alimentary canal is a tube that extends from the mouth to the anus.

_____ 23. Each lung is divided into two lobes.

_____ 24. Veins carry blood away from the heart.

_____ 25. Arteriosclerosis is more commonly known as hardening of the arteries.

_____ 26. Flat bones are the small, cube-shaped bones of the wrists, ankles, and toes.

_____ 27. The longest portion of a long bone is called the shaft.

_____ 28. Fibromyalgia is chronic pain in muscles and the fibrous tissue that surrounds them.

_____ 29. Lymph does not contain white blood cells.

_____ 30. Red bone marrow is generally found in infant bones and in the flat bones of adults.

_____ 31. The symptoms of trichomoniasis are the same in women and in men.

_____ 32. Ciliary muscles are used for focusing the eyes.

_____ 33. Hypoglycemia cannot be controlled with dietary changes.

_____ 34. Phalanges are the bones of the fingers and the toes.

_____ 35. The cerebellum is the area of the brain of conscious decision-making.

_____ 36. The lunula is the white portion of the eyeball.

_____ 37. Amphiarthroses are joints that do not move, such as the fibrous joints between the skull bones.

_____ 38. Ossicles are small, specially shaped bones in the middle ear.

_____ 39. Although not located within the GI tract, the liver performs many digestive functions.

_____ 40. The sigmoid colon is the first of four parts of the large intestine.

_____ 41. Otitis externa is an inflammation of the external ear canal.

_____ 42. Crohn's disease affects only the small intestine.

Fill in the Blank

Write the word (or words) that best completes the sentence in the blank provided.

43. A fibrous membrane called the _____ covers the outside of the bone.

44. _____ is one of two pancreatic enzymes that assist in digestion.

45. The _____ cuts the body into two parts, left and right.

46. _____ is swayback or an abnormal inward curvature of the lumbar vertebrae.

47. The three parts of a neuron are _____, _____, and _____.

48. _____ kill parasites and help control inflammation and allergic reactions.

49. _____ is the flow of blood between the heart and the lungs.

Name _____ Date _____

50. _____ convert complex proteins, sugars, and fat molecules into simpler substances that can be used by the body.

51. The skull or cranial bones join at points called _____.

52. Blood enters each kidney through the _____.

53. _____ is a degenerative disease of the motor neurons leading to the loss of muscular control and death.

54. The basic structures of the cell are the _____, _____, and _____.

55. The lining of the stomach is relatively thick, with many folds of mucous tissue called _____.

56. The nervous system consists of _____, _____, and _____.

57. Digestion of food begins in the mouth with chewing or _____.

58. Nails are plates made of _____ that cover the _____ surface of the _____ bone of the fingers and toes.

59. The two lower arm bones are the _____ and the _____.

60. Chickenpox is a common childhood disease caused by the _____ virus.

61. _____ secretions control metabolism and blood calcium concentrations.

62. A _____ fracture is a break in which the bone is fragmented or shattered.

63. Lymph nodes contain special cells known as _____ that devour foreign substances.

64. _____ expands and contracts allowing the body to move.

65. Skin and linings of internal organs such as the intestines are _____.

66. The _____ is an eight-foot section of the small intestine that continues the digestive process.

67. _____ or black lung is caused by coal dust in the lung.

68. A _____ is a localized, pus-producing infection, originating in a hair follicle.

69. The _____ is a passageway for both air and food.

70. _____ is chronic, recurrent seizure activity.

Multiple Choice

Circle the letter that best answers the question or completes the statement.

71. Another name for red blood cells is
a. leukocytes.
b. thrombocytes.
c. erythrocytes.
d. monocytes.

72. Myocardial infarction is also known as
a. stroke.
b. heart attack.
c. anemia.
d. congestive heart failure.

73. All of the following are glands *except:*
a. sudoriferous.
b. diaphoresis.
c. sebaceous.
d. exocrine.

74. Rubella is also known as
a. mumps.
b. varicella zoster.
c. chicken pox.
d. German measles.

75. All of the following are parts of the female reproductive system *except:*
a. flagellum.
b. cervix.
c. uterus.
d. hymen.

76. Which of the following is the narrowed bottom of the stomach?
a. fundus.
b. rugae.
c. cardiac.
d. pylorus.

77. Morbid obesity is considered to be _____ pounds over your ideal body weight.
a. 50
b. 75
c. 100
d. 25

78. All of the following are layers that make up the meninges *except:*
a. neuro mater.
b. pia mater.
c. arachnoid membrane.
d. dura mater.

79. Inflammation of the brain that results from a viral infection or from the spread of an infection to the brain is called
    a. meningitis.
    b. encephalitis.
    c. epilepsy.
    d. Tourette's syndrome.

80. Paralysis on one side of the body, usually from a stroke, is referred to as
    a. paraplegia.
    b. quadriplegia.
    c. hemiplegia.
    d. none of the above.

81. The pineal gland, located superior and posterior to the pituitary gland, releases
    a. melatonin.
    b. thyroxine.
    c. glucagons.
    d. prolactin.

82. The bones formed in a tendon near joints are called
    a. cancellous.
    b. irregular.
    c. spongy.
    d. sesamoid.

83. All of the following are sections of the vertebrae *except*
    a. cervical.
    b. scapula.
    c. thoracic.
    d. lumbar.

84. All of the following are bones located in the human leg *except*
    a. femur.
    b. ilium.
    c. tibia.
    d. patella.

85. Which of the following is commonly called the kneecap?
    a. fibula.
    b. tarsal.
    c. patella.
    d. carpal.

86. The muscular system is made up of over _____ individual muscles.
    a. 600
    b. 400
    c. 700
    d. 300

87. The protective sac covering the heart is called the
    a. endocardium.
    b. myocardium.
    c. epicardium.
    d. pericardium.

88. _____ destroy large unwanted particles in the bloodstream.
    a. Neutrophils.
    b. Monocytes.
    c. Lymphocytes.
    d. Eosinophils.

89. Failure of the bone marrow to produce enough red blood cells results in
    a. pernicious anemia.
    b. iron deficiency anemia.
    c. aplastic anemia.
    d. sickle cell anemia.

90. Groups of cells that work together to perform the same task are called
    a. organ.
    b. cytoplasm.
    c. tissue.
    d. muscles.

Labeling

In the space provided, write the word(s) that identifies the corresponding part on the diagram.

91. Label the cell parts in the figure below.

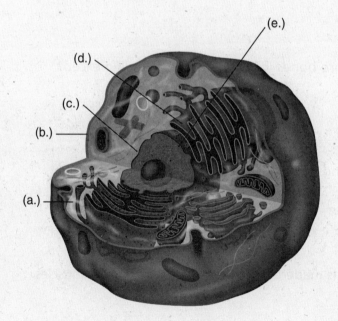

(a.) _____   (d.) _____

(b.) _____   (e.) _____

(c.) _____

92. Label the body cavities in the figure below.

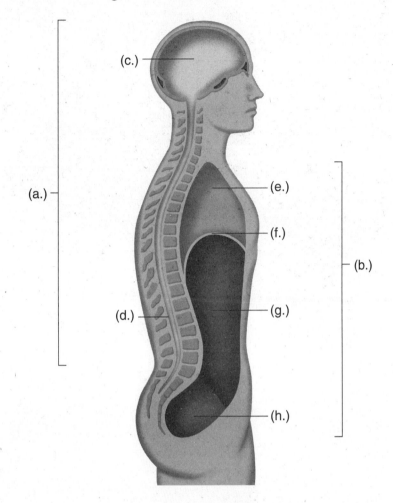

(a.) _____   (e.) _____

(b.) _____   (f.) _____

(c.) _____   (g.) _____

(d.) _____   (h.) _____

Name _____ Date _____

93. Label the directional terms in the figure below.

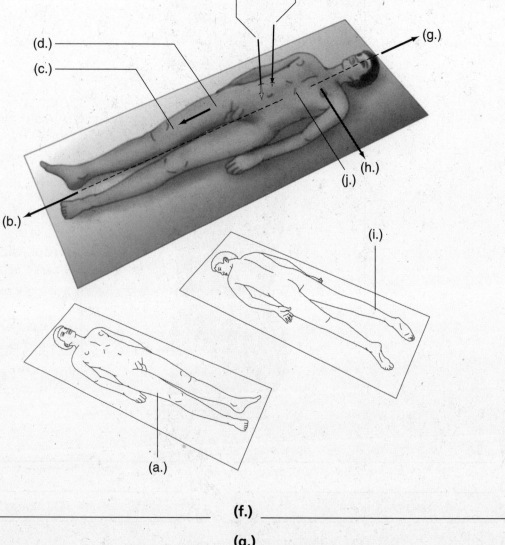

(a.) _____   (f.) _____

(b.) _____   (g.) _____

(c.) _____   (h.) _____

(d.) _____   (i.) _____

(e.) _____   (j.) _____

Human Growth and Development

Reinforcement Activities

Matching

Write the letter of the phrase that best matches each numbered item in the blank provided.

_____ 1. Alzheimer's disease

_____ 2. Cephalocaudal

_____ 3. Fertilization

_____ 4. Genes

_____ 5. Geriatric

_____ 6. Menarche

_____ 7. Osteoarthritis

_____ 8. Puberty

_____ 9. Synapse

_____ 10. Wellness

a. The onset of menstruation.

b. Nerve connection in the brain.

c. Middle age arthritis characterized by degeneration in bone & cartilage.

d. Quality or state of being in good health, especially as an actively sought goal.

e. Degenerative disease of central nervous system characterized by premature senile mental deterioration.

f. Factor in the chromosomes responsible for the transmission of hereditary characteristics.

g. Health care that deals with the problems & diseases of old age & aging people.

h. Maturation that takes place "head to tail."

i. Joining of egg and sperm in fallopian tube.

j. Period when a person begins to develop secondary sex characteristics and becomes capable of reproduction.

True/False

Write "T" in the blank provided if the statement is true. Write "F" if the statement is false.

_____ 11. Thinning and wrinkling skin is due to a decreased amount of collagen and elastin in the dermis.

_____ 12. Women in Western cultures begin to experience menopause age between 45 to 50.

_____ 13. The soft, downy hair on a newborn is called milia.

_____ 14. The imagination of the three-year old may lead to unfounded worries and fears, especially at night.

_____ 15. Around age 50, the brain begins to shrink, mostly due to water loss.

_____ 16. As one ages, the short-term memory seems to remain intact, and long-term memory may be less acute.

_____ 17. Boys are usually about a year and a half ahead of girls with their small muscle coordination.

Fill in the Blanks

Write the word (or words) that best completes the sentence in the blank provided.

18. The acronym which best recalls the five stages of grieving is _____.

19. A child is better able to grasp concepts of time as he or she approaches the age of _____.

20. Another term for curvature of the spine is _____.

21. One sign of aging is a decreased number of _____, which protect against ultraviolet light.

22. The waxy white substance in the folds of the skin on a newborn is called _____.

23. At eight weeks of life, the developing infant is now called a _____.

24. From birth to one month, the infant is referred to as a _____.

25. Neonatal jaundice is due to the accumulation of _____.

26. Newborns sleep approximately _____ of the time.

27. At _____ of age, an infant can follow simple directions.

28. At age _____, the child is able to draw and recognize simple shapes.

29. In America and most Western cultures, the onset of puberty occurs in females at _____ years of age.

30. Males may continue to grow in height until _____ of age.

31. Clients who suffer from _____ have an abnormal preoccupation with their weight and may starve themselves because they believe they will look better.

Multiple Choice

Circle the letter that best answers the question or completes the statement.

32. All of the following are STD (sexually transmitted diseases) *except*
    a. chlamydia.
    b. gonorrhea.
    c. cephalocaudal.
    d. syphilis.

33. Another term for farsightedness is
    a. morula.
    b. presbyopia.
    c. kyphosis.
    d. menarche.

34. The startle reflex is also known as
    a. babinski reflex.
    b. grasp.
    c. rooting.
    d. moro reflex.

35. Most deaths from SIDS (sudden infant death syndrome) occur between _____ and _____ months of age.
    a. 2 and 4
    b. 1 and 3
    c. 2 and 5
    d. 4 and 6

36. The umbilical cord "stump" is expected to fall-off by around the _____ day of life.
    a. 5th
    b. 10th
    c. 15th
    d. 7th

37. At 4-years-of-age, the vocabulary is about _____ words.
    a. 500
    b. 800
    c. 1600
    d. 1000

38. Cardiac, respiratory, and digestive functions are approaching their adult stages by the ages of
    a. 9 to 13 years.
    b. 14 to 19 years.
    c. 7 to 13 years.
    d. 15 to 20 years.

39. Quinceanera is an Hispanic tradition celebrating a girl's coming of age that occurs at age
    a. 15 years.
    b. 12 years.
    c. 16 years.
    d. 19 years.

40. Bone density loss may begin in a female as early as
    a. 25 years.
    b. 40 years.
    c. 30 years.
    d. 35 years.

Name _____ Date _____

Labeling

41. Determine the height measurements for the following height bars. Convert to feet and inches.

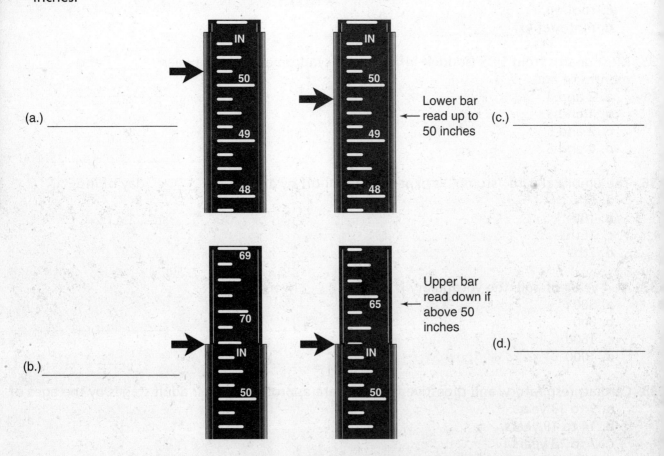

(a.) _____

(b.) _____

(c.) _____

Lower bar read up to 50 inches

Upper bar read down if above 50 inches

(d.) _____

42. Determine the weight measurement for the following weight bars.

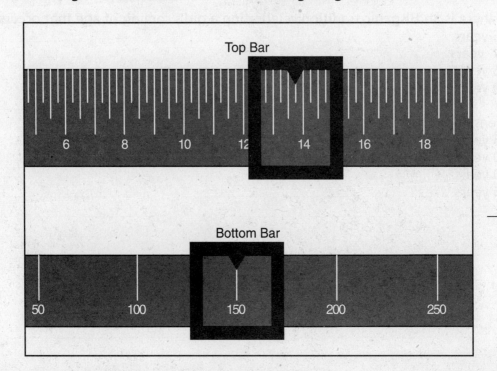

Top Bar

Bottom Bar

_____

Human Growth and Development

PROCEDURE 7A:
Measuring the Infant

PROCEDURE ASSESSMENT

Procedure Steps	Suggested Points	Self Practice	Peer Practice	Peer Testing	Final Testing	Total Earned
PREPROCEDURE						
1. Gather needed equipment.	4					
2. Place disposable scale sheet on scale.	3					
3. Balance the scale at zero.	3					
PROCEDURE						
4. Identify client and get parent's permission to weigh infant.	2					
5. Wash hands and follow infection control guidelines.	5					
6. Explain procedure to parent.	5					
7. Ask parent to undress infant.	3					
• Leave diaper on until ready to weigh infant.						
• For male infant, leave diaper over lower body until ready to read scale.						
8. Place infant face up on scale.	3					
9. Keep one hand on infant at all times to avoid a fall.	2					
10. Move lower weight to right and place at highest number that doesn't cause balance indicator to drop to bottom.	3					
11. Move upper weight slowly to right until balance bar is centered at middle mark.	3					
• Adjust gently as necessary.						
12. Add two weights together to obtain infant's weight.	2					
• Keep weight in mind until you can safely record it.						
13. Remove infant from scale; place him on table or in parent's arms.	5					
• Don't ever leave infant unattended while on scale.						
14. To measure infant's length:						
• On scale, proceed to Option A.						
• On table, proceed to Option B.						
Option A: Measuring Length on the Scale with Height (Length) Bar						
• Move infant to top of scale until head touches height bar.	3					
• Have parent hold infant by shoulders in this position.	2					

Procedure Steps	Suggested Points	Self Practice	Peer Practice	Peer Testing	Final Testing	Total Earned
• Keep head in place, hold ankles and gently extend legs.	4					
• Slide bottom bar to touch soles of feet.	3					
• Note infant's length.	3					
• Release ankles, but don't let go of infant.	2					
• Remove infant from scale and place him in parent's arms.	3					
Option B: Measuring Length on the Examination Table						
• Put infant on table and hold shoulders.	4					
• Place stiff piece of cardboard against infant's crown.	3					
• Mark table paper where infant's crown meets cardboard.	3					
• Keep head in place and hold ankles with knees extended.	2					
• Mark table paper where heels meet paper.	3					
• Release ankles, but don't let go of infant.	2					
• Return infant to parent.	2					
• Measure distance between two marks on table paper with tape measure.	3					
POSTPROCEDURE						
15. Record infant's weight and length:						
• Record weight in pounds and ounces, or to nearest tenth of kilogram.	3					
• Record length in inches or centimeters.	3					
16. Return weights to left side of scale, or move table's length bar back into place.	2					
17. Clean and replace all equipment.	3					
18. Wash hands.	4					
TOTAL POSSIBLE POINTS	**100**					

Comments:

_____

_____

_____

_____

_____

Signatures: _____   **Date:** _____

SCORING *See Preface for scoring instructions.*

Human Growth and Development

PROCEDURE 7B:
Measuring Head Circumference

PROCEDURE ASSESSMENT

Procedure Steps	Suggested Points	Self Practice	Peer Practice	Peer Testing	Final Testing	Total Earned
PREPROCEDURE						
1. Gather needed equipment.	6					
PROCEDURE						
2. Explain procedure to parent.	7					
3. Wash hands and follow infection control guidelines.	8					
4. Place infant on table.	6					
• If necessary, measure while parent holds infant.						
5. Starting at forehead, wrap tape measure around infant's head.	6					
• Adjust so tape measure fits around head at largest circumference.	6					
• Adjust so tape measure is positioned evenly around head.	6					
6. Overlap tape measure and read at 1-inch or 1-centimeter mark.	6					
7. Make mental note of number.	6					
POSTPROCEDURE						
8. Return infant to parent or put infant in safe location.	8					
9. Subtract 1 from number obtained during measurement.	6					
10. Record head circumference.	7					
11. Put away equipment.	6					
12. Dispose of tape measure.	8					
13. Wash hands.	8					
TOTAL POSSIBLE POINTS	**100**					

Comments: _____

_____

_____

_____

Signatures: _____ Date: _____

SCORING   *See Preface for scoring instructions.*

Human Growth and Development

PROCEDURE 7C:
Measuring the Toddler

PROCEDURE ASSESSMENT

Procedure Steps	Suggested Points	Self Practice	Peer Practice	Peer Testing	Final Testing	Total Earned
PREPROCEDURE						
1. Gather needed equipment.	5					
2. Ensure scale is in balance:	5					
• Move all weights to left side of balance beam.	2					
• Indicator should be level with middle mark.	2					
3. If using scale that measures either kilograms or pounds:						
• Ensure it is set on desired units.	2					
• Ensure that upper and lower weights show same units.	2					
4. Put disposable towel or scale sheet on scale.	6					
PROCEDURE						
5. Identify client and get parent's permission to weigh toddler.	4					
6. Wash hands and follow infection control guidelines.	6					
7. Explain procedure to parent.	5					
Weight						
• Ask parent to hold toddler and step on scale. Record weight.	5					
• Ask parent to hand child to staff or family member.	4					
• Record parent's weight	4					
• Subtract parent's weight from combined weight to determine child's weight.	5					
• Record child's weight on chart to nearest quarter pound or tenth of kilogram.	5					
Height						
• Ask child to stand on scale with his back to balance beam.	4					
a. Ask child to look straight ahead and stand up straight.	4					
b. Move height bar so that it touches crown of child's head.	6					
c. Don't hit child's head with height bar.						
• Record height in inches or feet and inches.	5					

PROCEDURE 7C: Measuring the Toddler *(continued)*

Procedure Steps	Suggested Points	Self Practice	Peer Practice	Peer Testing	Final Testing	Total Earned
POSTPROCEDURE						
8. Return height and weight bars to starting position.	4					
9. Assist parent and child to safety as necessary.	5					
10. Discard paper towel or scale sheet.	4					
11. Wash hands.	6					
TOTAL POSSIBLE POINTS	100					

Comments:

_____

_____

_____

_____

_____

_____

_____

_____

_____

_____

Signatures: _____ **Date:** _____

SCORING *See Preface for scoring instructions.*

Human Growth and Development

PROCEDURE 7D:
Measuring the Adult

·········· P R O C E D U R E   A S S E S S M E N T ··········

Procedure Steps	Suggested Points	Self Practice	Peer Practice	Peer Testing	Final Testing	Total Earned
PREPROCEDURE						
1. Gather needed equipment.	4					
2. Ensure scale is in balance:	4					
• Move all weights to left side of balance beam.	2					
• Indicator should be level with middle mark.	1					
3. If using scale that measures either kilograms or pounds:						
• Ensure it is set on desired units.	2					
• Ensure that upper and lower weights show same units.	1					
4. Put disposable towel or scale sheet on scale.	6					
PROCEDURE						
5. Introduce yourself and identify client.	4					
6. Wash hands and follow infection control guidelines.	6					
Weight						
• Ask client to remove shoes and heavy coat. Use same procedure for all weights.	3					
a. When weighing a hospitalized client, weigh at same time, with same amount of clothing, on same scale. Make note of this information.						
b. Before you use a bed or wheelchair scale, review manufacturer's instructions and ensure scale is balanced.						
• Assist client onto scale, if necessary. Provide for safety.	6					
• Move lower weight bar to highest number that doesn't cause balance indicator to drop to bottom.	4					
• Move upper weight bar slowly to right until balance bar is centered at middle mark. Adjust as necessary.	4					
• Add amounts of two bars to obtain client's weight.	4					
• Record client's weight on chart to nearest quarter of pound or tenth of kilogram.	5					

PROCEDURE 7D: Measuring the Adult *(continued)*

Procedure Steps	Suggested Points	Self Practice	Peer Practice	Peer Testing	Final Testing	Total Earned
Height						
• Ask client to stand erect on scale with back to balance beam and look straight ahead.	3					
• Raise height bar above client's head and swing out extension.	4					
• Lower height bar until extension rests on top of client's head, at center of crown. Don't hit client with bar.	6					
• Hold height bar in place and ask client to step off scale.	3					
a. Read measurement.	3					
b. Assist client as necessary.	3					
• Read height bar:	4					
a. If client is less than 50 inches tall, read height on bottom part of ruler.						
b. If client is more than 50 inches tall, read height on top movable part of ruler.						
c. Be sure to read height in correct direction.						
• Record client's height in inches or feet and inches.	4					
POSTPROCEDURE						
7. Return weights and height bar to starting positions.	3					
8. Assist client with shoes and belongings, if necessary. Return hospitalized client to bed, wheelchair, room, or dining room.	3					
9. Discard paper towel or scale paper. If you used a lift sheet for bed scales, place with dirty linens.	3					
10. Wash hands.	5					
TOTAL POSSIBLE POINTS	**100**					

Comments: _____

_____

_____

_____

_____

_____

Signatures: _____ **Date:** _____

SCORING *See Preface for scoring instructions.*

Nutrition

Reinforcement Activities

Matching
Write the letter of the phrase that best matches each numbered item in the blank provided.

_____ 1. Amino acids
_____ 2. Cholesterol
_____ 3. Osteoporosis
_____ 4. Dietary fiber
_____ 5. Calories
_____ 6. Antioxidants
_____ 7. Malnutrition

a. Units for measuring energy from nutrient.
b. Condition resulting from severe nutrient deficiencies.
c. Substances that help protect cells from damage.
d. A condition of porous bones.
e. Building blocks of proteins.
f. Waxy substance that is part of cells.
g. A plant substance that the body can't digest.

Multiple Choice
Circle the letter that best answers the question or completes the statement.

8. Which of the following foods do not contain carbohydrates?
   a. fruit.
   b. bread.
   c. eggs.
   d. squash.

9. Over a lifetime, what you eat affects your chances of developing
   a. anemia.
   b. a chronic disease.
   c. malnutrition.
   d. foodborne illness.

10. The nutrients in the foods you eat
    a. supply energy.
    b. regulate body processes.
    c. build and repair tissues.
    d. all of the above.

11. Eating too much of which type of fat can increase your chances of heart disease?
    a. cholesterol.
    b. unsaturated fat.
    c. saturated fat.
    d. all of the above.

12. Which is not a fat-soluble vitamin?
    a. vitamin A.
    b. vitamin E.
    c. vitamin D.
    d. vitamin B12.

13. Recommended Dietary Allowances (RDAs) are
    a. the amounts of nutrients needed by individuals of all ages.
    b. the amounts of nutrients found in foods.
    c. the figures used on food labels.
    d. the food group servings needed by individuals.

14. About how many calories do most children, teen girls, active women, and less active men need each day?
    a. 1,600
    b. 2,200
    c. 2,500
    d. 2,800

15. Your daily energy, or calorie, needs depend on which factors?
    a. age.
    b. gender.
    c. how active you are.
    d. all of the above.

Fill in the Blank

Write the word (or words) that best completes the sentence in the blank provided.

16. Plant chemicals, called _____, are produced naturally by plants and may help protect you from health problems, such as heart disease and some types of cancer.

17. About 55 percent of your daily calories should come from _____.

18. The USDA Food Guide shows you how to put the _____ into practice.

19. Foods that contribute a significant amount of several nutrients compared with the calories they contain are considered _____.

20. When your food choices don't supply enough of the nutrients you need over a period of time, a _____ may result, causing poor health and lack of energy.

True/False

Write "T" in the blank provided if the statement is true. Write "F" if the statement is false.

_____ 21. If you eat a variety of nutritious foods on most days, you are likely getting enough of the nutrients your body needs and probably don't need a dietary supplement.

_____ 22. Women are more likely than men to have an iron deficiency.

_____ 23. Minerals supply energy and help protect your cells from damage.

_____ 24. Plant sources of protein supply all the essential amino acids your body needs.

_____ 25. Anemia, which makes you feel weak and tired, can be caused by a deficiency of iron.

Name _____ Date _____

Labeling

In the space provided, write the word(s) that identifies the corresponding part on the diagram.

26. Label the pie chart with the correct percentages of fats, proteins, and carbohydrates.

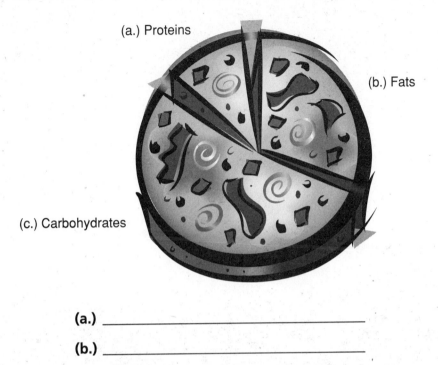

(a.) Proteins

(b.) Fats

(c.) Carbohydrates

(a.) _____

(b.) _____

(c.) _____

27. Using the USDA Food Guide, determine a healthy meal plan for yourself for one day.

Breakfast

_____

_____

_____

Lunch

_____

_____

_____

Dinner

_____

_____

_____

Snacks

_____

_____

_____

Nutrition

PROCEDURE 8A:
Create a Sample Meal Plan

PROCEDURE ASSESSMENT

Procedure Steps	Suggested Points	Self Practice	Peer Practice	Peer Testing	Final Testing	Total Earned
PREPROCEDURE						
1. Gather needed materials.	9					
2. Use Table 8-4 to determine your approximate daily calorie needs.	9					
3. Next, check Table 8-6 for the number of servings from each food group you need each day based on your energy needs.	8					
4. Write your personal serving goals next to each food group.	8					
PROCEDURE						
5. Write down what you eat on a typical day.	9					
• Divide your food group serving goals among your usual meals.	9					
6. Write down examples of foods you might eat and amounts that match the food group serving goals.	10					
• Use Food Guide serving sizes from each food group as a guide.						
7. Continue writing down foods and amounts for all your meals and snacks.	9					
• Include a few extras to add flavor and pleasure.						
POSTPROCEDURE						
8. Compare the sample meal plan with how you usually eat.	10					
• Do you usually eat more servings from any of the food groups?						
• Do you come up short on servings from any food groups?						
9. Think about how often you eat foods that are high in fats and/or added sugars.	9					
• Are there places you could cut back or eat healthier alternatives?						
10. Follow your sample meal plan for a day.	10					
• Think about changes you can make to meet your goals.						
TOTAL POSSIBLE POINTS	**100**					

PROCEDURE 8A: Create a Sample Meal Plan *(continued)*

Comments: _____

_____

_____

_____

_____

_____

_____

_____

_____

Signatures: _____   **Date:** _____

SCORING   *See Preface for scoring instructions.*

Vital Signs

Reinforcement Activities

Fill in the Blank

Write the word (or words) that best completes the sentence in the blank provided.

1. Write the expected ranges for vital signs for the following clients.

   a. 6 month old baby T _____ or _____

   P _____

   b. 10 year old boy   P _____

   c. 35 year old woman P _____ BP _____

   RR _____

2. _____ is the term you will use to document a client with fever, and _____ will be the term used to document a client without fever.

3. Invasive assessments such as a rectal temperature should be performed _____, while non-invasive assessments such as observing respirations should be performed _____.

4. When taking a tympanic temperature, gently pull the pinna of the ear _____ for adults and _____ for children.

5. Write the order of the following vital signs as if you are charting them on the client's record. Blood pressure: 126/62, pulse 69, temperature 97.9 degrees Fahrenheit, and respirations 18.

   _____

6. One "lub-dub" of the heart sounds is equal to _____ apical pulse beat.

7. The blood pressure cuff should fit snugly about _____ above the pulse site to be used.

8. When initially releasing the air in the blood pressure cuff, the point at which the sounds first appear will be the _____ blood pressure.

9. The last sound heard when taking the blood pressure will be the value for the _____ blood pressure.

10. Write an **E** for conditions causing an elevation in the vital sign, or write a **D** for conditions causing a decrease in the value of the vital sign(s).

    a. _____ T   stress or infection

    b. _____ T   exposure to the cold

    c. _____ P   crying infant

    d. _____ P   low blood pressure

e. _____ P   physically fit athlete

f. _____ RR   exercise

g. _____ RR   fever

h. _____ RR   alcohol intoxication

i. _____ RR   pain medication

11. Write the correct medical term for the following conditions.

a. client with fever _____

b. an abnormal condition where the temperature is below the normal range

_____

c. low heart rate _____

d. irregular heart rate _____ or _____

e. increased respiratory rate _____

f. difficulty breathing _____

g. no breathing _____

h. low blood pressure _____

i. high blood pressure _____

j. heart attack _____

k. damage to the brain caused by bleeding _____

True/False

Write "T" in the blank provided if the statement is true. Write "F" if the statement is false.

_____ 12. When recording an axillary temperature, always add one degree to the value.

_____ 13. Blue tipped glass thermometers measure body temperature more accurately than red tipped glass thermometers.

_____ 14. Report any abnormal vital sign values to the appropriate healthcare provider.

Labeling

In the space provided, write the word(s) that identifies the corresponding part on the diagram.

15. Label the pulse sites on the figure below.

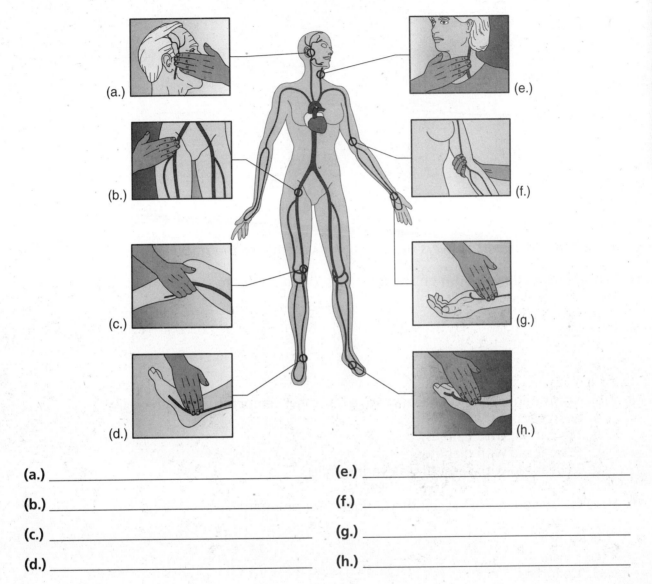

(a.) _____   (e.) _____

(b.) _____   (f.) _____

(c.) _____   (g.) _____

(d.) _____   (h.) _____

16. On the figure below, draw an arrow to each of the intercostal spaces (ics) on the left side of the chest and to the point where an apical pulse can best be heard.

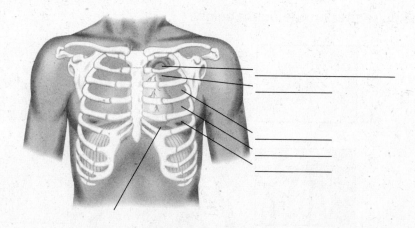

Multiple Choice

Circle the letter that best answers the question or completes the statement.

17. Which button do you push on the tympanic thermometer to remove the temperature probe from the thermometer?
   a. scan.
   b. eject.
   c. start.
   d. off.

18. Which of the following clients may have his or her temperature taken orally?
   a. two year old child.
   b. 18 year old with epilepsy.
   c. 55 year old with diabetes.
   d. 35 year old with fever and shivering chills.

19. How far do you insert a rectal thermometer for an infant?
   a. ½ inch.
   b. ¼ inch.
   c. 1 inch.
   d. 1½ inches.

20. How far do you insert a rectal thermometer for an adult?
   a. 1½ inches.
   b. ¼ inch.
   c. 1 inch.
   d. ½ inch.

21. How far do you insert a rectal thermometer for an child?
   a. ½ inch.
   b. ¼ inch.
   c. 1 inch.
   d. 1½ inches.

22. How long must you wait to take a temperature on a client who has just had a cup of coffee?
    a. 5 minutes.
    b. 15 minutes.
    c. 1 hour.
    d. waiting is not necessary.

23. If a pulse is irregular, how long do you count the rate?
    a. 15 seconds.
    b. 30 seconds.
    c. 1 minute
    d. 2 minutes.

24. If you counted 10 respirations in 30 seconds, what would be the RR? Is it normal or abnormal for an adult?
    a. 20; normal.
    b. 10; normal.
    c. 20; abnormal.
    d. 30; normal.

25. If you counted 20 beats in 15 seconds what would be the P? Is it normal or abnormal for an adult?
    a. 40; abnormal.
    b. 60; normal.
    c. 80; abnormal.
    d. 80; normal.

Vital Signs

PROCEDURE 9A:
Measuring and Recording Oral Temperature with a Glass Thermometer

PROCEDURE ASSESSMENT

Procedure Steps	Suggested Points	Self Practice	Peer Practice	Peer Testing	Final Testing	Total Earned
PREPROCEDURE						
1. Gather needed equipment.	2					
2. Introduce yourself to client.	3					
3. Identify client by asking his name and/or checking ID bracelet.	3					
4. Explain procedure to client.	3					
5. Provide for client privacy.	3					
6. Wash your hands.	5					
7. Put on gloves.	5					
8. Make sure client can hold thermometer in mouth and breath through nose.	5					
9. If client has been eating, drinking, or smoking, wait 15 minutes.	2					
PROCEDURE						
10. Hold handle of thermometer and shake until mercury level is below 95°F or 35°C.	3					
11. If using plastic sheath on thermometer, apply it now.	5					
12. Place bulb of thermometer under client's tongue, toward side of mouth.	3					
13. Ask client to gently close mouth, with lips holding thermometer. Teeth shouldn't be used to hold thermometer.	5					
14. Ask client to hold thermometer for 2 to 3 minutes.	3					
15. Hold handle of thermometer, ask client to open mouth, and remove thermometer.	3					
16. Remove sheath, turn it inside out, and discard it.	5					
17. Read thermometer:	4					
• Hold thermometer up to light.	3					
• Roll it between thumb and first finger.	3					
• Look for silver bar to appear.	3					
• Hold thermometer so you can see bar and numbers clearly. The number that marks where bar ends is the temperature.	3					
18. Record the temperature.	4					
• Include degree of temperature and unit of measurement (F or C).	2					
• Include method of measurement (oral).	2					

PROCEDURE 9A: Measuring and Recording Oral Temperature with a Glass Thermometer *(continued)*

Procedure Steps POSTPROCEDURE	Suggested Points	Self Practice	Peer Practice	Peer Testing	Final Testing	Total Earned
19. Wash thermometer with soapy, room-temperature water; rinse with cool water.	5					
20. Shake thermometer gently and store in clean, dry case.	3					
• If disinfection is needed, store thermometer in 70% isopropyl alcohol.	2					
21. Remove gloves and wash hands.	5					
22. Report to supervisor if temperature is a significant change from previous result or is outside normal range.	3					
TOTAL POSSIBLE POINTS	100					

Comments:

_____

_____

_____

_____

_____

_____

_____

_____

_____

Signatures: _____   Date: _____

SCORING   *See Preface for scoring instructions.*

Vital Signs

PROCEDURE 9B:
Measuring and Recording Tympanic Temperature

········· **P R O C E D U R E   A S S E S S M E N T** ·········

Procedure Steps	Suggested Points	Self Practice	Peer Practice	Peer Testing	Final Testing	Total Earned
PREPROCEDURE						
1. Gather needed equipment.	4					
2. Introduce yourself to client.	5					
3. Identify client by asking name and checking ID bracelet.	5					
4. Explain procedure to client.	6					
5. Provide for client privacy.	4					
6. Wash your hands.	7					
PROCEDURE						
7. Remove thermometer from charging base and snap disposable cover onto tip of probe.	3					
8. Hold outer edge of ear (pinna) with free hand.	6					
• For adults, lift pinna up.	5					
• For children, pull pinna down.	5					
9. Gently place probe tip into ear canal, directing it toward face.	5					
10. Press scan button. Be sure not to press probe eject button. Within 2 to 5 seconds, thermometer should beep or flash.	7					
11. Remove probe from ear and note reading.	4					
POSTPROCEDURE						
12. Press eject button and discard probe cover.	4					
13. Return thermometer to charging base.	4					
14. Wash your hands.	7					
15. Record measurement.	5					
• Include degree of temperature and unit of measurement (°F or °C).	4					
• Include method of measurement (tympanic).	4					
16. Report to supervisor if temperature is a significant change from previous result or is outside normal range.	6					
TOTAL POSSIBLE POINTS	100					

Comments: _____
_____
_____
_____
_____
_____
_____
_____
_____

Signatures: _____   Date: _____

SCORING   *See Preface for scoring instructions.*

Vital Signs

PROCEDURE 9C:
Measuring and Recording Axillary Temperature

--------- P R O C E D U R E   A S S E S S M E N T ---------

Procedure Steps	Suggested Points	Self Practice	Peer Practice	Peer Testing	Final Testing	Total Earned
PREPROCEDURE						
1. Gather needed equipment.	3					
2. Introduce yourself to client.	4					
3. Identify client by asking name and checking ID bracelet.	5					
4. Explain procedure to client.	5					
5. Provide for client privacy.	5					
6. Wash your hands.	7					
PROCEDURE						
7. Apply plastic sheath or probe cover to thermometer.	7					
8. Lift client's arm and place tip of thermometer into middle of armpit (axilla).	4					
9. Put arm back down.	4					
• Ensure tip of thermometer is completely covered with skin.	3					
10. Leave glass thermometer in place for 5 to 9 minutes. Electronic thermometer will signal when done.	4					
11. Lift up client's arm and remove thermometer.	3					
12. Note reading.	3					
POSTPROCEDURE						
13. Remove plastic sheath or eject probe cover and discard.	7					
14. Clean and return thermometer to its location.	7					
15. Wash your hands.	7					
16. Record measurement.	6					
• Include degree of temperature and unit of measurement (°F or °C).	5					
• Include method of measurement (axillary).	5					
17. Report to supervisor if temperature is a significant change from previous result or is outside normal range.	6					
TOTAL POSSIBLE POINTS	**100**					

PROCEDURE 9C: Measuring and Recording Axillary Temperature *(continued)*

Comments: _____
_____
_____
_____
_____
_____
_____
_____
_____

Signatures: _____   Date: _____

SCORING   *See Preface for scoring instructions.*

Vital Signs

PROCEDURE 9D:
Measuring and Recording Rectal Temperature

······· P R O C E D U R E   A S S E S S M E N T ·······

Procedure Steps	Suggested Points	Self Practice	Peer Practice	Peer Testing	Final Testing	Total Earned
PREPROCEDURE						
1. Gather needed equipment.	2					
2. Introduce yourself to client.	3					
3. Identify client by asking name and checking ID bracelet. Identify infant or child by asking parent.	3					
4. Explain procedure to client or parent.	3					
5. Provide for client privacy.	3					
6. Wash hands and put on gloves.	4					
PROCEDURE						
7. Apply plastic sheath or probe cover to thermometer.	4					
8. Place small amount of lubricant on paper towel and lay thermometer tip into lubricant.	4					
9. Assist client into side-lying position with knees bent. Left-side lying is best because of anatomy of anal canal.	3					
10. When taking temperature of young child or infant:	3					
• Place client on stomach with assistant pressing hips and thighs down.	2					
• Or place client on back and lift and hold legs securely.	2					
11. Insert thermometer, avoiding unnecessary exposure:	3					
• ½ inch for infants.	2					
• 1 inch for children.	2					
• 1½ inch for adults.	2					
12. Never force insertion of thermometer.	4					
• Ask client to take deep breaths to relax sphincter muscle. If you have difficulty, obtain assistance.	2					
13. Hold thermometer in place and lay your hand on buttocks. If client moves, your hand will move with buttocks and prevent further insertion of probe.	3					

PROCEDURE 9D: Measuring and Recording Rectal Temperature *(continued)*

Procedure Steps	Suggested Points	Self Practice	Peer Practice	Peer Testing	Final Testing	Total Earned
PROCEDURE						
14. Leave glass thermometer in place for 3 to 5 minutes.	3					
• Electronic thermometer will signal when done.						
15. Remove probe gently; tell client you are removing it.	3					
16. Note reading.	2					
POSTPROCEDURE						
17. Remove plastic sheath or probe cover and discard.	4					
• If you didn't use sheath or cover, wipe thermometer from tip to bulb.	2					
• Discard thermometer in proper receptacle.	2					
18. Wipe excess lubricant from buttocks.	4					
19. Return client to safe and comfortable position.	4					
20. Clean and return thermometer to its location.	4					
21. Remove your gloves.	4					
22. Wash your hands.	4					
23. Record measurement.	3					
• Include degree of temperature and unit of measurement (°F or °C).	2					
• Include method of measurement (rectal).	2					
24. Report to supervisor if temperature is a significant change from previous result or is outside normal range.	3					
TOTAL POSSIBLE POINTS	**100**					

Comments: _____

_____

_____

_____

_____

_____

_____

_____

Signatures: _____   Date: _____

SCORING *See Preface for scoring instructions.*

Vital Signs

PROCEDURE 9E:
Measuring and Recording Temperature with an Electronic Thermometer

········· **P R O C E D U R E   A S S E S S M E N T** ·········

Procedure Steps	Suggested Points	Self Practice	Peer Practice	Peer Testing	Final Testing	Total Earned
PREPROCEDURE						
1. Gather needed equipment.	4					
2. Introduce yourself to client.	5					
3. Identify client by asking name and checking ID bracelet.	6					
4. Explain procedure to client.	6					
5. Provide for client privacy.	5					
6. Wash hands and put on gloves for oral and/or rectal temperatures.	8					
PROCEDURE						
7. Position client as needed for method of measurement.	5					
8. Remove unit from base.	3					
9. Remove probe from unit.	3					
10. Insert probe into probe cover until it snaps into place.	4					
• If using small, battery-operated thermometer, apply plastic sheath.	3					
11. Perform procedure for obtaining measurement.	5					
12. Thermometer will beep or flash when done.	4					
13. Remove probe and eject or remove cover.	5					
14. Read digital display before returning probe to holder. Reinserting probe may clear the display.	5					
POSTPROCEDURE						
15. Place probe back into holder.	4					
16. Place holding unit back into base for recharging.	5					
17. Remove gloves and wash your hands.	8					
18. Document temperature, unit of measurement and location where temperature was taken.	6					
19. Report to supervisor if temperature is a significant change from previous result or is outside normal range.	6					
TOTAL POSSIBLE POINTS	**100**					

Comments: _____

_____

_____

_____

_____

_____

_____

_____

_____

Signatures: _____ Date: _____

SCORING *See Preface for scoring instructions.*

Vital Signs

PROCEDURE 9F:
Measuring and Recording Pulse and Respirations

············ P R O C E D U R E   A S S E S S M E N T ············

Procedure Steps	Suggested Points	Self Practice	Peer Practice	Peer Testing	Final Testing	Total Earned
PREPROCEDURE						
1. Gather needed equipment.	3					
2. Introduce yourself to client.	4					
3. Identify client by asking name and checking ID bracelet.	4					
4. Explain procedure: "I'm going to take your vital signs. We'll start by checking your pulse." Don't tell client that you're counting respirations.	5					
5. Wash your hands.	6					
PROCEDURE						
6. Ask client to sit or lie down in a comfortable position.	3					
7. Have client place arm on table or bed or on your hand.	4					
• Client's palm should be facing downward.	3					
• You may want to lay client's arm over his chest in order to feel chest movements.	3					
8. Position yourself so you can observe chest wall movement.	3					
9. Place 2 or 3 fingers on radial pulse.	4					
• Don't use thumb to take pulse.	3					
• Find radial bone and put your fingers in groove on inside of wrist to find radial pulse.	3					
10. Count pulse for 15 to 30 seconds, if regular.	4					
• Count for a full minute if irregular.	3					
• Remember the number.	3					
11. Don't let go of wrist, but begin observing respiratory rate.	4					
12. Count respiratory rate for a minute.	4					
13. When you are done, let go of wrist.	3					

PROCEDURE 9F: Measuring and Recording Pulse and Respirations *(continued)*

Procedure Steps POSTPROCEDURE	Suggested Points	Self Practice	Peer Practice	Peer Testing	Final Testing	Total Earned
14. Immediately write down two numbers.	5					
15. If pulse and respirations were counted for full minute, record numbers.	4					
• If you counted pulse for less than a minute, find beats per minute. Example: If you counted for 15 seconds, multiply number you obtained by 4 to get number of beats in 60 seconds.	3					
16. Document pulse rate, volume, and rhythm.	4					
17. Document respiratory rate, rhythm, volume, and effort.	4					
18. Wash your hands.	6					
19. Report to supervisor any findings that are a significant change from previous results or are outside normal range.	5					
TOTAL POSSIBLE POINTS	**100**					

Comments: _____

_____

_____

_____

_____

_____

_____

_____

_____

_____

_____

Signatures: _____   Date: _____

SCORING   *See Preface for scoring instructions.*

Vital Signs

PROCEDURE 9G:
Measuring and Recording Apical Pulse

PROCEDURE ASSESSMENT

Procedure Steps	Suggested Points	Self Practice	Peer Practice	Peer Testing	Final Testing	Total Earned
PREPROCEDURE						
1. Gather needed equipment.	4					
2. Introduce yourself to client.	5					
3. Identify client by asking name and checking ID bracelet.	4					
4. Explain procedure to client.	5					
5. Provide for client privacy.	4					
6. Wash your hands.	7					
PROCEDURE						
7. Ask client to sit or lie down	4					
8. To be able to hear apical pulse:	5					
• Give infant pacifier or calm him so he doesn't cry.	4					
• Ask adult clients not to speak.	4					
9. Place stethoscope tips in your ear canals, pointing forward toward eardrums.	5					
10. Place warmed diaphragm of stethoscope directly on skin over apex of heart.	5					
• Apex of heart is 2 to 3 inches left of sternum, right below nipple.	3					
11. Listen for "lub-dub" sounds; each one equals one apical pulse.	5					
12. Count pulse for 1 full minute.	5					
13. Note rhythm.	5					
POSTPROCEDURE						
14. Record rate, rhythm, date, time, and method of assessment (apical).	5					
• If you have taken apical pulse and radial pulse, note as A78/P78.	4					
• If there is pulse deficit, note as A78/P74 Pulse deficit 4.	4					
15. Wash your hands.	7					
16. Report to supervisor any findings that are a significant change from previous results or are outside normal range.	6					
TOTAL POSSIBLE POINTS	**100**					

PROCEDURE 9G: Measuring and Recording Apical Pulse *(continued)*

Comments: _____

_____

_____

_____

_____

_____

_____

_____

_____

Signatures: _____   Date: _____

SCORING   *See Preface for scoring instructions.*

Vital Signs

PROCEDURE 9H:
Measuring and Recording Blood Pressure

PROCEDURE ASSESSMENT

Procedure Steps	Suggested Points	Self Practice	Peer Practice	Peer Testing	Final Testing	Total Earned
PREPROCEDURE						
1. Gather needed equipment.	2					
2. Introduce yourself to client.	2					
3. Identify client by asking name and checking ID bracelet.	3					
4. Explain procedure to client.	3					
• If possible, have client sit quietly for 5 minutes before procedure.	1					
• Stay calm and reassure client.	2					
5. Provide privacy, if needed.	3					
6. Clean stethoscope earpieces, bell, and diaphragm with disinfectant.	4					
7. Wash your hands.	4					
PROCEDURE						
8. Ask client to sit or lie down.	3					
• Client's arm should be close to level of heart and relaxed.	1					
• Palm should be up.	1					
• Raise sleeve above level of pulse site.	1					
9. Choose appropriate-sized cuff.	3					
10. Turn valve of cuff to left (open position) and squeeze cuff until it's flat.	3					
11. Place cuff directly on skin of extremity.	3					
• Push client's sleeve up to shoulder level, if necessary.	1					
12. Wrap cuff snugly around extremity	3					
• Pulse site should be in middle of bladder of cuff.	1					
• Allow about an inch below cuff for placement of diaphragm.	1					
13. Palpate artery with your first and second fingers.	2					
14. Place earpieces of stethoscope in your ears, facing toward eardrums.	2					
15. Turn valve completely to right until it stops.	3					
• Loosen valve slightly so it can easily be turned back.	1					
16. Pump bulb, while watching sphygmomanometer indicator rise, until you no longer feel pulse.	3					
• At this point, no blood is flowing through the artery.						

Procedure Steps	Suggested Points	Self Practice	Peer Practice	Peer Testing	Final Testing	Total Earned
17. Quickly note number at which pulse disappears (approximation of systolic pressure).	3					
18. Quickly turn valve to left and allow air to fully escape cuff.	3					
19. Remove and replace cuff or wait 1 to 2 minutes before reinflating cuff.	3					
20. Position diaphragm of stethoscope directly over artery.	3					
• Reinflate cuff about 20 to 30 mm Hg above point at which pulse disappeared.	1					
21. Release valve to left, allowing indicator to fall slowly, about 2 to 4 mm Hg per second.	2					
22. Listen for beginning of sounds.	2					
• Number at which first sound is heard is systolic pressure.						
23. Number at which last sound is heard is diastolic pressure.	2					
24. Once last sound is heard, quickly release remaining air from bladder.	3					
POSTPROCEDURE						
25. Remove cuff from arm, and expel excess air from bladder.	2					
26. Record measurement as fraction (systolic number/diastolic number).	3					
27. Return client to safe and comfortable position.	4					
28. Clean earpieces, bell, and diaphragm of stethoscope and replace equipment.	3					
29. Wash your hands.	4					
30. Report to supervisor any findings that are a significant change from previous results or are outside normal range.	3					
• A change of 30 or more mm Hg in either systolic or diastolic reading should be recorded.	3					
TOTAL POSSIBLE POINTS	**100**					

Comments: _____

_____

_____

_____

_____

Signatures: _____   Date: _____

SCORING *See Preface for scoring instructions.*

Name _____ Date _____

Vital Signs

PROCEDURE 9I:
Measuring and Recording Vital Signs Electronically

PROCEDURE ASSESSMENT

Procedure Steps	Suggested Points	Self Practice	Peer Practice	Peer Testing	Final Testing	Total Earned
PREPROCEDURE						
1. Gather needed equipment.	3					
2. Introduce yourself to client.	4					
3. Identify client by asking name and checking ID bracelet.	3					
4. Explain procedure to client.	5					
5. Provide for client privacy, if needed.	3					
6. Wash your hands.	6					
PROCEDURE						
7. Ask client to sit or lie down.	4					
• Client's arm should be close to level of heart and relaxed.	3					
• Palm should be up.	3					
• Raise sleeve above level of pulse site.	3					
8. Remind client that cuff will become tight.	4					
9. Choose appropriate-sized cuff.	3					
10. Position extremity so it's slightly flexed, relaxed, and at level of heart.	4					
11. Push power button on face of machine.	3					
12. Push start button. Cuff will begin to inflate.	3					
13. Since machine is very sensitive to movement, ask client to stay still.	4					
• If client moves, and cuff starts inflating again, press stop button, remove cuff, and allow extremity to rest 1 to 2 minutes before starting process again.	4					
14. Systolic and diastolic readings will appear in boxes on machine screen.	4					
15. Pulse rate is recorded and will be displayed on screen.	4					
16. Machine will automatically release air from bladder.	4					
• Remove cuff and turn power off.	3					

PROCEDURE 9I: Measuring and Recording Vital Signs Electronically (continued)

Procedure Steps	Suggested Points	Self Practice	Peer Practice	Peer Testing	Final Testing	Total Earned
POSTPROCEDURE						
17. Record blood pressure, pulse, and other measurements.	4					
18. Return machine to proper location and plug into outlet or place on charging base.	4					
19. Wash your hands.	6					
20. Report to supervisor any findings that are a significant change from previous results or are outside normal range.	5					
• A change of 30 or more mm Hg in either systolic or diastolic reading should be recorded.	4					
TOTAL POSSIBLE POINTS	100					

Comments: _____

_____

_____

_____

_____

_____

_____

_____

_____

_____

Signatures: _____   Date: _____

SCORING   See Preface for scoring instructions.

Pharmacology

Reinforcement Activities

Matching

Write the letter of the phrase that best matches each numbered item in the blank provided.

_____ **1.** Pharmacognosy

_____ **2.** Antibiotics

_____ **3.** Sublingual

_____ **4.** Foxglove

_____ **5.** Vasoconstriction

_____ **6.** Histamine

_____ **7.** Hypertension

_____ **8.** MOA

_____ **9.** Pharmacokinetics

_____ **10.** Beta-2 agonists

a. A narrowing of blood vessels.

b. High blood pressure.

c. Drugs that produce the same effect in the lungs as the naturally occurring epinephrine.

d. These are used to kill bacteria that are growing in the body.

e. The study of four processes—absorption, distribution, transformation and elimination—that affect how the dosage of a drug is determined.

f. The study of drugs that are naturally derived from plants or animals.

g. The plant source of digitalis, which is used to treat congestive heart failure.

h. A chemical that is released from mast cells when a person is exposed to an allergen.

i. Mechanism of action.

j. Medication placed under the tongue.

Fill in the Blank.

Write the word (or words) that best completes the sentence in the blank provided.

11. _____ and _____, both used to treat pain, come from the seeds of the poppy.

12. _____ was originally an extract taken from the bark of willow trees.

13. Until 1980, diabetics used insulin extracted from _____ or _____.

14. _____ occur before a drug is absorbed into the bloodstream.

15. _____ are naturally occurring pain relievers produced by our bodies.

16. _____ describes an injection into the fatty layer just beneath the skin.

17. The _____ is the most widely used measurement system in pharmacy.

18. The _____ system includes units such as the fluid ounce and pound.

19. The _____ of measurement includes those used in the kitchen, such as teaspoon and tablespoon.

20. Most drugs are eliminated primarily in the _____.

Multiple Choice

Circle the letter that best answers the question or completes the statement.

21. The abbreviation for decigrams is
   a. dag.
   b. dc.
   c. dg.
   d. dec.

22. One teaspoon is equivalent to
   a. 5 mL.
   b. 5 mg.
   c. 5 L.
   d. 5 gm.

23. One kilogram (kg) is equivalent to
   a. 2 lbs.
   b. 1.2 lbs.
   c. 2.5 lbs.
   d. 2.2 lbs.

24. A parenteral route of medication is
   a. metered-dose inhaler.
   b. injection.
   c. transdermal patch.
   d. a, b, and c.

25. The chemicals produced in the body that cause pain and swelling associated with inflammation are called
   a. endorphins.
   b. prostaglandins.
   c. analgesics.
   d. statins.

26. One of the first drugs that did not come from a plant or animal was
   a. penicillin.
   b. aspirin.
   c. insulin.
   d. codeine.

27. All of the following are examples of antihistamines *except*
   a. benadryl.
   b. brethine.
   c. Claritin.
   d. Zertec.

28. The word pharmacy comes from a _____ word meaning medicine or drug.
   a. Latin
   b. French
   c. Greek
   d. German

29. Of the parenteral routes of medication, which has the longest onset of action?
    a. intramuscular.
    b. transdermal patch.
    c. rectal.
    d. buccal.
30. Plants remained the main source of medicine until
    a. the mid-1900s.
    b. 1850.
    c. 1890.
    d. the early 1900s.

Calculations

The order reads: Amoxicillin 500 mg PO QID. The client has 250 mg capsules on hand.

31. How many tablets would you give the client for one dose? _____

32. How many tablets would you give the client in one day? _____

Legal and Ethical Responsibilities

Reinforcement Activities

Matching

Write the letter of the phrase that best matches each numbered item in the blank provided.

_____ **1.** Laws

_____ **2.** Informed consent

_____ **3.** Privileged communication

_____ **4.** Standard of care

_____ **5.** Liability

_____ **6.** Reciprocity

a. Accountability under the law.

b. Rules of conduct enacted and enforced by a controlling authority.

c. A professional license obtained in one state is valid in another state without reexamination.

d. The client's right to receive all information about his or her condition.

e. A level of performance expected of a health care worker in carrying out his or her professional duties.

f. Information received within the context of the health care provider-client relationship.

True/False

Write "T" in the blank provided if the statement is true. Write "F" if the statement is false.

_____ **7.** Unethical behavior is always illegal.

_____ **8.** Unlawful acts are always unethical.

_____ **9.** Physicians are licensed by the state in which they wish to practice.

_____ **10.** Once granted, a health care practitioner's license cannot be revoked.

_____ **11.** Licensure is a mandatory process, established by law and required of certain health care practitioners.

_____ **12.** Negligence is a criminal charge.

_____ **13.** The durable power of attorney is not specifically a medical document, but it may serve that purpose.

_____ **14.** It is illegal for clients admitted to hospitals to specify that they do not want to be resuscitated if their hearts stop.

Multiple Choice

Circle the letter that best answers the question or completes the statement.

15. As a health care worker, which of the following doctrines will apply to you?
    a. the law of agency.
    b. the 3 Ds of negligence.
    c. standard of care or scope of practice.
    d. all of the above.

16. Which of the following statements is *not* a result of a health care practitioner's being accused of unethical conduct?
    a. being subjected to peer council review.
    b. having his or her medical license revoked.
    c. being expelled from the medical society.
    d. perhaps losing clients as word gets around.

17. What does the government enact to keep society running smoothly?
    a. laws.
    b. codes of ethics.
    c. morals.
    d. torts.

18. Statutes enacted in all 50 states to govern the practice of medicine are called
    a. occupational statutes.
    b. medical practice acts.
    c. the Bill of Rights.
    d. medical licensing boards.

19. Health care practitioners may be charged with negligence under
    a. the law of agency.
    b. reciprocity.
    c. the standard of care for their profession.
    d. licensure.

20. Confidentiality may be waived
    a. when a client sues a physician for malpractice.
    b. when a client signs a waiver.
    c. when a third party requests a medical examination and pays the physician's fee.
    d. all of the above.

21. Informed consent implies that the client understands
    a. the proposed modes of treatment.
    b. the reasons the treatment is necessary.
    c. the risks involved in the proposed treatment.
    d. all of the above.

22. A professional code of ethics
   a. is enforceable by law.
   b. exists only for physicians.
   c. serves as a guideline for moral conduct for members of a profession.
   d. originated in the twentieth century in Great Britain.

23. Which of the following is NOT considered a client's right?
   a. the right to refuse to pay a bill for medical care.
   b. the right to considerate and respectful care.
   c. the right to current and understandable information concerning diagnosis, treatment and prognosis.
   c. the right to know the immediate and long-term costs of treatment choices.

24. Client responsibilities include
   a. providing information about past illnesses, hospitalizations and medications.
   b. releasing medical information to anyone who asks for it.
   c. researching symptoms of an illness before seeing a physician.
   d. personally filing insurance forms for health care reimbursement.

Fill in the Blank

Write the word (or words) that best completes the sentence in the blank provided.

25. If a client wants to make his or her end-of-life wishes known, he or she completes an

_____ .

26. Successful health care workers must learn to _____ effectively in order to communi-cate well with clients.

27. _____ are derived from the influence of family, culture and society.

28. Health care practitioners who breach a client's _____ may be sued.

29. Medical malpractice is another term for charges of _____ .

30. Medical records must never be released without the _____ of the client.

Legal and Ethical Responsibilities

PROCEDURE 11A:
Recording Information on a Client's Medical Record

PROCEDURE ASSESSMENT

Procedure Steps	Suggested Points	Self Practice	Peer Practice	Peer Testing	Final Testing	Total Earned
PREPROCEDURE						
1. Gather needed equipment.	1					
2. Make sure you have correct medical records (existing record) or forms (new record).	2					
3. If you must transcribe a doctor's notes, do it as soon as possible, and enter notes into client's record.	2					
PROCEDURE						
When recording information, include:						
4. Client's basic information:	3					
• Full name.	2					
• Social Security number.	2					
• Birth date.	2					
• Full address.	2					
• Home and work telephone numbers.	2					
• Marital status.	2					
• Employer's name and address.	2					
5. Client's medical history:	3					
• Spell out names of disorders, diseases, medications and medical terms, and add abbreviations.	2					
6. Dates and times of client's arrival for appointments.	2					
7. Description of client's symptoms and reason for making appointment.	2					
8. The exam performed by the physician.	2					
9. Physician's notes:	3					
• Assessment.	2					
• Diagnosis.	2					
• Recommendations.	2					
• Treatment prescribed.	2					
• Progress notes.	2					
• Instructions given to client.	2					
10. X-rays and all other test results.	2					
11. A notation for each time:	3					
• Client phoned the medical facility.	2					
• Client was phoned by the medical facility.	2					
• Listing date.	2					
• Reason for call.	2					
• Resolution.	2					

Procedure Steps	Suggested Points	Self Practice	Peer Practice	Peer Testing	Final Testing	Total Earned
PROCEDURE						
12. A notation of copies made of medical record, including date copied and to whom copy was sent.	3					
13. Copies of all prescriptions and notes on refill authorizations.	2					
14. Documentation of informed consent, when necessary.	2					
15. Name of guardian or legal representative to be contacted if client is unable to give informed consent.	2					
16. Other documentation, including:	3					
• Complete written descriptions.	2					
• Photographs.	2					
• Samples of body fluids.	2					
• Foreign objects.	2					
• Clothing.	2					
• All items should be labeled and preserved.	2					
17. Condition of client at time of termination of treatment and reasons for termination.	3					
• If termination happened before treatment was completed, this should be explained.						
POSTPROCEDURE						
18. Read over all entries for omissions or mistakes.	2					
• Check with supervisor if you have questions.						
19. Ensure that you have dated and initialed each entry added to record.	3					
20. Ensure that you have included all pertinent data.	3					
21. Return client's file to filing system as quickly as possible.	2					
TOTAL POSSIBLE POINTS	100					

Comments:

_____

_____

_____

_____

_____

Signatures: _____   Date: _____

SCORING   *See Preface for scoring instructions.*

Employability Skills   Reinforcement Activities

Matching

Write the letter of the phrase that best matches each numbered item in the blank provided.

_____ **1.** Networking
_____ **2.** Objective
_____ **3.** Feedback
_____ **4.** Empathy
_____ **5.** Aphasia
_____ **6.** Passive
_____ **7.** Confidentiality
_____ **8.** Interference

a. Puts needs of others before needs of self.
b. Building mutually helpful relationships.
c. Ability to feel what someone else feels.
d. Communication disorder associated with stroke.
e. Anything that makes communication difficult.
f. Just the facts.
g. Only revealing information to authorized people.
h. Tells the sender if the message was received.

Short Answer

Answer the questions in the space below.

9. Discrimination against employees is prohibited based on what characteristics?

_____

_____

10. How much advanced notice is generally considered sufficient when leaving a job?

_____

_____

11. What is the standard mathematical system used in health care technology?

_____

_____

Fill in the Blank

Write the word (or words) that best completes the sentence in the blank provided.

12. Stress management requires that you _____ work with enjoyable outside activity.

13. The _____ is an opportunity for employees to get formal feedback about things they do well and about areas needing improvement.

14. _____ is the ability to influence others to accomplish goals.

True/False

Write "T" in the blank provided if the statement is true. Write "F" if the statement is false.

_____ 15. Verbal communication is limited to spoken messages.

_____ 16. A closed question has limited options for an answer.

_____ 17. Sexual harassment can include any unwanted communication or act of a sexual nature.

_____ 18. Someone with an aggressive personality usually looks out for the needs of others.

_____ 19. Someone with an assertive personality is often disrespectful toward others.

_____ 20. You should shout at people who don't hear well so that they will understand.

_____ 21. Use fairly closed questions for people who have aphasia.

_____ 22. It is possible to practice for an interview by developing generic questions.

Matching

Write the letter of the phrase that best matches each numbered item in the blank provide.

_____ 23. Resources skills   **a.** Reading, writing, math.

_____ 24. Subjective   **b.** Working with others to achieve shared goals.

_____ 25. Non-verbal communication   **c.** Concise document presenting your qualifications.

_____ 26. Basic skills   **d.** Ability to allocate people, time, materials.

_____ 27. Teamwork   **e.** Ability to work with others, teach, lead.

_____ 28. Thinking skills   **f.** Accompanies the résumé.

_____ 29. Cover letter   **g.** Includes personal perception, not just facts.

_____ 30. Résumé   **h.** Learning, reasoning, solving problems.

_____ 31. Interpersonal skills   **i.** Sends a message without speaking or writing.

Emergency Medical Services

Reinforcement Activities

Matching

Write the letter of the phrase that best matches each numbered item in the blank provided.

_____ **1.** Amniotic sac

_____ **2.** Crowning

_____ **3.** Mechanism of injury

_____ **4.** Oral airway

_____ **5.** Sign

_____ **6.** Symptom

_____ **7.** Nasal cannula

a. Head of baby protruding through vagina.

b. A curved plastic device placed in the mouth.

c. Something that the client tells you.

d. Evidence of a disease physically observed.

e. Bag of water that surrounds the fetus.

f. Forces that cause an injury.

g. Device used to deliver low concentrations of oxygen.

Multiple Choice

Circle the letter that best answers the question or completes the statement.

8. An oropharyngeal airway of the proper size will extend from the corner of the client's mouth to the
   a. tip of the earlobe on the same side of the client's face.
   b. angle of the lower jaw bone (mandible).
   c. tip of the nose.
   d. the chin.

9. When inserting the oropharyngeal airway into an adult client's mouth, position it so that the tip is pointing toward the
   a. corner of the client's mouth.
   b. roof of the client's mouth.
   c. client's tongue.
   d. client's chin.

10. When inserting a nasopharyngeal airway, lubricate the outside of the tube with
   a. petroleum jelly.
   b. water-based lubricant.
   c. a silicon-based lubricant.
   d. an oil-based lubricant.

11. Oxygen cylinders should never be allowed to be depleted below the safe residual. The safe residual for an oxygen cylinder is when the pressure gauge reads
   a. 125 psi.
   b. 145 psi.
   c. 180 psi.
   d. 200 psi.

12. All of the following statements are *true* except
    a. Never use oxygen around an open flame.
    b. Never leave an oxygen cylinder standing upright without being secured.
    c. Never use adhesive tape to protect an oxygen cylinder nor use adhesive tape to mark it.
    d. Never use nonferrous metal wrenches for changing regulators and gauges, or adjusting flow rates.

13. For an additional margin of safety, at what level do most EMS or First Responder agencies change oxygen tanks?
    a. 500 psi
    b. 200 psi
    c. 800 psi
    d. 2000 psi

14. A pressure regulator provides a safe working pressure of
    a. 20-80 psi.
    b. 30-70 psi.
    c. 40-80 psi.
    d. 50-90 psi.

15. The percent of oxygen delivered from a nonrebreather mask is
    a. 50-60
    b. 60-80
    c. 70-90
    d. 80-90

16. A nasal cannula has a flow rate of
    a. 1-2 liters per minute.
    b. 2-4 liters per minute.
    c. 1-6 liters per minute.
    d. 2-8 liters per minute.

17. A nonrebreather mask has a flow rate of
    a. 2-4 liters per minute.
    b. 2-6 liters per minute.
    c. 8-12 liters per minute.
    d. 12-15 liters per minute.

18. Which of the following clients would probably need supplemental oxygen?
    a. 2-year-old with the measles
    b. 10-year-old with scoliosis
    c. 15-year-old with Tourette's syndrome
    d. 20-year-old overdosed on illegal drugs

19. Examples of mechanism of injury would include *all but* which of the following
    a. a laceration on the forehead.
    b. a star burst pattern on the windshield.
    c. a damaged dashboard.
    d. a ladder lying beside the client.

20. Personal protective equipment which assists in Body Substance Isolation Precautions would be
   a. disposable latex or vinyl gloves.
   b. impervious gown.
   c. face shield.
   d. all of these.

21. The first step to take in the Initial Assessment is
   a. form a general impression of the client.
   b. establish the level of responsiveness.
   c. open and maintain the airway.
   d. assess for signs of circulation.

22. During the Initial Assessment, EMTs assess the client's "ABCs." What does "C" stand for?
   a. check pulse.
   b. check for breathing.
   c. circulation.
   d. check airway.

23. When in the process of assessing a client, you encounter a life-threatening problem involving airway, breathing, or circulation, you should
   a. continue with the survey and return to the problem later.
   b. stop the assessment and correct the problem immediately.
   c. stop the assessment of the client and seek immediate transport.
   d. stop the assessment and take the client's vital signs.

24. Which of the following clients would most likely need manual stabilization?
   a. heart attack victim
   b. motor vehicle accident victim
   c. stroke victim
   d. shock victim

25. The proper way to open the airway of an unresponsive trauma client
   a. head tilt-chin lift.
   b. use an oral pharyngeal airway.
   c. jaw thrust.
   d. jaw lift.

26. When communicating with an injured client, which of the following would be the correct way to address an elderly male client?
   a. Sir
   b. Gramps
   c. Bob
   d. Mr. Smith

27. A quick physical assessment of the client to quickly detect life-threatening injuries is called
   a. scene size-up.
   b. initial assessment.
   c. rapid physical exam.
   d. physical assessment.

28. When asking a responsive client the "SAMPLE" questions, what does the "P" stand for?
    a. previous medications taken.
    b. pertinent medical history.
    c. prior history of traumatic injuries.
    d. provokes.

29. The most reliable sign of spinal injury in a client who is conscious is
    a. deformity.
    b. paralysis.
    c. pain.
    d. shock.

30. If the mechanism of injury and observation indicate a neck or spinal injury, the first step of care after ensuring an open airway is
    a. quickly assess sensory and motor functions of the client's extremities.
    b. immediately provide manual immobilization of the neck.
    c. perform a rapid physical exam.
    d. splint the entire body.

31. When the AED is analyzing a client, you should
    a. continue providing CPR.
    b. continue providing ventilation.
    c. not touch the client.
    d. none of these.

32. If you are touching a client while a shock is being delivered, which of the following will occur?
    a. the client will be the only one who feels the shock.
    b. you will block the shock from being delivered.
    c. you will also receive a shock.
    d. the shock will not be delivered.

33. The use of an AED is not appropriate for which of the following?
    a. the client is less than 8 years old and appears to weigh less than 55–65 pounds.
    b. the client weighs 90 pounds or more.
    c. the client has suddenly collapsed for no apparent reason.
    d. the client has no spontaneous breathing or signs of circulation.

34. When using an AED, you will occasionally encounter a male client whose chest is too hairy to ensure good contact of the AED pads. What is the best course of action?
    a. tape the pads to the chest of the client.
    b. apply the pads as best you can. It makes no difference.
    c. hold the pads tight against the client while delivering the shock.
    d. quickly shave the client's chest with a razor and apply the pads.

35. Under which of these conditions would you not defibrillate a client?
    a. the client is wet.
    b. the client has no pulse or is not breathing.
    c. the client is older than 8.
    d. the client weighs more than 55 pounds.

36. If you receive a "No shock" message when using an AED and there is no pulse, then you should
   a. resume CPR for 1 minute.
   b. re-analyze the client.
   c. reposition the pads and re-analyze.
   d. turn off the AED and stop CPR.

37. The nine-month period of pregnancy is divided into three _____.
   a. gestations.
   b. trimesters.
   c. months.
   d. semesters.

38. The muscular organ that protects the unborn infant is the
   a. placenta.
   b. cervix.
   c. uterus.
   d. vagina.

39. The organ for exchange between the mother's blood and that of the developing unborn baby is the
   a. placenta.
   b. cervix.
   c. uterus.
   d. vagina.

40. While developing, the fetus is protected by a bag of water called the _____ sac
   a. placenta.
   b. amniotic.
   c. cervical.
   d. vaginese.

41. When the head of the baby first bulges from the vaginal opening, this is called
   a. bloody show.
   b. crowing.
   c. crowning.
   d. presentation.

42. The first stage of labor begins with
   a. delivery of the infant.
   b. crowning of the infant.
   c. contraction of the uterus.
   d. rupture of the bag of water.

43. One clue for knowing when the time of birth is nearing is
   a. labor pains.
   b. contractions are ten minutes apart.
   c. the bag of water ruptures.
   d. the mother expresses a need to have a bowel movement.

44. What occurs during the second stage of labor?
    a. beginning of regular contractions
    b. entrance of the baby into the birth canal
    c. delivery of the infant
    d. delivery of the placenta

45. What occurs during the third stage of labor?
    a. beginning of regular contractions
    b. entrance of the baby into the birth canal
    c. delivery of the embryo
    d. delivery of the placenta

46. Which of the following would *not* be described as a duty of a First Responder?
    a. transporting the client to the hospital.
    b. safely gaining access to the client.
    c. lifting or moving the client only if required, and without causing further injury to the client.
    d. determining what is wrong with the client and providing emergency care using a minimum amount of equipment.

47. Which of the following levels of certification would be considered the highest level in the EMS systems?
    a. First Responder
    b. EMT-Basic
    c. EMT-Intermediate
    d. EMT-Paramedic

48. The chief concern of EMS providers at all times should be which of the following?
    a. assisting rescuers with a high level of certification at the scene.
    b. knowing how to contact and initiate the EMS system.
    c. the safety of the client.
    d. personal safety.

True/False

Write "T" in the blank provided if the statement is true. Write "F" if the statement is false.

_____ **49.** First Responders transport clients to a hospital.

_____ **50.** First Responders can be firefighters, law enforcement officers, or industry workers.

_____ **51.** The career of an EMT is physically strenuous as well as stressful.

_____ **52.** EMT-Basics provide advanced life support skills such as starting IV lines and giving medications.

_____ **53.** EMT-Intermediates perform advanced airway techniques and interpret electrocardiograms.

_____ **54.** Paramedic training takes two or more years.

_____ **55.** Noting whether a client fell from a ladder is called determining the mechanism of injury.

_____ 56. A bent steering wheel might suggest a head injury.

_____ 57. If the client appears unresponsive, gently shake the client to determine his or her level of responsiveness.

_____ 58. It is important to correct any problems of the airway, breathing and circulation during the initial assessment.

_____ 59. The greatest threats to our airway are foreign bodies.

_____ 60. The nasopharyngeal airway is most effective on unresponsive clients with no gag reflex.

_____ 61. A correctly sized oropharyngeal airway will extend from the corner of the client's mouth or lips to the bottom of the earlobe or the angle of the jaw.

_____ 62. The oropharyngeal is the best airway to use for clenched teeth.

_____ 63. Never allow smoking in an area where oxygen is used.

_____ 64. Oxygen can be directly connected to a Bag-Valve Mask device to assist clients who are not breathing.

_____ 65. The nonrebreather mask delivers high concentrations of oxygen, up to 80-90% at a flow rate of 6-12 liters per minute.

_____ 66. For the AED to perform its job, the First Responder must attach adhesive electrode pads to the client's chest.

_____ 67. It is okay to touch the client when the Defibrillator is analyzing the client's rhythm.

_____ 68. The most common causes of spinal injury to children include automobile accidents and falls.

_____ 69. Common signs and symptoms of spinal injury include pain with or without movement.

_____ 70. The minimum standard for BSI of an EMT is a face shield.

_____ 71. A mechanism of injury is shortness of breath.

_____ 72. A gag reflex causes vomiting when something is placed deep inside the mouth.

_____ 73. PSI is a measurement of breathing capacity.

Short Answer

Answer the questions that follow in the space provided.

74. If you are using either an oral or a nasal airway, what type of body substance isolation precautions will you use?

_____

_____

75. Which airway is best suited for the unconscious unresponsive client?

_____

_____

_____

76. When should the nasopharyngeal airway be used?

_____

_____

_____

77. How do you measure the correct length for an oropharyngeal airway?

_____

_____

_____

78. Provide one example of a sign.

_____

_____

_____

79. Provide one example of a symptom.

_____

_____

_____

Name _____ Date _____

80. Name and describe the event which occur for each of the three stages of labor.

_____

_____

_____

_____

_____

81. Name two types of airways.

_____

_____

_____

82. The letters of the word SAMPLE represent questions to ask the client about his or her problem. What does each letter represent?

_____

_____

_____

_____

_____

_____

_____

83. What are the seven steps of the client assessment process?

_____

_____

_____

_____

_____

_____

_____

84. Name 8 conditions that require oxygen therapy.

_____

_____

_____

_____

_____

_____

_____

_____

85. Name two devices that may be used to provide oxygen to a client.

_____

_____

_____

Emergency Medical Services

PROCEDURE 13A1:
Inserting an Oropharyngeal Airway Adjunct

PROCEDURE ASSESSMENT

Procedure Steps	Suggested Points	Self Practice	Peer Practice	Peer Testing	Final Testing	Total Earned
PREPROCEDURE						
1. Gather needed equipment.	10					
2. Check for responsiveness:	8					
• Tap client on shoulder and shout, "Are you OK?"						
3. Open airway using appropriate maneuver for given situation.	8					
4. Select correct size OPA; place airway to side of the face.	9					
• A correctly sized airway will extend from corner of mouth to bottom of earlobe.						
PROCEDURE						
5. Open client's mouth using cross-finger technique:	10					
• Cross forefinger and thumb of one hand, place them on upper and lower teeth at corner of mouth, and spread fingers apart to open mouth.						
6. Insert airway upside down, with tip facing roof of mouth.	9					
7. Slide airway along roof of mouth until you meet resistance.	9					
8. Carefully rotate airway 180 degrees so that tip of airway is pointing down pharynx.	9					
9. To insert airway in infant:	10					
• Don't insert airway with tip pointing toward roof of mouth.						
• Use tongue depressor to hold tongue down.						
• Insert airway following natural curvature of tongue.						
10. Continue inserting airway until flange rests on client's teeth or lips.	10					
• If airway isn't correct size, remove it and insert correct size.						
POSTPROCEDURE						
11. Observe client. If client gags, remove airway immediately.	8					
TOTAL POSSIBLE POINTS	100					

PROCEDURE 13A1: Inserting an Oropharyngeal Airway Adjunct (continued)

Comments: _____

_____

_____

_____

_____

_____

_____

_____

Signatures: _____ Date: _____

SCORING *See Preface for scoring instructions.*

Emergency Medical Services

PROCEDURE 13A2:
Inserting a Nasopharyngeal Airway Adjunct

P R O C E D U R E   A S S E S S M E N T

Procedure Steps	Suggested Points	Self Practice	Peer Practice	Peer Testing	Final Testing	Total Earned
PREPROCEDURE						
1. Gather needed equipment.	13					
2. Choose correct size airway.	10					
• A correctly sized airway will extend from corner of mouth to bottom of earlobe.						
3. Apply water-based lubricant to outside tip of airway.	10					
• DO NOT use petroleum-based jelly such as Vaseline.						
PROCEDURE						
4. Gently push tip of client's nose upward.	12					
5. Insert airway with beveled side toward base of nostril or toward septum.	12					
6. Advance airway until flange rests against client's nostril.	12					
• Don't force airway.						
• If you encounter resistance, remove airway and try other nostril.						
POSTPROCEDURE						
7. Monitor placement of airway.	10					
8. Monitor client's airway and breathing.	10					
9. If needed, provide rescue breaths using a bag-valve mask.	11					
• If breathing of client is sufficient, but condition requires oxygen, give oxygen by a nonrebreather mask.						
TOTAL POSSIBLE POINTS	**100**					

Comments: _____

_____

_____

_____

_____

_____

Signatures: _____   **Date:** _____

SCORING   *See Preface for scoring instructions.*

Name _____   Date _____

Emergency Medical Services

PROCEDURE 13B:
Operating the Semiautomatic Defibrillator

PROCEDURE ASSESSMENT

Procedure Steps	Suggested Points	Self Practice	Peer Practice	Peer Testing	Final Testing	Total Earned
PREPROCEDURE						
1. Gather needed equipment.	4					
2. Verify client's unresponsiveness.	3					
3. Phone EMS or 911 and get the AED.	3					
4. If there are two First Responders or EMTs:	2					
• One phones 911.						
• The other stays and performs CPR.						
5. Return to client.	2					
6. Open client's airway using head tilt-chin lift.	5					
• Use jaw-thrust if you suspect trauma.						
7. Check for breathing using Look, Listen, and Feel method.	3					
8. If breathing is poor or absent, give 2 slow breaths.	3					
• Use pocket mask or other barrier device.						
9. Check for signs of circulation. If there are none, bare client's chest and start CPR.	3					
PROCEDURE						
10. Attach AED electrode pads to client's chest in proper position.	4					
• See troubleshooting box if client has excessive hair on chest.						
11. Attach lead wires to AED if not already attached.	3					
12. Turn on AED.	2					
13. Press analyze button.	5					
• Some AEDs will analyze automatically.						
• Don't touch client while AED analyzes.						
14. If client is to receive a shock, the AED will automatically charge.	2					
15. A voice prompt or message on LED screen will warn you to stand clear.	2					
16. Make sure no one touches client.	4					
17. When all are clear of client and AED is charged, press shock button.	3					
18. After delivering shock, press analyze button.	3					
• Some AEDs will analyze automatically.						

PROCEDURE 13B: Operating the Semiautomatic Defibrillator (continued)

Procedure Steps PROCEDURE	Suggested Points	Self Practice	Peer Practice	Peer Testing	Final Testing	Total Earned
19. If AED gives a "shock indicated" message:						
• AED will charge a second time if another shock is needed. Make sure all are clear and that AED is charged before pressing shock button.	4					
• Repeat analyze button a third time. If another shock is needed, AED will charge. Stand clear and press shock button.	3					
• After third shock, check for signs of circulation, including pulse. If you find none, start CPR and continue for 1 minute. If there is pulse, check for breathing. If there is none, give rescue breaths every 5 seconds. If client is breathing and has pulse, put client in recovery position and monitor breathing and circulation. Get client to hospital immediately.	4					
• After 1 minute of CPR for clients with no signs of circulation, press analyze button.	3					
• If shock is needed, AED will charge. Make sure everyone is clear and press shock button. You may give up to 2 more shocks if AED so indicates. In all, up to 6 shocks may be given.	3					
• After total of 6 shocks OR total of 3 consecutive no shocks, continue with CPR when there are no signs of circulation until help arrives or client is transported.	3					
20. If AED gives a "No shock indicated" message:						
• Should AED not charge, or it indicates no shock is needed, check for signs of circulation.	4					
• If there are no signs of circulation, perform CPR for 1 minute.	4					
• After 1 minute of CPR, press analyze button. If shock is needed, AED will charge.	3					
• If no shock is needed, perform 1 minute of CPR.	3					
• After 1 minute of CPR, analyze again. If AED indicates no shock is needed, continue CPR for 1 minute and analyze again.	4					

PROCEDURE 13B: Operating the Semiautomatic Defibrillator (continued)

Procedure Steps	Suggested Points	Self Practice	Peer Practice	Peer Testing	Final Testing	Total Earned
PROCEDURE						
• If AED indicates no shock is needed, continue CPR until help arrives or transport client to hospital, continuing CPR on the way.	3					
POSTPROCEDURE						
21. Monitor client until safely transported to hospital.	3					
TOTAL POSSIBLE POINTS	100					

Comments: _____

_____

_____

_____

_____

_____

_____

_____

_____

_____

Signatures: _____   Date: _____

SCORING   See Preface for scoring instructions.

Nursing

Reinforcement Activities

True/False

Write "T" in the blank provided if the statement is true. Write "F" if the statement is false.

_____ 1. Separating of clients with infections from others is the most important procedure for prevention of disease transmission.

_____ 2. Elastic stockings are used for clients to help prevent thrombophlebitis.

_____ 3. Some medications and disease processes can upset the fluid balance in the body.

_____ 4. Dialysis technicians must obtain a license to practice.

_____ 5. Clients who are upset should be left alone because they have the right to feel however they want.

_____ 6. Surgical technicians always work in an acute care setting because this is where surgeries take place.

_____ 7. Health care providers should explain the procedures they are performing to unconscious clients.

_____ 8. Unlicensed personnel are allowed to perform nail care for clients only after a licensed health care provider has assessed the client for safety.

_____ 9. Grooming is an important aspect of client care.

_____ 10. Advanced practice nurses work independently without the help of the rest of the health care team.

Fill in the Blank

Write the word (or words) that best completes the sentence in the blank provided.

11. Unlicensed personnel work under the _____ of a licensed person.

12. The highest priority for any health care provider is _____ safety.

13. Dialysis technician work requires frequent contact with _____ products.

14. Becoming a surgical technician is not the profession for someone who does not like the sight of _____.

15. LPN/LVNs work under supervision from a/an _____ or a/an _____.

16. Work as an RN requires _____ stability.

17. Clients have the right to _____ regarding their health care records.

18. To help prevent injury when transferring a client from bed to a wheelchair the proper use of _____ are necessary.

19. Performance of _____ must be done in a manner that protects client dignity.

20. _____ is the act of walking.

Multiple Choice

Circle the letter that best answers the question or completes the statement.

21. Nurses who have continued their education in a specific field are called
  a. Registered Nurses.
  b. Licensed Practical Nurses.
  c. Advanced Practice Nurses.
  d. Licensed Vocational Nurses.

22. Actions that are taken by health care workers to reduce the risk of disease transmission are called
  a. standard precautions.
  b. isolation.
  c. range of motion.
  d. dialysis.

23. Facilities that provide care for clients who are not ill but cannot live alone are called
  a. acute care facilities.
  b. respiratory care facilities.
  c. long-term care facilities.
  d. ambulatory care facilities.

24. To ensure accurate measurement of output fluid one should
  a. read the measurement lines on the collection bag.
  b. pour the liquid into a measurement cylinder and look at it at eye level.
  c. use the measurement device that is placed in the toilet.
  d. use a syringe to draw the liquid up and add the amount of times you have to fill the syringe.

25. When assisting a client with one sided weakness to get undressed you should start with
  a. their weak side.
  b. their strong side.
  c. their pants.
  d. their shirt.

26. When should routine oral care be performed?
  a. morning, bedtime, and after meals.
  b. one time a day.
  c. every eight hours for unconscious clients.
  d. when a client is admitted.

27. How many should you have to assist you when transferring an unconscious patient from a
bed to a stretcher?
    a. two
    b. three
    c. four
    d. one

28. When performing perineal care on a female client you should clean
    a. back to front.
    b. the cleaning direction does not matter.
    c. in a circular motion.
    d. front to back.

29. After shaving a client one should dispose of the safety razor
    a. in the trash can.
    b. in a sharps container.
    c. outside of the facility.
    d. don't dispose save it for later use.

30. The procedure to mechanically filter wastes and fluids from the blood is called
    a. dialysis.
    b. endoscopy.
    c. cholecystectomy.
    d. catheterization.

Matching

Write the letter of the phrase that best matches each numbered item in the blank provided.

_____ **31.** Ambulation	**a.** Mechanical filtering of the blood.
_____ **32.** Decubitus ulcer	**b.** Friction between skin and linen.
_____ **33.** Fluid balance	**c.** Precautions to reduce disease transmission.
_____ **34.** Thrombophlebitis	**d.** Prevents normal movement in a joint or muscle.
_____ **35.** Contracture	**e.** A tube inserted into the bladder.
_____ **36.** Shear force	**f.** Loss of self-control of bladder or bowels.
_____ **37.** Incontinent	**g.** Inflammation of a vein.
_____ **38.** Standard precautions	**h.** Pertaining to psychological factors.
_____ **39.** Dialysis	**i.** Sore that can be caused by pressure.
_____ **40.** Psychosocial	**j.** Walking.
	k. Regulation of fluids in the body.

Name _____ Date _____

Labeling

In the space provided, write the number that identifies the corresponding part on the diagram.

41. Identify how much liquid is in each of the measuring devices shown.

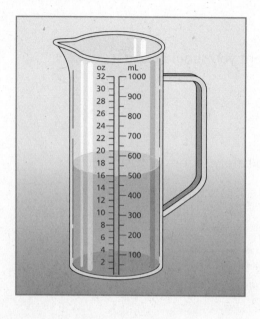

_____

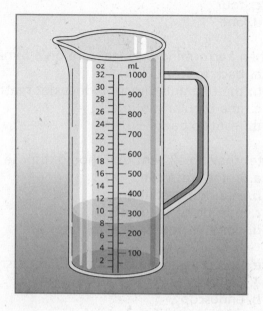

_____

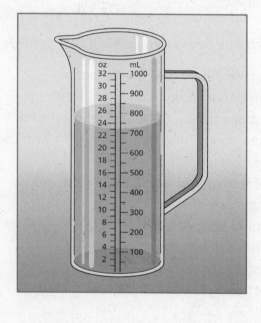

_____

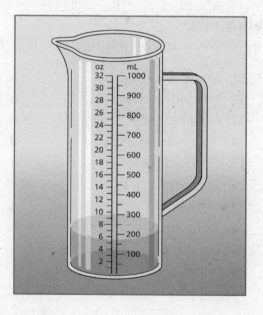

_____

Name _____ Date _____

42. Identify each of the positions shown below.

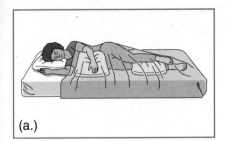

(a.)

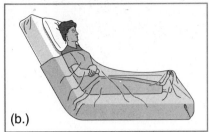

(b.)

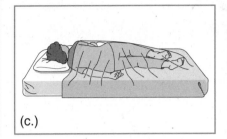

(c.)

(a.) _____ **(c.)** _____

(b.) _____

Name _____   Date _____

Nursing

PROCEDURE 14A:
Admitting a Client

---------- **P R O C E D U R E   A S S E S S M E N T** ----------

Procedure Steps	Suggested Points	Self Practice	Peer Practice	Peer Testing	Final Testing	Total Earned
PREPROCEDURE						
1. Gather needed equipment.	2					
2. Determine how client will arrive at facility: walking, in wheelchair or on stretcher?	1					
3. Wash your hands.	3					
4. Position bed according to client needs.	3					
• If client is ambulatory or in wheelchair, put bed in lowest position.	2					
• If client is on stretcher, raise bed to appropriate height for patient transfer.	2					
5. Open bed to make access easy; fan-fold top linens to bottom of bed.	1					
6. Lay out hospital gown for client, if applicable.	1					
7. Unpack client admittance packet and put supplies in correct location.	1					
8. Ensure initial paperwork is in room.	2					
• May include history and physical form, clothing inventory, valuables list, vital signs record.	1					
• Put blood pressure cuff, stethoscope, and thermometer in room.	1					
9. Attach call light to linens.	3					
10. Wash your hands.	3					
11. Record/report as necessary.	2					
PREPROCEDURE						
12. Wash your hands.	3					
13. Greet client by name.	2					
• Ask client how he/she likes to be addressed.	1					
• Note preference on chart.	1					
14. Introduce yourself and explain each task before you begin.	2					
15. If there is a roommate, introduce them to each other.	1					
16. Help client into bed or to a chair.	2					
17. Ensure client has privacy.	2					
• If there is a roommate, close curtain between beds.	1					
• Ask client if he/she would like his/her family to leave room, if applicable.	1					

PROCEDURE 14A: Admitting a Client (continued)

Procedure Steps	Suggested Points	Self Practice	Peer Practice	Peer Testing	Final Testing	Total Earned
• If family leaves, tell them where to wait and how long you'll be.	1					
18. If client has to change clothes, help him/her with gown.	2					
19. Ensure client's comfort in bed or chair.	2					
20. Complete procedure for handling client's possessions.	2					
• Fill out clothing inventory.	1					
• Put clothing away, or pack for family to take home.	1					
21. Fill out valuables list and put valuables in container.	2					
• Some facilities allow clients to keep small amount of money with them.						
22. Help client arrange personal possessions.	1					
23. Ask client whether he/she brought medications.	3					
• Take medications to nurse or handle as facility's policy requires.	2					
24. Perform other admissions procedures required by facility.	2					
25. If urine sample is required, follow facility's policy for collection.	3					
• Use standard precautions.	1					
26. If client can drink, ensure pitcher is filled with ice water.	2					
• If client can't drink or eat, explain this to client and follow facility's policy for posting of signs and charting.	1					
27. Explain following to client and ask if he/she has questions:	2					
• How to use call light.	3					
• How to use bed controls.	3					
• What is in bedside table.	3					
• How to operate TV, radio, lights, and phone.	1					
• When mealtimes are, how to find out menu, and how to order from menu, if applicable.	1					
• Visiting policies.	1					
• How nursing system works, who nurse is, what time new shifts arrive, and which team members will be involved with his/her care.	1					
28. Complete all items on admission checklist.	2					

PROCEDURE 14A: Admitting a Client (continued)

Procedure Steps	Suggested Points	Self Practice	Peer Practice	Peer Testing	Final Testing	Total Earned
POSTPROCEDURE						
29. Unscreen client, if appropriate.	2					
30. Take urine specimen, medication, clothing list, valuables, and admission checklist to nurses' station or proper location.	2					
31. Wash your hands	3					
32. Find family members, explain what you just did, and familiarize them with facility.	2					
• Ask them if they have questions.	1					
33. Ensure client has a call light within easy reach and room is neat.	1					
34. Record/report as necessary	2					
TOTAL POSSIBLE POINTS	100					

Comments: _____

_____

_____

_____

_____

_____

_____

_____

_____

_____

Signatures: _____ Date: _____

SCORING *See Preface for scoring instructions.*

Name _____ Date _____

Nursing

PROCEDURE 14B:
Transferring a Client

PROCEDURE ASSESSMENT

Procedure Steps PREPROCEDURE	Suggested Points	Self Practice	Peer Practice	Peer Testing	Final Testing	Total Earned
1. Gather needed equipment.	3					
2. Ensure new unit is ready for client by contacting unit or asking your supervisor.	3					
3. Help client pack his or her belongings.	2					
• If client is going to another facility, ensure valuables are kept secure.	3					
4. Find out how client will be moved and ensure appropriate transportation is available.	2					
PREPROCEDURE						
5. Identify client.	4					
6. Tell client where he or she is going and why.	4					
7. Wash your hands.	5					
8. Collect client's belongings and put them on transportation cart on in client's lap.	2					
9. Ask client whether he/she wants to say goodbye to anyone in unit.	3					
10. Transport client to new location in wheelchair or on stretcher.	4					
• If using stretcher, get help to transfer client from bed to stretcher and move stretcher to new room.	2					
• Use safety equipment (side rails, etc.) during transfer.	5					
11. Introduce client to new staff and roommate, if applicable.	3					
12. Provide new staff with client's chart.	4					
13. Ensure client has privacy to get settled in new room.	3					
14. Assist client to comfortable position.	3					
15. Tell client where you are putting his/her belongings.	3					
16. Unscreen client, if necessary.	2					
17. Ensure client doesn't need anything.	2					
18. Ensure call light is within easy reach of client.	5					
19. Wash your hands.	5					
20. Report to appropriate person:	4					
• That client has arrived.	3					
• How client has tolerated transfer.	3					

PROCEDURE 14B: Transferring a Client *(continued)*

Procedure Steps	Suggested Points	Self Practice	Peer Practice	Peer Testing	Final Testing	Total Earned
• Whether client is anxious, confused, sleepy, angry, etc.	3					
• Any pertinent information about client's care.	3					
POSTPROCEDURE						
21. Return to your unit and clean client's old room according to facility's policy.	3					
22. Wash your hands.	5					
23. Record/report as necessary.	4					
TOTAL POSSIBLE POINTS	**100**					

Comments: _____

_____

_____

_____

_____

_____

_____

_____

_____

_____

_____

Signatures: _____   **Date:** _____

SCORING   *See Preface for scoring instructions.*

Nursing

PROCEDURE 14C:
Discharging a Client

PROCEDURE ASSESSMENT

Procedure Steps	Suggested Points	Self Practice	Peer Practice	Peer Testing	Final Testing	Total Earned
PREPROCEDURE						
1. Gather needed equipment.	3					
2. Ensure all paperwork is completed before client is discharged.	3					
3. If equipment/supplies are going home with client, ensure they're ready.	2					
PREPROCEDURE						
4. Identify client.	3					
5. Provide privacy, if necessary.	2					
6. Explain process to client and ask whether he/she has questions.	3					
7. Wash your hands.	5					
8. Help client dress.	3					
9. Help client pack his or her belongings.	4					
• Check clothes against clothing list.	3					
• Ask client to sign list.	3					
10. Return valuables according to facility's policy.	3					
• Check valuables against list made when client was admitted.	2					
11. Report to supervising nurse that client is ready for discharge so nurse can give instructions and/or prescriptions.	3					
12. Depending on client's condition, bring wheelchair or stretcher to client's room, and help him/her transfer to it.	3					
• Check facility's regulations to see if client is allowed to walk, if able.	2					
13. Put client's belongings on a cart or in his/her lap.	2					
14. Help client remove ID bracelet according to your facility's policy.	2					
15. Take client to front door of facility and safely escort him/her out.	5					
16. Help client into car.	3					
• Lock wheels on wheelchair or stretcher before transferring client.	4					
17. Help client with luggage and belongings.	3					
18. Say goodbye and ask client if he/she has questions.	3					

PROCEDURE 14C: Discharging a Client (continued)

Procedure Steps	Suggested Points	Self Practice	Peer Practice	Peer Testing	Final Testing	Total Earned
POSTPROCEDURE						
19. Return wheelchair or stretcher to unit. Clean and store it.	2					
20. Return to client's room, strip linens off bed, and put in proper receptacle.	2					
21. Wash your hands.	5					
22. Tell housekeeping that room needs to be cleaned.	3					
23. Tell supervising nurse:	4					
• Time client was discharged.	3					
• Whether wheelchair or stretcher was used.	3					
• Who was with client when he/she was discharged.	3					
• How client tolerated the procedure.	3					
• Any other important information.	3					
TOTAL POSSIBLE POINTS	**100**					

Comments: _____

_____

_____

_____

_____

_____

_____

_____

_____

_____

Signatures: _____ **Date:** _____

SCORING   *See Preface for scoring instructions.*

Nursing

PROCEDURE 14D1:
Making an Open or Closed Bed

······· P R O C E D U R E   A S S E S S M E N T ·······

Procedure Steps	Suggested Points	Self Practice	Peer Practice	Peer Testing	Final Testing	Total Earned
PREPROCEDURE						
1. Gather needed equipment.	3					
2. Wash your hands; put on gloves if used linens are contaminated.	4					
3. Identify client and introduce yourself.	3					
4. Collect linen and put in clean, convenient location. Stack in order of use from top to bottom:	2					
• Mattress pad.	1					
• Bottom sheet.	1					
• Plastic bed protector.	1					
• Lift or turning sheet.	1					
• Top sheet.	1					
• Bedspread or blanket.	1					
• Pillowcase.	1					
5. Don't let clean linens touch your uniform. Carry them away from body.	4					
6. Raise bed to a level for best body mechanics.	4					
• You shouldn't have to bend to place linens.						
• Usually, higher is better.						
7. Before making closed bed, ensure housekeeping has cleaned mattress.	2					
PREPROCEDURE						
8. Remove bedspread and put in clean area if it will be reused.	2					
• Bedspreads are changed if bed is closed.						
9. Remove soiled linen and place in soiled linen cart or other location.	2					
10. Place mattress pad even with top of mattress.	2					
11. Unfold bottom contour sheet without shaking it and place on bed so hem stitching is toward the mattress.	4					
12. Put top and bottom corners of sheet over corners of mattress. If sheet doesn't have elastic fitted corners, make a mitered corner:	2					
• Tuck top or bottom end of sheet evenly under mattress.	1					

PROCEDURE 14D1: Making an Open or Closed Bed *(continued)*

Procedure Steps	Suggested Points	Self Practice	Peer Practice	Peer Testing	Final Testing	Total Earned
• Lift side edge of sheet 1 foot from mattress corner and hold at right angle to mattress.	1					
• Tuck in bottom edge of sheet hanging below mattess.	1					
• Drop top edge of sheet and tuck it under mattress.	1					
13. If plastic bed protector is used, put in middle of bed.	2					
14. Put lift sheet over plastic protector. Ensure protector is completely covered.	2					
• Tuck draw sheet under mattress on side nearest you.	1					
15. Unfold top sheet without shaking it and place so center crease is in middle of bed and large hem is even with top of mattress.	4					
16. Open top sheet, but don't tuck it in.	2					
• Hemstitching should be to outside (away from client) when he/she gets into bed.	1					
17. Put blanket on bed so center crease is in middle and upper hem is 6 to 8 inches from top of bed.	2					
• Pull blanket out flat, on your side of the bed.	1					
18. Put bedspread on bed so center crease is in middle.	2					
• Unfold your side and ensure it is even and covers other linen.	1					
19. Tuck bedspread, blanket, and top sheet together smoothly and tightly at bottom bed corner near you and make a mitered corner.	2					
20. Go to other side and pull bottom contour sheet corners over corners of bed so there are no wrinkles.	2					
21. Pull lift sheet and plastic bed protector tight. Tuck them in so there are no wrinkles.	2					
22. Straighten all top linen from top to bottom.	2					
• Tuck in linen at bottom and make a mitered corner.	1					
23. For closed bed, linens should be flat to top of bed or folded down 6 inches.	2					
• Check policy at facility.						
24. Change pillowcase. Use approved method to avoid contamination. One is:	3					
• Grasp closed end of pillowcase in middle on outside.	2					

PROCEDURE 14D1: Making an Open or Closed Bed *(continued)*

Procedure Steps	Suggested Points	Self Practice	Peer Practice	Peer Testing	Final Testing	Total Earned
• Turn pillowcase inside out and grasp pillow, with hand holding pillowcase in middle on one end. You should be holding pillow by short end, with end of pillowcase between pillow and your hand.	2					
• Using other hand, pull case right side out over pillow. Don't shake pillow into case.	4					
25. Put pillow on bed so open end is away from door and seam is toward head of bed.	2					
26. Attach call light to bed and lower bed to lowest position.	4					
27. Place used linen in appropriate place.	2					
POSTPROCEDURE						
28. Wash your hands.	4					
29. To open bed, fan-fold linens to foot of bed.	2					
• To fan-fold, fold sheet back and forth on top of itself in equal parts.	1					
TOTAL POSSIBLE POINTS	**100**					

Comments: _____

_____

_____

_____

_____

_____

_____

_____

_____

_____

Signatures: _____ Date: _____

SCORING   *See Preface for scoring instructions.*

Nursing

PROCEDURE 14D2:
Making an Occupied Bed

PROCEDURE ASSESSMENT

Procedure Steps	Suggested Points	Self Practice	Peer Practice	Peer Testing	Final Testing	Total Earned
PREPROCEDURE						
1. Gather needed equipment.	2					
2. Explain procedure to client and draw curtain closed or close door.	2					
3. Arrange clean linen and soiled linen hamper conveniently.	1					
• Place linens in order of use.	1					
• Place used linens on chair or other location, but not on floor.	3					
PREPROCEDURE						
4. Wash hands; put on gloves if linens are contaminated.	3					
5. Raise side rails and bed to provide proper body mechanics for you.	3					
• Lower head of bed to make bed as flat as possible.	1					
• Check client's condition.	1					
• In some cases, you won't be able to make head of bed completely flat.						
6. Lower side rail on side of bed where you are working.	1					
7. Loosen top linens from foot of bed.	2					
• Place spread and blanket (if used) in hamper separately or in clean location if they will be reused.	1					
8. Provide privacy for client with top sheet or bath blanket.	2					
• Have client hold top of sheet or bath blanket while you remove soiled sheet underneath.	1					
9. Position client on his/her side on side of bed away from you.	2					
• Put pillow under client's head.	1					
• Ensure side rail on opposite side of bed is up and secure.	1					
10. Loosen bottom linens.	2					
• Separately fan-fold linens to be changed toward client and tuck them under client.	1					
11. If mattress pad is changed, put clean pad on side of bed near you and fan-fold pad toward client.	2					
• Ensure there are no wrinkles.	3					

PROCEDURE 14D2: Making an Occupied Bed (continued)

Procedure Steps	Suggested Points	Self Practice	Peer Practice	Peer Testing	Final Testing	Total Earned
• Ensure soiled linens don't touch clean linens.	1					
12. Place bottom fitted sheet on mattress pad so stitching is away from client.	2					
• Pull nearest corners into place and fan-fold sheet toward client.	1					
• Smooth any wrinkles.	3					
13. If plastic protector is used, put it on middle of bed and fan-fold toward client.	1					
• Tuck it under mattress and smooth any wrinkles.	3					
14. If cotton draw sheet is used, put it on middle of bed and fan-fold toward client.	2					
• Tuck it under mattress and smooth any wrinkles.	1					
15. Raise side rail, and go to other side of bed and lower side rail.	3					
16. Help client roll toward opposite side of bed.	2					
• Tell client he/she will roll over a "hump" of linens.	1					
• Position client facing side rail.	1					
• Adjust pillow for comfort and provide privacy.	1					
17. Remove bottom linens individually and put them in hamper.	1					
18. Pull mattress pad toward you and smooth any wrinkles.	3					
19. Pull clean bottom sheet toward you, pull corners into place, and smooth wrinkles.	3					
20. Pull plastic protector and cotton draw sheet toward you, tuck under mattress, and smooth wrinkles.	3					
21. Position client in supine position in middle of bed and adjust pillow.	1					
22. Unfold top sheet without shaking it and place so center crease is in middle of bed, large hem is even with top of mattress, and hem stitching is to outside.	3					
23. Have client hold top sheet or tuck it under his/her shoulders.	2					
• Remove privacy cover and put in hamper.	1					
24. Put blanket on bed so center crease is in middle and upper hem is 6 to 8 inches from top of bed.	2					
• Unfold blanket and cover client.	1					
25. Put bedspread on bed so center crease is in middle.	2					
• Unfold your side and ensure it's even and covers client.	1					

PROCEDURE 14D2: Making an Occupied Bed *(continued)*

Procedure Steps	Suggested Points	Self Practice	Peer Practice	Peer Testing	Final Testing	Total Earned
26. Turn top sheet and blanket top edges down over spread to make cuff.	1					
27. Before tucking in bottom sheets, ensure client's feet have room to move. Make a toe pleat by making a fold in bed coverings across foot of bed near feet.	3					
28. Tuck bedspread, blanket (if used), and top sheet together at bottom corner near you and make a mitered corner.	1					
29. Raise side rail, go to other side of bed, lower side rail, and smooth top linens over client.	1					
30. Tuck top linens under mattress and make a mitered corner.	1					
31. Change pillowcase, using an approved method to avoid contamination.	3					
32. Position side rails as instructed, attach call signal, and put bed in lowest position.	2					
• Ensure client is comfortable.	1					
POSTPROCEDURE						
33. Put soiled linens in proper area.	1					
34. Wash your hands.	3					
35. Record and report as necessary.	2					
TOTAL POSSIBLE POINTS	**100**					

Comments: _____

_____

_____

_____

_____

_____

_____

_____

_____

_____

Signatures: _____   Date: _____

SCORING   *See Preface for scoring instructions.*

Name _____   Date _____

Nursing

PROCEDURE 14E1:
Measuring Oral Fluid Intake

·········· P R O C E D U R E   A S S E S S M E N T ··········

Procedure Steps	Suggested Points	Self Practice	Peer Practice	Peer Testing	Final Testing	Total Earned
PREPROCEDURE						
1. Gather needed equipment.	6					
2. Identify client.	7					
3. Introduce yourself and explain procedure.	7					
PREPROCEDURE						
4. Wash your hands.	8					
Method 1						
• If you're using a measuring device, pour leftover liquid from tray into device.	5					
• Put measuring device on flat surface at eye level and read fluid level.	5					
• Determine how much fluid was on tray to begin with by determining how much fluid each container holds.	5					
• Subtract leftover amount from total amount of fluid. The difference is amount of fluid taken in by client.	5					
Method 2						
• Determine total amount of fluid each container on meal tray contained at outset by checking containers. Convert ounces, teaspoons, and tablespoons to milliliters.	5					
• A facility intake and output chart will list amount that bowls, cups, and glasses hold. If chart isn't available, measure amount in each container when full.	5					
• Determine how much is gone from each container and subtract that amount from total amount.	5					
• Add each amount together. Don't forget to include spoonfuls of fluids such as Jell-O®, broth, and soup.	5					
5. Record total amount of fluid client took in for meal.	6					
6. If client drinks something between meals, measure amount using either of above methods.	6					

PROCEDURE 14E1: Measuring Oral Fluid Intake *(continued)*

Procedure Steps	Suggested Points	Self Practice	Peer Practice	Peer Testing	Final Testing	Total Earned
POSTPROCEDURE						
7. Clean measuring device and store it.	6					
8. Wash your hands.	8					
9. Record and report as necessary.	6					
TOTAL POSSIBLE POINTS	100					

Comments: _____

_____

_____

_____

_____

_____

_____

_____

_____

Signatures: _____ **Date:** _____

SCORING   *See Preface for scoring instructions.*

Nursing

PROCEDURE 14E2:
Measuring Urinary Fluid Output

············· **P R O C E D U R E   A S S E S S M E N T** ·············

Procedure Steps	Suggested Points	Self Practice	Peer Practice	Peer Testing	Final Testing	Total Earned
PREPROCEDURE						
1. Gather needed equipment.	7					
2. Identify client.	8					
3. Introduce yourself and explain procedure.	8					
PREPROCEDURE						
4. Wash hands and put on gloves.	10					
5. Collect urine:	7					
• For females, either put collection device in toilet or use bedpan.	7					
• For males, help them use a handheld urinal.	7					
• Even if these devices have measuring marks, measure with a cylinder for accuracy.	7					
6. If client has catheter, drain collection bag into cylinder for measurement.	7					
7. Put cylinder on flat surface at eye level; read fluid level in container.	7					
POSTPROCEDURE						
8. Clean and store cylinder.	7					
9. Wash your hands.	10					
10. Record and report as necessary.	8					
TOTAL POSSIBLE POINTS	100					

Comments: _____

_____

_____

_____

_____

_____

_____

_____

Signatures: _____   **Date:** _____

SCORING   *See Preface for scoring instructions.*

Nursing

PROCEDURE 14F:
Positioning Clients

PROCEDURE ASSESSMENT

Procedure Steps	Suggested Points	Self Practice	Peer Practice	Peer Testing	Final Testing	Total Earned
PREPROCEDURE						
1. Gather needed equipment.	1					
2. Identify client.	2					
3. Explain procedure to client.	2					
4. Provide for client's privacy.	1					
5. Wash your hands.	3					
6. Adjust bed to comfortable working height.	3					
PREPROCEDURE						
Semi-Side-Lying or Side-Lying Positions						
• Raise rail on side of bed opposite side where you are working.	3					
• Help client to side of bed opposite side he/she will face when turned.	2					
• Apply padding and/or splints as ordered.	2					
• Turn client on his/her side.	2					
• Firmly tuck support pillow behind client's back, with long side parallel to client.	1					
• Position pillow to support head and neck in level position.	2					
• Adjust client's lower shoulder to prevent direct body pressure from bearing on it.	2					
a. Position lower shoulder slightly forward or behind client, depending on position.	1					
• Straighten client's lower leg.	1					
• Flex upper leg and place it in front of lower leg on pillow(s) to prevent contact with lower leg and also to keep it level from hip to foot.	2					
a. For semi-side-lying position, put straightened upper leg behind lower leg, supported on pillow(s).	1					
• Put lower arm with elbow flexed and palm up or with elbow straight and arm alongside body.	2					
• Support upper arm with pillow, in front of body for side-lying or behind body for semi-side-lying.	1					
• Ensure client is comfortable and in correct body alignment.	2					

PROCEDURE 14F: Positioning Clients *(continued)*

Procedure Steps	Suggested Points	Self Practice	Peer Practice	Peer Testing	Final Testing	Total Earned
Supine Position						
• Center client on flat mattress with his/her arms and legs extended.	2					
• Position pillow to support client's head and neck in level position.	1					
• Apply padding and/or splints as ordered.	2					
• Place Trochanter rolls to prevent external rotation of hips, if necessary.	3					
a. A Trochanter roll is rolled towels or foam.						
• Separate client's legs with pillow or abduction wedge, if needed.	2					
a. An abduction wedge is a small triangular pillow.						
• Support feet with a foot board and/or pillow to prevent plantar flexion.	2					
• Place pad or towel under knees or elevate knee section of bed to prevent knee flexion.	2					
• Place hand rolls in client's hands if this is included in plan of care.	1					
• Ensure client's comfort.	2					
Fowler's Position						
• Center client on mattress, in supine position with hip joints directly above joint or bend in bed frame.	2					
• Apply padding and/or splints as ordered.	2					
• Raise head of bed to 45- to 60-degree angle.	2					
• Position pillow behind client's head to prevent neck flexion.	1					
• Separate client's legs with pillows or abduction wedges, if needed.	2					
• Support feet with foot board and/or pillow to prevent plantar flexion.	1					
• Place pad or towel under knees or elevate knee section of bed to prevent knee flexion.	2					
• Support client's arms on pillows, keeping shoulders level.	1					
• Ensure client's comfort.	2					
Sims' Position						
• Raise side rail on side where you are not working.	3					
• Apply padding and/or splints as ordered.	3					
• Help client to right side of bed.	2					
• Have client gently tuck his/her left arm under his/her body with palm of hand down.	1					

PROCEDURE 14F: Positioning Clients *(continued)*

Procedure Steps	Suggested Points	Self Practice	Peer Practice	Peer Testing	Final Testing	Total Earned
• Turn client onto his/her left side. Left arm will be behind body.	2					
• Adjust left shoulder and arm for comfort.	1					
• Sharply flex or bend right leg and support it on pillow.	2					
• Position pillow to support head and neck in level position.	1					
• Support right arm on pillow in comfortable position.	1					
• Ensure client's comfort.	2					
a. Sims' position may need to be modified for some clients.						
b. Check with your supervisor for directions.						
POSTPROCEDURE						
7. Place call light within client's reach.	3					
8. Lower or raise side rails, as ordered.	3					
9. Return bed to lowest horizontal position.	3					
10. Remove privacy screen.	1					
11. Wash your hands.	3					
12. Report and record as necessary.	1					
TOTAL POSSIBLE POINTS	**100**					

Comments: _____

_____

_____

_____

_____

_____

_____

_____

_____

_____

Signatures: _____ Date: _____

SCORING *See Preface for scoring instructions.*

Name _____ Date _____

Nursing

PROCEDURE 14G1:
Moving a Client Up in Bed with the Client's Assistance

PROCEDURE ASSESSMENT

Procedure Steps	Suggested Points	Self Practice	Peer Practice	Peer Testing	Final Testing	Total Earned
PREPROCEDURE						
1. Gather needed equipment.	3					
2. Identify client.	4					
3. Explain procedure to client.	4					
4. Determine client's ability to assist with move.	3					
• Client should be able to follow directions.						
• Client should have some strength in his/her arms and legs.						
5. Provide for client's privacy.	4					
6. Lock bed wheels.	5					
PREPROCEDURE						
7. Wash your hands.	5					
8. Raise side rail on side of bed opposite from where you will be working.	5					
• Then go to side of bed where you will be working.	2					
9. Adjust bed to comfortable working height, with head of bed as flat as client can tolerate.	5					
• Check orders, because some clients aren't allowed to have bed flat.	2					
10. Place pillow against headboard to protect client's head.	3					
11. Have client bend his or her knees with feet flat on mattress.	3					
12. Place one arm under client's shoulder blades and other arm under buttocks.	3					
13. Stand sideways in lunge position with knees and hips flexed and body weight over rear leg.	5					
14. Instruct client, on count of 3, to push himself/herself to head of bed by pushing his/her feet into mattress and using his/her hands on mattress or side rails.	3					
15. On count of 3, shift your body weight from rear leg to front leg, keeping your shoulders in line with hips.	5					
• Don't lift client.						
• Just allow client to slide up sheet on your forearms.						
16. Repeat steps 11 to 15 until proper position is achieved.	3					

PROCEDURE 14G1: Moving a Client Up in Bed with the Client's Assistance (continued)

Procedure Steps	Suggested Points	Self Practice	Peer Practice	Peer Testing	Final Testing	Total Earned
17. Replace pillow under client's head and arrange linens.	3					
18. Ensure client's comfort.	4					
POSTPROCEDURE						
19. Lower bed to lowest horizontal position.	5					
20. Place call light within reach.	5					
21. Lower or raise side rails as ordered.	5					
22. Remove privacy screen.	2					
23. Wash your hands.	5					
24. Report and record as necessary.	4					
TOTAL POSSIBLE POINTS	**100**					

Comments: _____

_____

_____

_____

_____

_____

_____

_____

_____

_____

_____

Signatures: _____ Date: _____

SCORING *See Preface for scoring instructions.*

Nursing

PROCEDURE 14G2:
Moving a Client Up in Bed Using a Turn or Lift Sheet

PROCEDURE ASSESSMENT

Procedure Steps	Suggested Points	Self Practice	Peer Practice	Peer Testing	Final Testing	Total Earned
PREPROCEDURE						
1. Gather needed equipment.	2					
2. Obtain assistance from at least one other staff member.	3					
3. Obtain a turn or lift sheet, if one isn't already on bed.	2					
• Turn sheets are used for clients who can't assist with move.						
4. Identify client.	3					
5. Explain procedure to client.	3					
6. Provide for client's privacy.	3					
7. Lock wheels on bed.	5					
PREPROCEDURE						
8. Wash your hands.	5					
9. Adjust bed to comfortable working height, with head of bed as flat as client can tolerate.	5					
10. Ensure that turn sheet is under client, positioned from shoulders to upper thighs.	2					
11. Place pillow against headboard to protect client's head.	2					
12. Bend client's knees to decrease weight of legs.	2					
13. Roll up turn sheet to side of body and grasp turn sheet at level of shoulder blades and top of thigh.	3					
• Each caregiver should do this step.	2					
14. Stand in sideways lunge position, with knees and hips flexed and body weight over rear leg.	5					
• Caregivers should face slightly toward head of bed.	2					
• Each caregiver should do this step.	2					
15. On count of 3, shift body weight from rear leg to front leg, keeping elbows at side and shoulders in line with hips.	5					
• Don't lift client.	2					
• Just allow client to slide up bed on sheet.	2					
• Be aware of sheer force applied to client's skin when he/she is moved in bed.	2					
• Each caregiver should do this step.	2					
16. Repeat steps 13 to 15 until proper position is achieved.	2					

PROCEDURE 14G2: Moving a Client Up in Bed Using a Turn or Lift Sheet (continued)

Procedure Steps	Suggested Points	Self Practice	Peer Practice	Peer Testing	Final Testing	Total Earned
17. Remove turn sheet.	2					
18. Replace pillow under client's head.	2					
19. Ensure client's comfort.	2					
POSTPROCEDURE						
20. Return bed to lowest horizontal position.	5					
21. Place call light within easy reach.	5					
22. Lower or raise side rails as ordered.	5					
23. Remove privacy screen.	2					
24. Put soiled linen in proper receptacle.	3					
25. Wash your hands.	5					
26. Record and report as necessary.	3					
TOTAL POSSIBLE POINTS	**100**					

Comments: _____
_____
_____
_____
_____
_____
_____
_____
_____
_____
_____

Signatures: _____   Date: _____

SCORING   See Preface for scoring instructions.

Nursing

PROCEDURE 14H1:
Transferring a Client Using a Mechanical Lift

PROCEDURE ASSESSMENT

Procedure Steps	Suggested Points	Self Practice	Peer Practice	Peer Testing	Final Testing	Total Earned
PREPROCEDURE						
1. Gather needed equipment.	2					
2. Obtain help if necessary.	4					
3. Identify client.	2					
4. Introduce yourself to client and explain procedure.	2					
5. Provide for client's privacy.	2					
PREPROCEDURE						
6. Wash your hands. Maintain standard precautions.	4					
7. Raise side rail on side of bed opposite from where you are standing.	4					
8. Center mechanical lift swing under client.	2					
• Usually two people are needed to do this.						
• Turn client as if you were making occupied bed.	1					
• Lower edge of sling should reach underneath client's knees.	1					
9. Place wheelchair or stretcher beside head of bed.	2					
• Lock wheels and ensure it's ready for client to be transferred.	4					
10. Put bed in lowest position and lock its wheels.	4					
11. Raise head of bed to sitting position.	2					
12. Close release valve on lift.	2					
13. Raise lift so it can be moved into position over client.	2					
14. Ensure legs of lift are spread and locked into position.	4					
15. Fasten sling to lift using the devices provided with lift.	2					
• Move hooks away from client to prevent injury.	4					
16. Attach sling to swivel bar.	2					
• Ensure that short side is attached to top of sling and long side to bottom.	2					
17. Cross client's arms over his/her chest or have client hold onto chain or straps.	2					
• To prevent injury, don't let client hold onto swivel bar.	4					

PROCEDURE 14H1: Transferring a Client Using a Mechanical Lift (continued)

Procedure Steps	Suggested Points	Self Practice	Peer Practice	Peer Testing	Final Testing	Total Earned
18. Raise lift slowly until it's clear of bed.	2					
• At each step, tell client what you're doing so he/she doesn't become anxious.	4					
19. Ask assistant to support client's legs.	4					
20. Turn client in sling so he/she is facing mast.	2					
• Mast is arm of lift that's attached to the base.						
21. Position lift so client's back is facing toward chair or stretcher.	1					
22. Position client over seat of chair or over stretcher.	2					
23. Warn client that you're going to let him/her down into chair or onto stretcher.	2					
24. Slowly open lift release valve.	2					
25. Lower lift enough that you can unhook swing and leave it under client.	1					
26. Position client in wheelchair and place slippers on his/her feet.	2					
• Or cover client on stretcher and raise side rails.	4					
27. If client will be left in room, place call bell within easy reach.	4					
POSTPROCEDURE						
28. Clean and store mechanical lift.	4					
29. Wash your hands.	4					
30. Report and record as necessary.	2					
TOTAL POSSIBLE POINTS	100					

Comments:

_____

_____

_____

_____

_____

_____

_____

_____

Signatures: _____ Date: _____

SCORING *See Preface for scoring instructions.*

Nursing

PROCEDURE 14H2:
Transferring a Client into a Wheelchair

··········· **P R O C E D U R E A S S E S S M E N T** ···········

Procedure Steps	Suggested Points	Self Practice	Peer Practice	Peer Testing	Final Testing	Total Earned
PREPROCEDURE						
1. Gather needed equipment.	2					
• A gait (transfer) belt is a wide belt placed around client's waist to hold client during transfer.	1					
2. Identify client and introduce yourself.	3					
3. Explain procedure to client.	3					
4. Provide for client's privacy.	3					
PREPROCEDURE						
5. Wash your hands.	4					
6. Put foot pedals in up position and remove them from wheelchair, if possible.	3					
7. Put wheelchair or chair on client's strongest side and parallel to bed.	3					
8. Lock wheelchair wheels and ensure chair is in good shape.	4					
• Lock wheels on bed and put it in lowest position.	3					
9. Ensure client is wearing nonslip footwear and appropriate clothing.	4					
10. Help client to sit on edge of bed.	3					
11. Apply gait belt and position client's feet shoulder width apart, flat on floor with knees slightly bent.	4					
12. Stand in front of client and grasp gait belt with both hands at each side of client.	3					
13. Ask client to put his/her hands on bed.	3					
14. Bend client's upper body so that head is over knees.	3					
• It may help to rock client to count of 3.						
15. Cue client to push off bed and upward with his/her hands, straightening knees.	3					
16. Ensure client's balance is good and keep client's body close to yours.	4					
17. Adjust your footing to allow client to pivot to chair.	3					
18. Cue client to turn slowly and reach for far arm of chair.	3					
19. Have client back up until back of his/her legs touch chair.	3					
20. Help client sit.	3					

PROCEDURE 14H2: Transferring a Client into a Wheelchair *(continued)*

Procedure Steps	Suggested Points	Self Practice	Peer Practice	Peer Testing	Final Testing	Total Earned
• Tell client to reach back for other chair arm and slowly lower the client to sitting position.	2					
• Use your weight to counterbalance client's weight.	2					
21. Replace foot pedals on wheelchair.	3					
22. Help client sit correctly in wheelchair.	4					
23. Remove gait belt.	3					
24. Apply positioning aids as ordered.	2					
25. Ensure client's comfort.	3					
POSTPROCEDURE						
26. Remove the privacy screen.	2					
27. Place call light within easy reach.	4					
28. Wash your hands.	4					
29. Report and record as necessary.	3					
TOTAL POSSIBLE POINTS	100					

Comments: _____

_____

_____

_____

_____

_____

_____

_____

_____

_____

Signatures: _____ **Date:** _____

SCORING   *See Preface for scoring instructions.*

Nursing

PROCEDURE 14H3:
Transferring a Conscious Client from the Bed to a Stretcher

PROCEDURE ASSESSMENT

Procedure Steps PREPROCEDURE	Suggested Points	Self Practice	Peer Practice	Peer Testing	Final Testing	Total Earned
1. Gather needed equipment.	3					
2. Identify client and introduce yourself and helpers.	4					
3. Explain procedure to client.	4					
4. Provide for client privacy.	4					
5. Choose one side of bed to work from, ensuring there is room to work.	3					
PREPROCEDURE						
6. Wash your hands.	6					
7. Raise bed so it's even with height of stretcher.	4					
8. Fan-fold top linens to foot of bed and provide for client privacy.	3					
9. Place a sheet or bath blanket over client.	3					
10. Lower side rail on side where stretcher will be placed.	3					
11. Move stretcher into position parallel with bed.	4					
• Ensure wheels are locked on both bed and stretcher.	6					
12. Position one person on each side of bed and stretcher and one at head of bed.	3					
• Lower side rails when someone is there to protect client.	3					
13. Ask person alongside bed to put his/her hands under client's back and lower legs.	4					
14. Ask person on far side of stretcher to put his/her hands under client's back and legs.	4					
15. Ask person at head of bed to put his/her hands under pillow and client's head.	4					
16. If necessary, move client closer to stretcher with one move.	3					
17. On count of three, move client to stretcher.	4					

PROCEDURE 14H3: Transferring a Conscious Client from the Bed to a Stretcher *(continued)*

Procedure Steps	Suggested Points	Self Practice	Peer Practice	Peer Testing	Final Testing	Total Earned
POSTPROCEDURE						
18. Fasten safety straps around client.	6					
19. Raise side rails of stretcher.	6					
20. Don't leave client unattended.	6					
21. Wash your hands.	6					
22. Report and record as necessary.	4					
TOTAL POSSIBLE POINTS	100					

Comments:

Signatures: **Date:**

SCORING   *See Preface for scoring instructions.*

Nursing

PROCEDURE 14H4:
Transferring an Unconscious Client from the Bed to a Stretcher

PROCEDURE ASSESSMENT

Procedure Steps	Suggested Points	Self Practice	Peer Practice	Peer Testing	Final Testing	Total Earned
PREPROCEDURE						
1. Gather needed equipment.	3					
2. Get 3 people to assist you.	6					
3. Identify client and introduce yourself and helpers.	3					
• Do this even if client doesn't respond.						
4. Explain procedure, even if client doesn't respond.	4					
5. Provide for client privacy.	3					
PREPROCEDURE						
6. Wash your hands.	6					
7. Choose one side of bed to work from, ensuring there's room to work.	3					
8. Raise bed even with height of stretcher.	3					
9. Fan-fold top linens to foot of bed.	3					
10. Place sheet or bath blanket over client.	4					
11. Lower side rail on side of bed where stretcher will be placed.	4					
12. Move stretcher into position parallel with bed.	3					
• Ensure wheels are locked on both bed and stretcher.	6					
13. Position one person on each side of bed and stretcher and one at foot of bed.	4					
• Lower bed side rails when someone is there to protect client.	3					
14. Roll in both sides of turning sheet next to client.	3					
15. Person at foot of bed should be in position to raise client's lower legs and feet.	4					
16. Ask person on far side of bed to hold turning sheet and be ready to raise it and lift client toward stretcher.	3					
17. Ask person on far side of stretcher to hold turning sheet with both hands and be ready to pull client toward stretcher.	3					
18. Ask person at head of bed to put his/her hands under client's shoulders and be ready to guide client toward stretcher.	4					
19. On count of 3, move client to stretcher.	3					
20. Position client in middle of stretcher and fasten restraints.	6					

PROCEDURE 14H4: Transferring an Unconscious Client from the Bed to a Stretcher *(continued)*

Procedure Steps	Suggested Points	Self Practice	Peer Practice	Peer Testing	Final Testing	Total Earned
POSTPROCEDURE						
21. Raise side rails on stretcher.	6					
22. Wash your hands.	6					
23. Record and report as needed.	4					
TOTAL POSSIBLE POINTS	100					

Comments: _____

_____

_____

_____

_____

_____

_____

_____

_____

_____

Signatures: _____ **Date:** _____

SCORING   *See Preface for scoring instructions.*

Nursing

PROCEDURE 14I1:
Assisting with a Bath or Shower

PROCEDURE ASSESSMENT

Procedure Steps	Suggested Points	Self Practice	Peer Practice	Peer Testing	Final Testing	Total Earned
PREPROCEDURE						
1. Gather needed supplies.	3					
2. Ensure tub or shower is clean.	5					
3. Place a nonslip mat on floor next to tub or shower.	5					
4. Identify client and introduce yourself.	3					
5. Explain procedure to client.	3					
6. Provide for client privacy.	3					
PREPROCEDURE						
7. Wash your hands.	5					
8. Help client to bathing area. Use a shower chair, if needed.	2					
9. For a bath, fill tub about ½ full of water between 105° and 110° F.	3					
• Test temperature to ensure water isn't too hot or cold.	5					
10. Help client remove his/her clothes.	3					
11. For a shower, turn water on and test it before helping client in.	5					
12. For a bath, help client into tub.	3					
13. If client is alone while bathing, ensure client can reach emergency signal light.	5					
• Check facility policy on whether clients can be left alone while bathing.	3					
• Check on client at least every 5 minutes.	5					
• Limit time in tub to 20 minutes.	3					
14. Knock on door before entering bathing room.	3					
15. If you can't leave client alone, let client wash as much as he/she can manage.	3					
• Offer assistance with back and as needed.	2					
16. When bathing is done, help client get out of tub or shower.	3					
17. Wrap towel around client and help client dry off.	2					
• Make sure to dry all areas of body.	4					
POSTPROCEDURE						
18. Help client apply deodorant if necessary.	2					
19. Offer and provide a back massage.	3					

PROCEDURE 14I1: Assisting with a Bath or Shower *(continued)*

Procedure Steps	Suggested Points	Self Practice	Peer Practice	Peer Testing	Final Testing	Total Earned
20. Help client dress.	2					
21. Clean bath area and put soiled linen in proper receptacle.	3					
22. Wash your hands.	5					
23. Report and record as necessary.	4					
TOTAL POSSIBLE POINTS	**100**					

Comments:

Signatures: _____   Date: _____

SCORING   *See Preface for scoring instructions.*

Nursing

PROCEDURE 1412:
Performing a Partial Bed Bath

PROCEDURE ASSESSMENT

Procedure Steps	Suggested Points	Self Practice	Peer Practice	Peer Testing	Final Testing	Total Earned
PREPROCEDURE						
1. Gather needed equipment.	2					
2. Identify client and introduce yourself.	3					
3. Explain procedure to client.	3					
4. Provide for client privacy.	3					
5. Wash your hands.	4					
6. Gather equipment and linen and place on towel on over-the-bed table.	2					
7. Adjust table to comfortable working height.	4					
8. Offer to let client use bedpan or urninal.	2					
9. Wear gloves if client has open sores.	4					
• Always wear gloves for perineal care.	3					
10. Help client with oral care.	2					
PREPROCEDURE						
11. Wash your hands.	4					
12. Cover client with bath blanket.	3					
• Ask client to hold blanket under chin.	2					
• Remove top linens from underneath bath blanket.	2					
13. Help client remove his/her clothing.	2					
14. Raise head of bed so client is sitting up as much as possible.	3					
15. Place water in basin.	3					
• Water temperature should be approximately 110°.	2					
16. Move table so client can reach it.	3					
17. Check facility's policy about leaving room while clients are bathing.	2					
• If you leave room, ensure client can easily reach call light.	4					
18. Wash your hands before leaving room.	4					
19. When you return, wash your hands and help client wash and dry any areas he/she was unable to reach.	4					
POSTPROCEDURE						
20. Offer and provide a back rub.	2					
21. Help client apply deodorant, if necessary.	2					
22. Help client dress; help with hair care.	2					

PROCEDURE 1412: Performing a Partial Bed Bath (continued)

Procedure Steps	Suggested Points	Self Practice	Peer Practice	Peer Testing	Final Testing	Total Earned
23. Change linens. If client can't get out of bed, follow procedure for making an occupied bed.	3					
24. Lower bed to lowest position.	4					
25. Ensure client's comfort.	3					
26. Clean area and put soiled linen in proper receptacle.	3					
27. Wipe off over-the-bed table.	2					
28. Remove gloves, if you have worn them.	2					
29. Wash your hands.	4					
30. Report and record as necessary.	3					
TOTAL POSSIBLE POINTS	100					

Comments: _____

_____

_____

_____

_____

_____

_____

_____

_____

_____

Signatures: _____ **Date:** _____

SCORING   *See Preface for scoring instructions.*

Nursing

PROCEDURE 1413:
Performing a Complete Bed Bath

············ P R O C E D U R E   A S S E S S M E N T ············

Procedure Steps	Suggested Points	Self Practice	Peer Practice	Peer Testing	Final Testing	Total Earned
PREPROCEDURE						
1. Gather needed equipment.	1					
2. Identify client and introduce yourself.	1					
3. Explain procedure to client.	1					
4. Provide for client privacy.	1					
5. Place water in basin.	2					
• Water temperature should be approximately 110°.	3					
• Test water with your elbow or use bath thermometer.	2					
PREPROCEDURE						
6. Wash your hands.	3					
7. Raise side rails of bed.	3					
8. Raise bed to comfortable working height and lock wheels.	3					
9. Adjust bed to as flat a position as possible.	1					
10. Lower side rail nearest you.	1					
11. Remove bedspread and place bath blanket over top sheet.	1					
12. Remove top sheet from under bath blanket without uncovering client.	2					
• Hold bath blanket at top or ask client to hold it, if he/she is able.	1					
• Pull sheet gently to foot of bed.	1					
13. Remove client's clothes.	1					
14. Put towel over client's chest.	1					
15. Wear gloves as needed.	3					
• If you or client has open skin areas, you must wear gloves.	1					
16. Wash eyes from nose toward ear.	3					
• Use different area of washcloth for each eye.	1					
• Don't use soap on face.	1					
17. Wash and rinse face, ears, and neck.	2					
18. Pat all areas dry.	1					
19. Reach under towel and fold bath blanket to waist.	2					
20. Lifting towel one part at a time, wash, rinse, and pat dry chest.	2					

PROCEDURE 1413: Performing a Complete Bed Bath *(continued)*

Procedure Steps	Suggested Points	Self Practice	Peer Practice	Peer Testing	Final Testing	Total Earned
• For female clients, check for redness under breasts.	1					
21. Fold bath blanket to pubic area.	1					
22. Wash abdomen and navel, rinse, and pat dry.	2					
23. Cover chest and abdomen with bath blanket.	1					
24. Place towel lengthwise under arm nearest you.	1					
25. Wash, rinse, and dry the hand, arm, armpit, and shoulder.	2					
26. Raise the side rail.	3					
27. Go to other side of bed, lower side rail, and repeat steps 24 to 25 on opposite arm.	2					
28. Place towel lengthwise under leg nearest you and wash, rinse, and dry leg and foot.	1					
29. Raise the side rail.	3					
30. Go to other side of bed, lower side rail, and repeat step 28 on opposite leg.	1					
31. Raise the side rail.	3					
32. Rinse bath basin and refill with clean water.	3					
33. Lower the side rail.	1					
34. Position client on his/her side facing away from you.	2					
• Keep client covered to protect privacy.	1					
35. Put on gloves, if not wearing them already.	3					
36. Use clean washcloth to wash, rinse, and pat dry back, back of neck, and buttocks.	2					
37. Wash, rinse, and pat dry anal area, from front to back.	2					
38. Rinse bath basin, remove gloves, and refill basin with clean water.	1					
39. Position client for perineal care.	1					
40. Put on gloves.	3					
41. Using clean washcloth, wash and pat dry genital area, following perineal procedure steps.	2					
POSTPROCEDURE						
42. Help client dress and groom.	1					
43. Return client to comfortable position.	1					
44. Lower bed to lowest position.	3					
• Leave side rails up or down, as ordered.	1					
45. Clean and put away equipment.	2					
46. Wash your hands.	3					
47. Report and record as necessary.	2					
TOTAL POSSIBLE POINTS	**100**					

PROCEDURE 14I3: Performing a Complete Bed Bath (continued)

Comments: _____
_____
_____
_____
_____
_____
_____
_____
_____

Signatures: _____ Date: _____

SCORING *See Preface for scoring instructions.*

Name _____ Date _____

Nursing

PROCEDURE 14J1:
Providing Denture Care

PROCEDURE ASSESSMENT

Procedure Steps	Suggested Points	Self Practice	Peer Practice	Peer Testing	Final Testing	Total Earned
PREPROCEDURE						
1. Gather needed equipment.	4					
2. Identify client.	4					
3. Instruct client on procedure.	4					
4. Provide for client privacy.	4					
PREPROCEDURE						
5. Wash your hands.	5					
6. Help client to a sitting position.	3					
7. Spread a face towel across client's chest.	3					
8. Put on gloves.	5					
9. Line an emesis basin with washcloth or paper towel.	3					
• Ask client to place dentures in basin.	2					
10. Ask client to remove his/her dentures.	3					
11. Help client remove dentures, if necessary.	3					
• Slip a finger under dentures and gently remove them.	2					
12. Take dentures to sink in emesis basin.	3					
13. Line bottom of sink with washcloth or paper towels.	5					
• Fill sink ⅓ full of water.	2					
• Be careful not to contaminate gloves.						
14. Apply toothpaste or denture cleaner to dentures.	3					
15. Hold dentures firmly and brush all surfaces until clean.	3					
16. Rinse dentures thoroughly under cool running water.	3					
17. Fill clean denture cup with cool water and dental soaking agent.	3					
• Ensure cup is marked with client's name and room number.	2					
• Ask client or check plan of care to ensure you're using correct soaking agent.	2					
18. Place dentures in cup to soak.	2					
19. Help client rinse his/her mouth with water or diluted mouthwash.	2					
20. Help client replace dentures in mouth, if appropriate.	3					
21. Clean client's face as needed.	2					
22. Help client to comfortable position.	3					

PROCEDURE 14J1: Providing Denture Care (continued)

Procedure Steps POSTPROCEDURE	Suggested Points	Self Practice	Peer Practice	Peer Testing	Final Testing	Total Earned
23. Clean equipment.	3					
24. Store equipment according to facility policy.	3					
25. Remove gloves.	3					
26. Wash your hands.	5					
27. Report and record as necessary.	3					
TOTAL POSSIBLE POINTS	100					

Comments:

_____

_____

_____

_____

_____

_____

_____

_____

_____

Signatures: _____   Date: _____

SCORING   See Preface for scoring instructions.

Nursing

PROCEDURE 14J2:
Assisting with Oral Care

PROCEDURE ASSESSMENT

Procedure Steps	Suggested Points	Self Practice	Peer Practice	Peer Testing	Final Testing	Total Earned
PREPROCEDURE						
1. Gather needed equipment.	5					
2. Identify client.	6					
3. Instruct client on procedure.	6					
4. Provide for client privacy.	6					
PREPROCEDURE						
5. Wash your hands.	7					
• Put on gloves, if you will be helping client brush teeth.	6					
6. Help wash client's hands.	5					
7. Help client put toothpaste on toothbrush and moisten toothbrush.	5					
8. Wait while client brushes his or her teeth.	5					
9. Help client rinse his or her mouth with water.	5					
• Tell client to spit water into sink.	4					
• If client is bedridden, have client spit in emesis basin.	4					
10. Help client use mouthwash, if client so wishes.	5					
• Dilute mouthwash if required for client.	4					
11. Help client dry his or her face with towel.	5					
POSTPROCEDURE						
12. Help client to a comfortable position.	5					
13. Remove gloves if used.	5					
14. Wash your hands.	7					
15. Report and record as necessary.	5					
TOTAL POINTS	100					

Comments:

_____

_____

_____

_____

_____

Signatures: _____   **Date:** _____

SCORING   *See Preface for scoring instructions.*

Name _____ Date _____

Nursing

PROCEDURE 14J3:
Performing Oral Care for a Helpless Client

PROCEDURE ASSESSMENT

Procedure Steps	Suggested Points	Self Practice	Peer Practice	Peer Testing	Final Testing	Total Earned
PREPROCEDURE						
1. Gather needed equipment.	4					
2. Identify client.	4					
3. Instruct client on procedure even if client doesn't respond.	4					
• Remember that client may be able to hear you.						
• Provide for client privacy.	4					
PREPROCEDURE						
4. Wash your hands.	6					
5. Raise bed to a comfortable working position.	6					
6. Lower side rail, if necessary.	4					
7. Position client in a side-lying position facing toward you.	3					
8. Place face towel under client's face and neck.	3					
9. Place emesis basin near client's mouth.	3					
10. Put on gloves.	6					
11. Dip toothette, glycerine swab, or toothbrush in cleaning solution.	3					
• Remove excess liquid by tapping gently over container.	3					
12. Separate upper and lower teeth with padded tongue blade.	6					
13. Clean entire mouth and all teeth.	3					
• Change and/or remoisten toothette, glycerine swab, or toothbrush as needed.	3					
14. Apply lubricant to lips if so instructed in plan of care.	3					
POSTPROCEDURE						
15. Clean client's face with a warm, wet cloth as needed.	3					
16. Clean equipment and store as directed.	4					
17. Position client as directed in plan of care.	3					
18. Return bed to lowest position and raise side rails, if ordered.	6					
19. Remove gloves.	6					
20. Wash your hands.	6					
21. Report and record as necessary.	4					
TOTAL POSSIBLE POINTS	**100**					

Comments:

_____
_____
_____
_____
_____
_____
_____
_____
_____
_____

Signatures: _____ **Date:** _____

SCORING   *See Preface for scoring instructions.*

Nursing

PROCEDURE 14K:
Nail Care

PROCEDURE ASSESSMENT

Procedure Steps	Suggested Points	Self Practice	Peer Practice	Peer Testing	Final Testing	Total Earned
PREPROCEDURE						
1. Gather needed equipment.	4					
2. Identify client.	4					
3. Instruct client on procedure.	4					
4. Provide for client privacy.	4					
PREPROCEDURE						
5. Wash your hands.	5					
6. Help client to a sitting position.	4					
7. Help client wash his/her hands.	5					
8. Soak nails for 10 to 20 minutes in warm water, if nails are brittle.	3					
9. Dry client's hands thoroughly.	4					
10. Clean under fingernails with orangewood stick.	4					
11. Push cuticles back toward fingers using orangewood stick.	4					
12. Clip fingernails straight across.	4					
13. File nails with emery board until they're smooth and corners are round.	4					
14. Apply lotion to client's hands.	4					
15. Wash client's feet as directed.	4					
16. Soak feet for 10 minutes in warm water.	4					
17. Clean under toenails with a new orangewood stick.	4					
18. File nails straight across with a new emery board until they're smooth.	4					
• Ensure that facility's policy allows this.	3					
19. Scrub callused areas of feet with washcloth.	4					
20. Apply lotion to feet.	4					
POSTPROCEDURE						
21. Remove gloves.	4					
22. Wash your hands.	5					
23. Report and record as necessary.	4					
• Make special note of any abnormalities on hands and/or feet.	3					
TOTAL POSSIBLE POINTS	**100**					

PROCEDURE 14K: Nail Care *(continued)*

Comments: _____
_____
_____
_____
_____
_____
_____
_____
_____
_____
_____

Signatures: _____ **Date:** _____

SCORING   *See Preface for scoring instructions.*

Nursing

PROCEDURE 14L1:
Shampooing a Bed-Bound Client's Hair

············ P R O C E D U R E   A S S E S S M E N T ············

Procedure Steps	Suggested Points	Self Practice	Peer Practice	Peer Testing	Final Testing	Total Earned
PREPROCEDURE						
1. Gather needed equipment.	3					
2. Identify client.	3					
3. Introduce yourself and explain procedure, even if client doesn't respond.	3					
4. Provide for client privacy.	3					
5. Place equipment on over-the-bed table.	4					
• Move table so it's in a comfortable working position.	3					
6. Raise side rails.	4					
7. Raise bed to comfortable working height.	4					
• Ensure bed wheels are locked.	3					
PREPROCEDURE						
8. Wash your hands.	4					
9. Remove client's pillow and put waterproof barrier under client's head.	2					
10. Put trough under client's head.	2					
11. Ensure there is a collection unit under drain for excess water.	2					
12. Loosen client's gown and fold it over at neck.	2					
13. Comb or brush client's hair.	3					
14. Have warm water (110° to 115°F) ready to use in a pitcher.	2					
15. Cover client's eyes with washcloth; put cotton balls in client's ears.	3					
• Client may hold washcloth, if able.						
16. Run water over client's hair until it's wet.	2					
17. Apply small amount of shampoo.	2					
18. Work up a lather, working from hairline to back of scalp.	2					
19. Gently massage scalp with your fingertips.	2					
20. Rinse with warm water.	3					
• Repeat the shampoo if necessary or if client asks you to.	2					
21. If client's hair needs conditioner, apply small amount and work it in.	2					
22. Rinse hair thoroughly.	2					

PROCEDURE 14L1: Shampooing a Bed-Bound Client's Hair *(continued)*

Procedure Steps	Suggested Points	Self Practice	Peer Practice	Peer Testing	Final Testing	Total Earned
23. Remove washcloth from eyes and pat client's face dry.	3					
24. Wrap client's hair with large towel.	2					
25. Remove trough and other equipment from bed.	2					
26. Change client's gown if it's wet.	3					
• Remove cotton from ears.	2					
• Remove sheets or padding that has become wet.	2					
27. Comb or brush client's hair.	3					
28. Dry hair with blow dryer on lowest setting.	3					
• Style hair as client chooses.						
POSTPROCEDURE						
29. Position client comfortably.	3					
30. Clean and put away all equipment.	3					
31. Wash your hands.	4					
32. Record and report as necessary.	3					
TOTAL POSSIBLE POINTS	**100**					

Comments: _____

_____

_____

_____

_____

_____

_____

_____

_____

_____

Signatures: _____   Date: _____

_____

SCORING   *See Preface for scoring instructions.*

Nursing

PROCEDURE 14L2:
Brushing or Combing a Client's Hair

····· P R O C E D U R E   A S S E S S M E N T ·····

Procedure Steps	Suggested Points	Self Practice	Peer Practice	Peer Testing	Final Testing	Total Earned
PREPROCEDURE						
1. Gather needed equipment.	4					
2. Identify client.	6					
3. Explain procedure to client.	6					
4. Provide for client privacy.	6					
5. Wash your hands.	8					
6. Obtain client's brush or comb.	4					
7. Help client to a sitting or Fowler's position.	6					
PREPROCEDURE						
8. If hair isn't tangled:						
• Brush or comb hair from scalp to hair ends.	5					
• Place towel over shoulders to prevent hair from getting on gown or bed.	5					
9. If hair is tangled:						
• Separate small locks of hair.	5					
• Grasp one lock firmly near scalp to prevent pulling on scalp.	5					
• Brush or comb from bottom of lock toward scalp as tangles are removed.	5					
10. If hair is kinky or curly, use a pick-style comb to gently comb hair.	4					
11. Arrange hair in style client chooses.	5					
POSTPROCEDURE						
12. Help client to comfortable position.	6					
13. Clean and put away brush or comb.	6					
14. Wash your hands.	8					
15. Record and report as necessary.	6					
TOTAL POSSIBLE POINTS	100					

Comments:

_____

_____

_____

_____

_____

_____

_____

_____

_____

Signatures: _____ **Date:** _____

SCORING *See Preface for scoring instructions.*

Nursing

PROCEDURE 14M:
Shaving

PROCEDURE ASSESSMENT

Procedure Steps	Suggested Points	Self Practice	Peer Practice	Peer Testing	Final Testing	Total Earned
PREPROCEDURE						
1. Gather needed equipment.	3					
2. Identify client and introduce yourself.	3					
3. Wash hands and put on gloves.	5					
4. Provide for client privacy.	3					
5. Put equipment on over-the-bed table.	5					
• Move table into comfortable working position.	2					
6. Raise head of bed to as high a level as client can tolerate.	3					
7. Cover client's chest with towel.	3					
PREPROCEDURE						
8. Place mirror so client can see his face.	3					
9. If razor is electric or a nondisposable safety razor, make sure it's clean.	4					
• If disposable safety razor is used, make sure it's new.	2					
10. If client is using electric razor, allow him to shave, if possible.	4					
• Or, assist client and shave face, chin, and neck.	2					
11. If safety razor is used, put warm water in basin.	4					
• Use washcloth to moisten areas to be shaved.	2					
12. Put shaving cream on areas to be shaved.	3					
13. Begin shaving one side of face next to ear.	3					
14. Hold skin taut and bring razor down cheek.	4					
• Repeat until shaving cream is gone.	2					
• Clean razor in water when it becomes full of shaving cream or hair.	2					
• If you lift razor off skin, rinse it before shaving another area.	2					
15. Shave between nose and upper lip, using short, downward strokes.	3					
16. Use clean washcloth to remove remaining shaving cream.	2					
17. Pat face dry.	3					
18. Apply shaving lotion as requested.	2					

PROCEDURE 14M: Shaving *(continued)*

Procedure Steps	Suggested Points	Self Practice	Peer Practice	Peer Testing	Final Testing	Total Earned
POSTPROCEDURE						
19. If nicks or cuts occurred, put pressure on area with gauze pad.	3					
• Report incident.	4					
20. Dispose of razor in proper container.	5					
21. Clean area and store equipment.	2					
22. Remove gloves.	2					
23. Help client to comfortable position.	2					
24. Wash your hands.	5					
25. Record and report as necessary.	3					
TOTAL POSSIBLE POINTS	**100**					

Comments: _____

_____

_____

_____

_____

_____

_____

_____

_____

_____

Signatures: _____ **Date:** _____

SCORING *See Preface for scoring instructions.*

Nursing

PROCEDURE 14N1:
Providing Female Perineal Care

· · · · · · · P R O C E D U R E   A S S E S S M E N T · · · · · · ·

Procedure Steps	Suggested Points	Self Practice	Peer Practice	Peer Testing	Final Testing	Total Earned
PREPROCEDURE						
1. Gather needed equipment.	2					
2. Identify client.	2					
3. Explain procedure to client.	2					
4. Provide for client privacy.	2					
5. Raise bed to comfortable working height.	4					
6. Lower side rail on working side.	2					
PREPROCEDURE						
7. Wash your hands.	4					
8. Cover client with bath blanket or sheet.	3					
9. Pull top linens to foot of bed.	1					
10. Position client on her back.	3					
11. Put waterproof pad or towel under buttocks.	2					
12. Drape client using this suggested method:	3					
• Put bath blanket in diamond shape, with one corner between client's legs, one corner on each side of bed, and one at head.	2					
• Help client raise legs with knees bent and feet flat on bed.	2					
• Wrap bath blanket corner on each side of bed around client's leg on that side of bed, tucking it under hip.	2					
• Place corner of bath blanket that is between client's legs so it provides privacy over perineal area.	2					
13. Fill wash basin with water.	4					
• Ensure water temperature is warm but not too hot.	2					
14. Uncover just enough of perineal area to provide care.	3					
15. Put on gloves.	4					
16. Separate labia (folds of skin around vaginal opening).	3					
17. Clean downward from front to back with one stroke.	3					
• Never wipe from back to front.	4					
• Never rewipe using same area of cloth.	2					
18. Repeat until clean, changing to clean area of cloth with each stroke.	1					
19. Rinse and pat dry.	2					

Procedure Steps	Suggested Points	Self Practice	Peer Practice	Peer Testing	Final Testing	Total Earned
20. Wash remainder of pubic and groin area.	1					
21. Rinse and pat dry.	2					
22. Fold bath blanket back between client's legs.	2					
23. Help client lower her legs.	3					
24. Turn client onto her side, facing away from you, and wash buttocks.	1					
25. Clean rectal area from front to back.	1					
26. Rinse buttocks and anal area.	2					
27. Pat areas dry.	2					
28. For clients who have indwelling catheters, see Procedure 14Q5.						
POSTPROCEDURE						
29. Remove gloves.	2					
30. Wash your hands.	4					
31. Help client to comfortable position.	1					
32. Return linens to proper position.	1					
33. Remove bath blanket.	1					
34. Raise side rail.	2					
35. Lower bed to lowest position.	2					
36. Wash your hands.	4					
37. Report and record as necessary.	3					
TOTAL POSSIBLE POINTS	**100**					

Comments: _____
_____
_____
_____
_____
_____
_____
_____
_____
_____

Signatures: _____   Date: _____

SCORING   *See Preface for scoring instructions.*

Nursing

PROCEDURE 14N2:
Providing Male Perineal Care

PROCEDURE ASSESSMENT

Procedure Steps PREPROCEDURE	Suggested Points	Self Practice	Peer Practice	Peer Testing	Final Testing	Total Earned
1. Gather needed equipment.	3					
2. Wash your hands.	4					
3. Cover client with bath blanket or sheet.	2					
4. Pull top linens to foot of bed.	2					
5. Position client on his back.	3					
6. Put on gloves.	4					
7. Put waterproof pad or towel under client's buttocks.	2					
8. Drape client using this suggested method:	2					
• Put bath blanket in diamond shape with one corner between client's legs, one corner on each side of bed, and one corner at his head.	1					
• Help client raise legs with knees bent and feet flat on bed.	1					
• Wrap bath blanket corner on each side of bed around client's leg on that side of bed, tucking it under hip.	1					
• Place corner of bath blanket that is between client's legs so it provides privacy over perineal area.	1					
9. Fill wash basin with water.	4					
• Ensure water temperature is warm but not too hot.	2					
10. Uncover just enough of perineal area to provide care.	2					
11. Retract the foreskin, if client is uncircumcised.	2					
12. Clean penis with circular motion.	3					
• Start at urethral opening and work outward.	2					
13. Repeat as needed, using clean area of cloth each time.	3					
14. Rinse with clean cloth and pat dry.	3					
15. Return foreskin to its natural position.	2					
16. Clean shaft of penis with firm downward strokes from top to base.	2					
17. Rinse all areas well.	2					
18. Clean scrotum, pubic, and groin areas.	2					
19. Rinse these areas.	2					

PROCEDURE 14N2: Providing Male Perineal Care *(continued)*

Procedure Steps	Suggested Points	Self Practice	Peer Practice	Peer Testing	Final Testing	Total Earned
20. Pat all areas dry.	3					
21. Fold bath blanket back between client's legs.	2					
22. Help client lower his legs.	2					
23. Turn client onto his side, facing away from you, and wash, rinse, and dry buttocks.	2					
24. Clean rectal area from front to back.	2					
25. Rinse these areas.	2					
26. Pat area dry.	3					
27. For clients who have indwelling catheters, see Procedure 14Q5.	2					
POSTPROCEDURE						
28. Remove gloves.	2					
29. Wash your hands.	4					
30. Help client to comfortable position.	2					
31. Return linens to proper position.	1					
32. Remove bath blanket.	1					
33. Raise side rail.	4					
34. Lower bed to lowest position.	4					
35. Wash your hands.	4					
36. Report and record as necessary.	3					
TOTAL POSSIBLE POINTS	100					

Comments:

_____

_____

_____

_____

_____

_____

_____

_____

_____

_____

Signatures: _____   **Date:** _____

SCORING   *See Preface for scoring instructions.*

Nursing

PROCEDURE 1401:
Changing a Client's Gown

PROCEDURE ASSESSMENT

Procedure Steps	Suggested Points	Self Practice	Peer Practice	Peer Testing	Final Testing	Total Earned
PREPROCEDURE						
1. Gather needed equipment.	4					
2. Identify client and introduce yourself.	5					
3. Explain procedure to client.	6					
4. Provide for client privacy.	5					
PREPROCEDURE						
5. Wash your hands.	7					
6. Help client turn to his/her side.	5					
• Untie gown.	4					
• If client cannot turn, reach under client's neck to untie gown.	4					
7. Loosen soiled gown from around client.	3					
8. Place clean gown over client's chest.	5					
• Unfold gown so it provides privacy when you remove soiled gown.	4					
9. Remove one arm at a time, starting with client's stronger side.	5					
• If client has an IV, you will need help to change gown because the IV might be dislodged during procedure.	4					
10. Help client to slide each arm through sleeve of gown.	5					
• Put weaker arm through sleeve first.	4					
11. Remove soiled gown from underneath clean gown.	5					
12. Help client to comfortable position and tie gown.	4					
13. Put soiled gown in proper container.	4					
POSTPROCEDURE						
14. Unscreen client.	4					
15. Wash your hands.	7					
16. Record and report as necessary.	6					
TOTAL POSSIBLE POINTS	100					

PROCEDURE 1401: Changing a Client's Gown *(continued)*

Comments: _____

_____

_____

_____

_____

_____

_____

_____

_____

Signatures: _____ **Date:** _____

SCORING   *See Preface for scoring instructions.*

Name _____ Date _____

Nursing

PROCEDURE 1402:
Undressing and Dressing a Client Who Has Limited Use of Limbs

PROCEDURE ASSESSMENT

Procedure Steps	Suggested Points	Self Practice	Peer Practice	Peer Testing	Final Testing	Total Earned
PREPROCEDURE						
1. Gather needed equipment.	3					
2. Identify client and explain procedure.	4					
3. Provide clothing or help client select clothing.	2					
4. Provide for client privacy.	4					
PREPROCEDURE						
5. Wash your hands.	5					
6. Explain procedure to client.	4					
To Undress a Client						
7. Help client to a supine or sitting position.	4					
• If possible, position yourself on client's strong side.	3					
8. If client has affected side, begin undressing on his/her strong side.	3					
9. Remove client's upper clothing, pulling off one sleeve at a time.	3					
10. Remove client's lower clothing, pulling off one pant leg at a time.	3					
11. Put removed clothing in laundry container or reuse.	4					
To Dress a Client						
12. If client has weak side, begin to dress on weak side.	4					
13. Help with underclothing as needed.	3					
14. Undo all fasteners of clothing to be put on.	3					
15. Help client put on pants:	3					
• Gather pant leg of the leg away from you, lift leg at ankle, and pull pant leg over foot.	2					
• Repeat above step for other leg.	2					
• Pull pants up legs as far as possible.	2					
• Ask client to lift buttocks or roll to side so you can pull pants to waist.	2					
• Fasten pants as necessary.	2					
16. Help client put on a top that opens at front:	3					
• Gather sleeve, grasp client's weak arm at wrist, and slide sleeve over arm.	2					

Procedure Steps	Suggested Points	Self Practice	Peer Practice	Peer Testing	Final Testing	Total Earned
• Ask client to roll toward you and tuck garment under back.	2					
• Ask client to roll away from you and pull garment through toward you.	2					
• Gather sleeve and place over client's arm.	2					
• Adjust garment and fasten as necessary.	2					
17. Help client put on pullover:	3					
• Place client's hands in sleeves, starting with weak side.	2					
• Pull garment up client's arms.	2					
• Pull neck opening over head.	2					
• Pull garment down over trunk, adjust, and fasten.	2					
18. Help client put on footwear (socks, stockings, shoes, slippers).	2					
POSTPROCEDURE						
19. Wash your hands.	5					
20. Record and report as necessary.	4					
TOTAL POSSIBLE POINTS	**100**					

Comments: _____

_____

_____

_____

_____

_____

_____

_____

_____

_____

Signatures: _____ **Date:** _____

SCORING *See Preface for scoring instructions.*

Nursing

PROCEDURE 14P:
Applying Elastic Stockings

PROCEDURE ASSESSMENT

Procedure Steps	Suggested Points	Self Practice	Peer Practice	Peer Testing	Final Testing	Total Earned
PREPROCEDURE						
1. Obtain correctly sized stockings.	5					
2. Identify client.	6					
3. Explain procedure to client.	6					
4. Raise bed to proper working height and lock wheels.	8					
PREPROCEDURE						
5. Wash your hands.	8					
6. Have client lie supine in bed with legs elevated or level with pelvis.	4					
7. Grasp stockings from top and turn them inside out to the ankle.	5					
• Or, bunch them with right side out.						
8. Slide stockings over toes, foot, and heel.	5					
• If client is able, ask him/her to push against you while you apply stockings.	4					
9. Regrasp remaining portion of stocking and pull up to knee.	4					
10. Release gently. Don't snap stocking.	5					
11. Ensure stockings are smooth and wrinkle-free.	8					
• Ensure client's toes are easily accessible and visible.	5					
POSTPROCEDURE						
12. Wash your hands.	8					
13. At least every 2 hours, check circulation of client's feet.	6					
• Check for swelling, tingling, and redness or blueness of skin.	5					
14. Report and record as necessary.	4					
15. Remove and reapply at least every 8 hours.	4					
TOTAL POSSIBLE POINTS	100					

PROCEDURE 14P: Applying Elastic Stockings *(continued)*

Comments: _____
_____
_____
_____
_____
_____
_____
_____
_____
_____

Signatures: _____ **Date:** _____

SCORING *See Preface for scoring instructions.*

Name _____   Date _____

Nursing

PROCEDURE 14Q1:
Providing a Bedpan

PROCEDURE ASSESSMENT

Procedure Steps	Suggested Points	Self Practice	Peer Practice	Peer Testing	Final Testing	Total Earned
PREPROCEDURE						
1. Gather needed equipment.	3					
2. Identify client.	4					
3. Explain procedure to client.	4					
4. Provide for client privacy.	4					
5. Wash your hands.	5					
6. Put on gloves.	5					
7. Raise bed to comfortable working position and lock wheels.	5					
8. Lower side rail, if necessary.	5					
• Don't leave client unattended with bed raised.						
PREPROCEDURE						
9. Warm bedpan if needed by running warm water over it.	3					
• Or, rub pan briskly with paper towel or washcloth.						
10. Dry bedpan with paper towels.	3					
11. Fold back top sheets so they're out of the way.	2					
12. Raise client's gown or pull pants or pajama bottoms down.	3					
• Maintain client privacy and warmth.						
13. Ask client to bend his or her knees, with feet flat on mattress.	3					
14. Ask client to raise his or her hips. Help client if necessary.	3					
15. Put protective pad and bedpan into position:	3					
• Fracture bedpans should be placed with small end toward client's head.	2					
• Regular bedpans should be placed with rounded end toward client's head.	2					
16. If client cannot raise his or her hips, roll client away from you and place bedpan under client.	3					
17. Place bedpan firmly against buttocks.	4					
18. Holding bedpan firmly in place, help client roll onto his/her back and bedpan.	3					
19. Replace covers over client.	3					

PROCEDURE 14Q1: Providing a Bedpan *(continued)*

Procedure Steps	Suggested Points	Self Practice	Peer Practice	Peer Testing	Final Testing	Total Earned
20. Raise head of bed so client is in comfortable sitting position, if he/she can sit.	4					
21. Put toilet tissue and call light within client's reach.	3					
POSTPROCEDURE						
22. Raise side rail if so ordered by physician.	5					
23. Lower bed to lowest position.	2					
24. Dispose of gloves.	2					
25. Wash your hands.	5					
26. Leave room to provide client privacy, if appropriate.	3					
27. Await the call light to assist with removing bedpan.	4					
TOTAL POSSIBLE POINTS	100					

Comments:

_____
_____
_____
_____
_____
_____
_____
_____
_____
_____
_____

Signatures: _____ **Date:** _____

SCORING *See Preface for scoring instructions.*

Nursing

PROCEDURE 14Q2:
Removing a Bedpan

PROCEDURE ASSESSMENT

Procedure Steps	Suggested Points	Self Practice	Peer Practice	Peer Testing	Final Testing	Total Earned
PREPROCEDURE						
1. Gather needed equipment.	4					
2. Wash your hands.	6					
3. Put on gloves.	6					
4. Raise bed to comfortable working position.	6					
• Lower head of bed, if necessary.						
PREPROCEDURE						
5. Help client raise his or her hips or roll client off pan.	5					
• Hold firmly onto pan while client is turned or lifting.	4					
6. Remove the pan.	4					
7. Clean client's perineal area with toilet tissue or warm washcloth, if necessary.	5					
8. Offer client a warm, wet washcloth for hand cleaning.	4					
9. Cover pan with appropriate cover.	4					
10. Measure and record urine measurement if so ordered.	5					
• Note color and quality.	4					
11. Note amount, color, and odor of feces.	5					
• Document findings according to facility policy.	4					
12. Empty pan in toilet.	3					
POSTPROCEDURE						
13. Clean bedpan according to facility procedure.	5					
14. Put bedpan away.	5					
15. Remove gloves.	5					
16. Wash your hands.	6					
17. Lower bed to lowest position.	5					
18. Report and record as necessary.	5					
TOTAL POSSIBLE POINTS	**100**					

PROCEDURE 14Q2: Removing a Bedpan *(continued)*

Comments: _____

_____

_____

_____

_____

_____

_____

_____

_____

_____

_____

Signatures: _____   Date: _____

SCORING   *See Preface for scoring instructions.*

Nursing

PROCEDURE 14Q3:
Providing a Urinal

PROCEDURE ASSESSMENT

Procedure Steps	Suggested Points	Self Practice	Peer Practice	Peer Testing	Final Testing	Total Earned
PREPROCEDURE						
1. Gather needed equipment.	6					
2. Identify client.	6					
3. Explain procedure to client.	6					
4. Provide for client's privacy.	6					
5. Wash your hands.	8					
6. Put on gloves.	8					
7. Raise bed to comfortable working position and lock wheels.	8					
8. Lower side rail if necessary.	8					
PREPROCEDURE						
9. Help client position urinal if necessary.	6					
10. Ask client to signal when he's done.	8					
• Put call light within easy reach.	5					
11. Leave room to provide privacy, if appropriate.	6					
POSTPROCEDURE						
12. Dispose of gloves.	5					
13. Wash your hands.	8					
14. Await the client call light to assist with removing the bedpan.	6					
TOTAL POSSIBLE POINTS	100					

Comments: _____

_____

_____

_____

_____

_____

_____

_____

_____

Signatures: _____   **Date:** _____

SCORING   *See Preface for scoring instructions.*

Nursing

PROCEDURE 14Q4:
Removing a Urinal

PROCEDURE ASSESSMENT

Procedure Steps	Suggested Points	Self Practice	Peer Practice	Peer Testing	Final Testing	Total Earned
PREPROCEDURE						
1. Gather needed equipment.	6					
2. Wash your hands.	8					
3. Put on gloves.	8					
4. Explain procedure to client.	6					
5. Raise bed to comfortable working height.	8					
PREPROCEDURE						
6. Remove urinal.	6					
• Offer client a warm, wet washcloth for hand cleaning.	4					
7. Cover the urinal.	4					
8. Lower bed to lowest position.	8					
9. Take urinal to bathroom.	4					
10. Check appearance of urine and measure amount.	4					
11. Empty urinal into toilet.	4					
POSTPROCEDURE						
12. Rinse the urinal.	5					
13. Replace equipment and store urinal.	6					
14. Remove gloves.	5					
15. Wash your hands.	8					
16. Report/record as necessary.	6					
TOTAL POSSIBLE POINTS	100					

Comments: _____
_____
_____
_____
_____
_____
_____
_____
_____

Signatures: _____ Date: _____

SCORING *See Preface for scoring instructions.*

Name _____   Date _____

Nursing

PROCEDURE 14Q5:
Indwelling Catheter Care

PROCEDURE ASSESSMENT

Procedure Steps	Suggested Points	Self Practice	Peer Practice	Peer Testing	Final Testing	Total Earned
PREPROCEDURE						
1. Gather needed supplies.	2					
2. Identify client.	2					
3. Explain procedure to client.	2					
4. Provide for client privacy.	2					
5. Adjust bed to comfortable working height and lock wheels.	4					
PREPROCEDURE						
6. Wash your hands.	4					
7. Drape and position client as you would for perineal care.	2					
8. Place a waterproof pad or towel under client.	2					
9. Put on gloves.	4					
For Female						
Care for catheter:						
• Separate labia with thumb and forefinger.	2					
• Using moist, soaped washcloth, gently wash down one side of meatus (opening to urethra) and catheter.	2					
• Wash from front to back.	2					
• Change to clean area of washcloth and wash down other side of meatus and catheter.	2					
• Anchor catheter between two fingers.	2					
• Wash from meatus down catheter tubing 4 inches with clean part of washcloth.	2					
• Rinse with clear water in same manner as you washed.	2					
For Male						
Care for catheter:						
• If client is uncircumcised, retract foreskin gently.	2					
• With moist, soaped washcloth, wash tip of penis in circular motion from meatus outward.	2					
• Change to clean area of washcloth to repeat.	2					
• Anchor catheter between two fingers.	2					

Procedure Steps	Suggested Points	Self Practice	Peer Practice	Peer Testing	Final Testing	Total Earned
• With clean area of washcloth, wash 4 inches of catheter from meatus down.	2					
• Rinse with clear water in same manner as you washed.	2					
• Return foreskin to original position.	2					
10. For all clients, wash rest of perineum and buttocks as you do for perineal care.	3					
• Use top half of folded towel to dry.	2					
11. Remove towel or pad.	2					
12. Ensure bed linen is dry and catheter tubing is secured to upper thigh.	2					
13. Reposition client and ensure client's comfort.	2					
14. Coil and secure catheter bag tubing to bed.	4					
POSTPROCEDURE						
15. Remove gloves.	2					
16. Wash your hands.	4					
17. Cover client with top linens and remove bath blanket.	2					
18. Use side rails as ordered.	4					
19. Return bed to lowest horizontal position.	4					
20. Place call light within client's reach.	4					
21. Remove privacy screen.	2					
22. Clean area:	2					
• Clean and store equipment.	1					
• Dispose of soiled linens as directed.	1					
23. Wash your hands.	4					
24. Report and record as necessary.	3					
TOTAL POSSIBLE POINTS	**100**					

Comments:

_____

_____

_____

_____

_____

_____

_____

Signatures: _____ **Date:** _____

SCORING *See Preface for scoring instructions.*

Nursing

PROCEDURE 14Q6:
Emptying a Catheter Drainage Bag

PROCEDURE ASSESSMENT

Procedure Steps	Suggested Points	Self Practice	Peer Practice	Peer Testing	Final Testing	Total Earned
PREPROCEDURE						
1. Gather needed equipment.	5					
2. Identify client.	6					
3. Explain procedure to client.	6					
4. Provide for client privacy.	6					
PREPROCEDURE						
5. Wash hands and put on gloves.	7					
6. If you set measuring container on floor, put it on paper towel.	7					
7. Position drain tube over container.	7					
• Make sure drain tube doesn't touch container.	5					
8. Open drain tube clamp and empty collection bag completely.	5					
9. Close clamp and replace tube in holder on bag, if one is present.	6					
10. Measure the urine.	5					
11. If urine has odor or looks abnormal, keep it and ask a licensed nurse to assess it.	6					
12. Empty urine as directed.	4					
POSTPROCEDURE						
13. Rinse and store measuring container properly.	6					
14. Remove gloves.	6					
15. Wash your hands.	7					
16. Report and record as necessary.	6					
TOTAL POSSIBLE POINTS	100					

Comments: _____

_____

_____

_____

_____

_____

Signatures: _____ Date: _____

SCORING   *See Preface for scoring instructions.*

Nursing

PROCEDURE 14Q7:
Assisting with the Bedside Commode

P R O C E D U R E   A S S E S S M E N T

Procedure Steps	Suggested Points	Self Practice	Peer Practice	Peer Testing	Final Testing	Total Earned
PREPROCEDURE						
1. Gather needed equipment.	2					
2. Identify client and introduce yourself.	2					
3. Explain procedure to client.	2					
4. Provide for client privacy.	2					
5. Wash your hands.	4					
6. Position commode close to bed and remove lid of commode.	2					
PREPROCEDURE						
7. Help client put on robe and nonskid footwear.	4					
8. Ensure brakes are set on commode and bed wheels are locked.	4					
9. Help client sit on side of bed.	2					
10. Transfer client to commode using same procedure used for transferring client to a wheelchair.	2					
11. Cover client with blanket if it's cool in room.	2					
12. Place toilet paper and call light within reach.	4					
• Tell client to call when ready.	2					
13. Wash your hands.	4					
14. Leave room and close door.	2					
15. Answer call signal immediately.	4					
• Announce your entry before you enter room.	2					
16. Wash your hands.	4					
17. Put on gloves.	4					
18. Help client with perineal care.	2					
19. Remove gloves and wash your hands.	4					
20. Transfer client into bed.	2					
21. Help client to comfortable position.	2					
22. Put on clean pair of gloves.	4					
23. Cover and remove collection container from commode.	2					
24. Take container to toilet.	4					
• Check urine and/or feces for color, odor, amount, and character.	2					
• Measure urine, if necessary.						

PROCEDURE 14Q7: Assisting with the Bedside Commode *(continued)*

Procedure Steps POSTPROCEDURE	Suggested Points	Self Practice	Peer Practice	Peer Testing	Final Testing	Total Earned
25. Clean container according to facility policy.	2					
26. Clean commode if necessary and replace container.	4					
• Store commode properly.	2					
27. Remove gloves.	2					
28. Help client wash his/her hands.	4					
29. Unscreen client.	2					
30. Clean the area and the equipment.	2					
31. Wash your hands.	4					
32. Report and record as necessary.	2					
TOTAL POSSIBLE POINTS	**100**					

Comments: _____

_____

_____

_____

_____

_____

_____

_____

_____

_____

Signatures: _____   Date: _____

SCORING   *See Preface for scoring instructions.*

The Physician's Office   Reinforcement Activities

Matching

Write the letter of the phrase that best matches each numbered item in the blank provided.

_____ **1.** Prescribe

_____ **2.** Pathogen

_____ **3.** Credential

_____ **4.** Diagnose

_____ **5.** Vial

_____ **6.** Biohazard

_____ **7.** Ampule

_____ **8.** Purulent

_____ **9.** Sterilize

_____ **10.** Competent

a. A small glass bottle with a rubber stopper for medications or chemicals.

b. Forming or containing pus.

c. That which entitles one to authority.

d. To make free of all microorganisms.

e. An order for dispensing and administering medications.

f. To determine the cause and nature of a condition.

g. Properly or sufficiently qualified or capable.

h. A disease-producing microorganism.

i. A small breakable glass container with medication solutions.

j. A condition that constitutes a threat to humans.

Matching

Write the letter of the phrase that best matches each numbered item in the blank provided.

_____ **11.** proximal

_____ **12.** distal

_____ **13.** palpation

_____ **14.** cytology

_____ **15.** allergy

a. Farthest away from the point of attachment.

b. The study of cells.

c. Closest to the point of attachment.

d. A reaction to something that is normally harmless.

e. To examine something by touching.

True/False

Write "T" in the blank provided if the statement is true. Write "F" if the statement is false.

_____ **16.** It is the responsibility of the physician who prescribes a medication to administer and dispense it.

_____ **17.** Physician assistants must work under the supervision of a physician and the physician must be in the immediate geographical area.

_____ **18.** The supine position requires that the client be lying flat, facing upward on the examination table.

_____ **19.** If in doubt about the sterility of a surgical instrument used during a minor office procedure, the item should be considered contaminated.

_____ **20.** The *Physicians' Desk Reference* is an excellent source to check for client allergies to specific medications.

Name _____ Date _____

Multiple Choice

Circle the letter that best answers the question or completes the statement.

21. Physician office employees, including the physician, must be able to communicate with a variety of people including
    a. clients.
    b. salespersons.
    c. pharmacists.
    d. all of the above.

22. Duties of the physician assistant may be limited according to
    a. the client.
    b. state law.
    c. federal law.
    d. the training of the assistant.

23. Formal MA programs include a clinical experience known as a/an:
    a. internship.
    b. residency.
    c. externship.
    d. clinical.

24. All of the following are clinical skills except
    a. administering medications.
    b. preparing the client for an examination.
    c. assembling the medical record.
    d. sanitizing and disinfecting surgical instruments.

25. A position in which the client is lying on one side with the superior leg brought forward and slightly bent is called
    a. Sims'.
    b. knee-chest.
    c. lithotomy.
    d. prone.

26. Vaginal specimens obtained during the gynecological exam are sent to the lab to check for abnormal
    a. bacteria.
    b. cells.
    c. bleeding.
    d. turbidity.

27. A streptococcal infection of the throat left untreated can cause a condition known as rheumatic fever which can ultimately damage
    a. heart valves.
    b. cardiac muscle.
    c. pharyngeal tissue.
    d. hepatic tissue.

28. When instructing the client on the procedure for obtaining a clean-catch urine specimen, the _____ of the client should be cleansed with an antiseptic wipe.
   a. hands.
   b. urethra.
   c. specimen container.
   d. urinary meatus.

29. Suture material that must be removed after several days is known as
   a. absorbable.
   b. nonabsorbable.
   c. approximated.
   d. sterile.

30. Purulent drainage contains
   a. blood.
   b. water.
   c. pus.
   d. tissue.

Fill in the Blank
Write the word (or words) that best completes the sentence in the blank provided.

31. Bandages should always be applied to an extremity from the _____ end to the _____ end of the extremity.

32. A _____ is a symptom or circumstance that indicates that a specific medication or treatment should not be administered.

33. A/An _____ is a small glass container that may be sealed and its contents sterilized.

34. _____ injections are made into the soft tissue beneath the skin.

35. The liquid added to a powder medication is called the _____.

Labeling

In the space provided, write the word(s) that identifies the corresponding part on the diagram.

36. Identify the instruments shown below by writing the correct name of the instrument beside the correct letter.

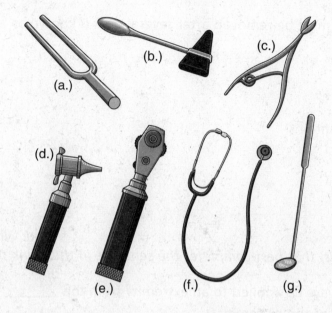

(a.) _____   (e.) _____

(b.) _____   (f.) _____

(c.) _____   (g.) _____

(d.) _____

37. In the first circle below, show how you would swab a culture plate after a throat culture specimen is obtained. In the next two circles below, show how you would inoculate a culture plate after you have swabbed the culture plate.

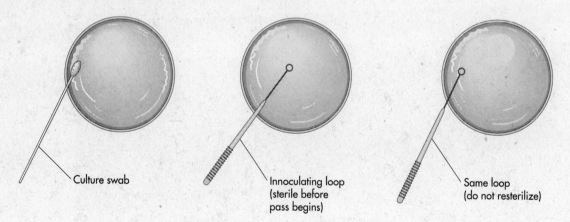

Short Answer

Answer the questions below in the space provided. Answers can be found in Lab Manual Part B.

38. What size of needle and syringe should be used for an intramuscular (IM) injection?

_____

_____

39. What size needle and syringe should be used for a subcutaneous (SC) injection.

_____

_____

40. What size needle and syringe are used for an intradermal (ID) injection?

_____

_____

41. When giving an injection you pull back the plunger and see blood. What should you do?

_____

_____

The Physician's Office

PROCEDURE 15A:
Positioning Clients for a Physical Examination

⋯⋯⋯⋯⋯⋯⋯⋯⋯ **PROCEDURE ASSESSMENT** ⋯⋯⋯⋯⋯⋯⋯⋯⋯

Procedure Steps	Suggested Points	Self Practice	Peer Practice	Peer Testing	Final Testing	Total Earned
PREPROCEDURE						
1. Gather equipment and wash your hands.	5					
2. Ensure client has been instructed on clothing removal.	3					
• Ensure client has been instructed on donning exam gown.	2					
3. Drape client for warmth and privacy.	3					
4. Position client only when physician is ready for exam.	2					
5. Explain to client how you want him/her positioned.	2					
6. Help client into and out of position as necessary.	2					
PROCEDURE						
Sitting:						
• Ask client to sit on side of exam table with his/her legs hanging down and back unsupported.	2					
• Place drape so it covers lower extremities.	2					
Supine:						
• Extend lower end of table if necessary.	2					
• Ask client to lie down, face up, with arms extended.	2					
• Place drape over body, covering chest, abdomen, and lower extremities.	2					
Dorsal recumbent:						
• Extend lower end of table if necessary.	2					
• Ask client to lie down, face up, in supine position and bring knees up.	3					
• Bottom of feet should be flat on exam table.	3					
• Place drape over abdomen and lower extremities.	2					
Lithotomy:						
• Extend stirrups at end of table about 12 inches from table.	2					
• Ask client to lie down, face up, and put feet in stirrups.	3					
• Ask client to bring buttocks down to end of table.	2					
• Place drape over abdomen and legs.	2					

PROCEDURE 15A: Positioning Clients for a Physical Examination *(continued)*

Procedure Steps	Suggested Points	Self Practice	Peer Practice	Peer Testing	Final Testing	Total Earned
Prone:						
• Extend lower end of table.	2					
• Ask client to lie down, face down, with head turned to side.	3					
• Place drape so it covers back, buttocks, and lower extremities.	2					
Sims':						
• Extend lower end of table.	2					
• Ask client to lie down on one side, usually left.	2					
• Client should bring top leg forward and bend it slightly.	4					
• Place drape so it covers client from neck to feet.	2					
Knee-Chest:						
• Ask client to lie face down on table with knees bent up onto table.	3					
• Thighs should be at 90 degree angle with table.	2					
• Feet should be 12 inches apart.	2					
• Head should be turned to side.	2					
• Place drape so it covers upper back, buttocks, and lower extremities.	2					
POSTPROCEDURE						
7. If client complains of dizziness after exam:	2					
• Have client lie back down on table.	5					
• Don't leave client on table unattended.	5					
8. Help client get dressed, if appropriate.	2					
9. Clean exam room after client leaves.	2					
• Dispose of gown and drape in proper receptacles.	3					
10. Wash your hands.	5					
TOTAL POSSIBLE POINTS	**100**					

Comments:

Signatures: _____   Date: _____

SCORING *See Preface for scoring instructions.*

The Physician's Office

PROCEDURE 15B:
Assisting with Gynecological Examinations

PROCEDURE ASSESSMENT

Procedure Steps	Suggested Points	Self Practice	Peer Practice	Peer Testing	Final Testing	Total Earned
PREPROCEDURE						
1. Gather needed equipment.	3					
2. Ensure exam table stirrups are in good working order.	4					
3. Assemble supplies on a Mayo stand, countertop, or other tray covered with paper towel.	3					
4. Wash your hands.	6					
5. Identify client by asking her full name.	4					
6. Tell client to remove all clothing, including underwear.	3					
• Tell client to put on gown with opening to the front.	3					
7. Ask client to sit in exam room with drape over lower extremities until physician is ready to begin.	3					
PROCEDURE						
8. Ask client to put feet in stirrups and bring buttocks down to end of table.	3					
9. Warm speculum by placing it in warm water, if doctor prefers.	4					
• Otherwise, no lubricant is used.						
10. When physician obtains specimen and puts smears on slides:						
• Put on clean gloves.	3					
• Gently spray slides with cytology fixative.	3					
• Hold can 6 inches from slide and lightly spray with back-and-forth motion.	3					
• Let slides dry completely.	4					
• With pencil, label frosted end of slides with client's name, the date, and where specimen was obtained.	3					
11. Apply lubricant to physician's gloved hand before digital exam.	4					
12. When exam is over, ask client to remove feet from stirrups and sit up.	3					
• Assist client as necessary.	4					
• Give client tissues to remove lubricant.	3					
13. Ask client to get dressed.	3					
• Explain how she will be told of lab results.	3					

PROCEDURE 15B: Assisting with Gynecological Examinations (continued)

Procedure Steps POSTPROCEDURE	Suggested Points	Self Practice	Peer Practice	Peer Testing	Final Testing	Total Earned
14. Wear exam gloves to clean exam room and equipment.	4					
• Sanitize, disinfect, and sterilize nondisposable vaginal speculums.	3					
• Dispose of disposable speculums in biohazard waste container.	4					
15. Store other supplies.	3					
16. Straighten exam room and discard used exam table paper.	4					
17. Prepare lab request.	3					
• Put specimen in container for transport to lab.	4					
18. Remove gloves and wash hands.	3					
TOTAL POSSIBLE POINTS	**100**					

Comments:

_____

_____

_____

_____

_____

_____

_____

_____

_____

Signatures: _____ **Date:** _____

SCORING *See Preface for scoring instructions.*

The Physician's Office

PROCEDURE 15C:
Obtaining a Throat Culture

P R O C E D U R E   A S S E S S M E N T

Procedure Steps	Suggested Points	Self Practice	Peer Practice	Peer Testing	Final Testing	Total Earned
PREPROCEDURE						
1. Gather needed supplies.	6					
PROCEDURE						
2. Wash hands and put on clean exam gloves.	6					
3. Identify client and explain procedure.	6					
4. Open applicator of Culturette or culture swab.	3					
• Don't contaminate it.	5					
• Don't put it on nonsterile surface.	5					
5. Turn on exam light and position it toward client's mouth.	3					
6. Have client face light source and open mouth wide.	4					
• Client may need to say, "Ah."	3					
7. Insert tongue depressor in mouth and hold tongue down.	4					
• View posterior pharynx.	3					
8. Insert sterile swab.	4					
• Don't touch inside of cheeks, lips, teeth or tongue with swab.	3					
9. Firmly rotate swab on back of throat and on either side.	4					
• Make sure to touch areas that are reddened or white.	3					
10. Quickly remove swab without touching teeth, lips, tongue, or uvula.	4					
11. Dispose of tongue depressor in biohazard container.	6					
12. Immediately perform rapid streptococcus test on specimen or inoculate culture plate or break transport medium capsule in Culturette system.	8					
13. Remove gloves and wash hands.	6					
POSTPROCEDURE						
14. Record results of test in client's record.	4					
• Or, put inoculated culture plate in incubator.	2					
• Or, prepare Culturette for transport to lab.	2					
15. Tell physician of test results.	4					
• Or, tell client how to obtain test results.	2					
TOTAL POSSIBLE POINTS	100					

PROCEDURE 15C: Obtaining a Throat Culture *(continued)*

Comments:

_____

_____

_____

_____

_____

_____

_____

_____

_____

Signatures: _____   Date: _____

SCORING   *See Preface for scoring instructions.*

The Physician's Office

PROCEDURE 15D:
Collecting a Clean-Catch Urine Specimen

PROCEDURE ASSESSMENT

Procedure Steps	Suggested Points	Self Practice	Peer Practice	Peer Testing	Final Testing	Total Earned
PREPROCEDURE						
1. Gather needed equipment.	5					
PROCEDURE						
2. Identify client by asking his/her full name.	6					
3. Write client's name on label and put label on specimen container.	4					
• Don't put label on lid, which could be separated from container.	3					
4a. Explain procedure to female client:	5					
• Remove lid from container without touching inside and put it face up on counter.	4					
• Expose urinary meatus by holding labia back with one hand.	2					
• Using antiseptic wipe, clean each side of meatus from front to back.	4					
• Without releasing labia, urinate a small amount into toilet.	2					
• Place sterile container under meatus.	2					
• Continue voiding into container. Filling it ⅓ to ½ full is enough.	3					
• Put lid on container and wipe area with tissue.	3					
• Tell health care worker if you are menstruating.	2					
4b. Explain procedure to male client:	5					
• Remove lid from container without touching inside and put it face up on counter.	4					
• Clean area around meatus with antiseptic wipe.	4					
• Urinate a small amount into toilet.	2					
• Stop flow and put container under meatus.	2					
• Don't touch inside of container.	4					
• Continue voiding into container. Filling it ⅓ to ½ full is enough.	3					
• Put lid on container and wipe area with tissue, if necessary.	3					
5. Give client directions for taking specimen for processing.	3					
• Or, complete testing ordered by physician.						

PROCEDURE 15D: Collecting a Clean-Catch Urine Specimen *(continued)*

Procedure Steps	Suggested Points	Self Practice	Peer Practice	Peer Testing	Final Testing	Total Earned
POSTPROCEDURE						
6. Put on clean gloves before handling specimen.	6					
7. Prepare lab request and put specimen in proper container for transport to outside lab.	5					
• Or, process specimen in physician's office as ordered.						
8. If you process specimen in office, discard container in biohazard receptacle when you're done.	4					
9. Remove gloves and wash hands.	6					
10. Document procedure in client's record.	4					
TOTAL POSSIBLE POINTS	**100**					

Comments:

_____

_____

_____

_____

_____

_____

_____

_____

_____

Signatures: _____   **Date:** _____

SCORING   *See Preface for scoring instructions.*

The Physician's Office

PROCEDURE 15E:
Applying Bandages

PROCEDURE ASSESSMENT

Procedure Steps	Suggested Points	Self Practice	Peer Practice	Peer Testing	Final Testing	Total Earned
PREPROCEDURE						
1. Wash hands and gather needed supplies.	6					
PROCEDURE						
2. Identify client by asking his/her full name.	3					
3. Inspect area where bandage will be applied.	5					
4. Have client hold extremity to be bandaged up and outward.	5					
• Get help if necessary.						
5. Starting at distal end of extremity, anchor bandage with two circular turns.	6					
6. Wrap extremity going in a proximal direction.	6					
• Unroll bandage in spiral motion.	4					
• Each spiral turn should overlap previous one by ½ width of bandage.	4					
7. When bandaging extremity that has a joint, use figure eight bandaging technique.	4					
8. Wrap bandage snugly, but not too tightly.	9					
9. When done, cut off excess bandage and secure with tape or metal clips.	4					
• Don't cut off excess of elastic roller bandage; instead, get proper size bandage and use entire bandage for procedure.	4					
POSTPROCEDURE						
10. Check circulation and instruct client on signs of impaired circulation, including:	7					
• Swelling of fingers or toes.	4					
• Numbness or tingling sensation in extremities.	4					
• Bluish discoloration of nail beds of affected extremity.	4					
11. Ensure client understands how to loosen bandage and reapply, if necessary.	6					
12. Wash your hands.	9					
13. Record procedure in client's medical record	6					
TOTAL POSSIBLE POINTS	**100**					

PROCEDURE 15E: Applying Bandages *(continued)*

Comments:
_____
_____
_____
_____
_____
_____
_____
_____
_____
_____

Signatures: _____   Date: _____

SCORING   *See Preface for scoring instructions.*

Mental Health

Reinforcement Activities

Labeling

1. Label the diagram below and on the line provided explain how "external noise" can interfere with the communication process in the field of mental health.

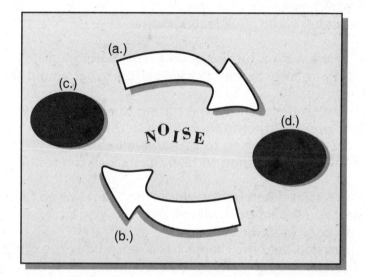

(a.) _____ (c.) _____

(b.) _____ (d.) _____

_____

_____

_____

Matching

Write the letter of the phrase that best matches each numbered item in the blank provided.

_____ 2. Autism
_____ 3. Mental health
_____ 4. Postmortem
_____ 5. Reflective listening
_____ 6. Geropsychology
_____ 7. Cerebral palsy
_____ 8. Interpersonal skills
_____ 9. Neuropsychology

a. After death.
b. Pertaining to elderly individuals mental health.
c. Self-centered mental state
d. Concerns both neurology and psychology.
e. Repeating a message to verify its meaning.
f. Emotional, personal, and spiritual well-being.
g. Characterized by mental retardation, epilepsy, and motor impairment.
h. Skills in relations between people.

Multiple Choice
Circle the letter that best answers the question or completes the statement.

10. You are a mental health aide in an acute care facility. Your duties include personal care and observation for the clients on the geriatrics ward. One male client is sitting in the corner, he appears sad. When you address him he looks at you and tells you to "Go fly a kite." What would your best response be?
    a. The wind is not blowing, a kite would not fly.
    b. You seem to be feeling sad, can I help?
    c. I will tell the activity director your want to fly a kite.
    d. I will come back later when your feeling better.

11. One of the clients on the ward is hitting other clients during lunch. You observe and see two other clients are trying to take the client's milk carton. What would the best course of action be?
    a. use wrist restraint on the client who is hitting to prevent injury.
    b. move the client who is hitting to their room so they can't hurt someone.
    c. talk to the clients who are trying to take the milk.
    d. restrict the clients who are trying to take the milk carton to their rooms.

12. There is a client who is near death on the ward. The client has no family or significant others to be with the client. You should do which of the following?
    a. shut the client's door so for privacy.
    b. sit with the client and hold the client's hand, encourage the client to talk if he or she feels like it.
    c. don't let the client talk about his or her impending death, because it is too morbid.
    d. tell all the other care providers to leave the client alone so no one disturbs him or her.

13. One of your clients is confused, the client does not know what day it is or where she is. This client usually recognizes you but does not now. What might be the most likely answer as to what is wrong?
    a. the client has suddenly developed Alzheimer's disease.
    b. the client is forgetful, people naturally forget sometimes.
    c. the client is being revengeful because you had a day off yesterday.
    d. the client may have developed an infection or illness that is affecting him.

14. One of your long-term clients has died. The family wants to spend an hour or two in the room to say good-bye. You are in a hurry because your shift is about to end.
    a. you should let the family have as much time as they want.
    b. you should tell them you have to finish your job, they can only spend about 10 minutes.
    c. you should loudly proclaim that some people have no consideration for others.
    d. you should go to the supervisor and complain about the family not letting you do your job.

True/False

Write "T" in the blank provided if the statement is true. Write "F" if the statement is false.

_____ 15. A mental health aide can change the treatment plan that has been established by a psychiatrist.

_____ 16. It is best if you speak quietly and slowly to a confused client.

_____ 17. A psychiatrist is a medical doctor who specializes in mental health care.

_____ 18. A counselor will not refer a client to a community service, because it is their responsibility to take care of all the client's needs.

_____ 19. Restraints are used when clients are a danger to themselves or others.

_____ 20. Mental health care providers must have a great deal of patience and understanding.

_____ 21. It does not matter what you do in postmortem care since the client is dead anyway.

_____ 22. It is important to use Standard Precautions any time there is a risk of contamination with body fluids.

_____ 23. A social worker may not perform counseling.

_____ 24. Client's emotional needs are not a consideration in mental health care.

Fill in the Blank

Write the word (or words) that best completes the sentence in the blank provided.

25. Mental health includes emotional, mental, and _____ well-being.

26. Confused clients respond best to being approached from the _____.

27. Chemical restraints are _____ that are used to sedate the client.

28. Psychologists hold a _____ degree.

Mental Health

PROCEDURE 16A:
Applying Physical Restraints

PROCEDURE ASSESSMENT

Procedure Steps	Suggested Points	Self Practice	Peer Practice	Peer Testing	Final Testing	Total Earned
PREPROCEDURE						
1. Gather needed equipment.	1					
2. Check to ensure there's a written order for restraints.	2					
• The order should be in plan of care of supervising nurse.						
• Remember: No order, no restraints.						
3. Wash your hands.	3					
4. Identify client.	3					
5. Introduce yourself to client.	2					
6. Provide privacy for client.	2					
• If client has visitors, explain to visitors that when they leave, you will apply restraints.	1					
• If visitors are close family, you can describe restraints to them.	1					
7. Ask visitors to let you know when they leave.	2					
• Explain importance of their informing you of their departure.	1					
8. Explain procedure to client and family, if appropriate.	2					
9. Raise bed to comfortable working height.	3					
10. Ensure client is in comfortable position.	1					
PREPROCEDURE						
Ankle or Wrist Restraint						
• Ensure soft edge of restraint is next to client's skin.	3					
a. If necessary, use padding under restraint.	1					
b. Wrap restraint around wrist or ankle.	1					
c. Ensure there are no wrinkles in restraint.	1					
• Pull tie straps through the fastening ring.	2					
• Put two fingers between wrist or ankle and restraint to ensure it's not too tight.	3					
• Place client's arm or leg into a comfortable position.	1					
• Secure straps to bed frame following facility policy.	3					
• Assess circulation, sensation, and motion of client's foot or hand.	3					

PROCEDURE 16A: Applying Physical Restraints *(continued)*

Procedure Steps	Suggested Points	Self Practice	Peer Practice	Peer Testing	Final Testing	Total Earned
Jacket Restraint						
• Help client sit up.	1					
• Put client's arms through jacket armholes and cross straps over client's chest.	2					
• Help client lie down in comfortable position.	1					
• Pull end of tie straps through slot in jacket. Ensure jacket is straight, without wrinkles.	3					
• Tie straps of jacket to bed frame.	3					
• Lower bed to lowest position.	3					
• Raise side rails, if so ordered.						
Safety Belt Restraint						
• Help client sit up.	1					
• Wrap safety belt in front of client, around waist.	1					
• Wrap ties around client's back and pull ties through slots in belt.	2					
• Ensure there aren't any wrinkles under belt or in belt.	3					
• Help client to lie down in comfortable position.	2					
• Tie straps from safety belt to bed frame.	3					
POSTPROCEDURE						
11. Make sure client is comfortable.	1					
12. Make sure you can insert 2 fingers between restraint and client.	3					
13. Lower bed to lowest position.	3					
• If side rails are ordered, raise them.						
14. Make sure client can reach signal bell.	3					
15. Wash your hands.	3					
16. Record procedure in client's record.	2					
17. Report to supervisor that you have done procedure.	2					
• Report any abnormal occurrence.						
18. Check on client frequently to ensure his/her safety.	3					
• Offer fluids, as necessary.	1					
• Check to see if client needs to use bathroom.	1					
19. Check frequently the circulation, or sensation, and motion of the hand or foot that is restrained and record your findings.	3					

PROCEDURE 16A: Applying Physical Restraints (continued)

Procedure Steps	Suggested Points	Self Practice	Peer Practice	Peer Testing	Final Testing	Total Earned
POSTPROCEDURE						
20. Loosen or remove restraint every 2 hours.	3					
• Check skin condition under restraint.	1					
• Ensure client is experiencing no harm from restraint.	1					
• Chart your activities and findings.	1					
21. Report any adverse findings to your supervisor immediately.	2					
TOTAL POSSIBLE POINTS	100					

Comments:

_____

_____

_____

_____

_____

_____

_____

_____

_____

_____

Signatures: _____ **Date:** _____

SCORING *See Preface for scoring instructions.*

Mental Health

PROCEDURE 16B:
Providing Reality Orientation

PROCEDURE ASSESSMENT

Procedure Steps PREPROCEDURE	Suggested Points	Self Practice	Peer Practice	Peer Testing	Final Testing	Total Earned
1. Gather needed equipment.	4					
2. If confused behavior is new for client, report to supervising nurse.	7					
3. If confused behavior is not new for client, chart behavior objectively.	5					
• Don't record how you feel about the behavior.						
4. Work with other team members to provide environmental objects to help clients with reality orientation. Things that might help include:	6					
• Marking off days on calendar.						
• Color-coding areas of room and equipment.						
• Ensuring client's watch or clock is set to correct time.						
• Ensuring client's eyeglasses are clean.						
• Ensuring client's hearing aid(s) work and are turned on.						
PREPROCEDURE						
5. Approach client from front and get client's attention.	7					
6. Speak quietly and calmly, in a friendly manner.	6					
7. Talk with client to assess his/her level of confusion.	5					
8. Validate client's thoughts and feelings.	6					
• Use a conversational tone.	5					
• Tell client where he/she is and what day it is.	5					
• Tell client what his/her name is (if necessary).	5					
• Tell client what weather is like and other information.	5					
9. Don't confront a client who seems confused.	7					
• Work with clients to help orient them.	5					
10. Record your findings objectively.	5					
• Describe client's behavior and how he/she reacted to reality orientation.	4					

PROCEDURE 16B: Providing Reality Orientation (continued)

Procedure Steps	Suggested Points	Self Practice	Peer Practice	Peer Testing	Final Testing	Total Earned
POSTPROCEDURE						
11. Check on client frequently to ensure his/her safety.	7					
12. Report any changes in your findings to supervising nurse immediately.	6					
TOTAL POSSIBLE POINTS	100					

Comments: _____

_____

_____

_____

_____

_____

_____

_____

_____

_____

Signatures: _____   Date: _____

SCORING   See Preface for scoring instructions.

Mental Health

PROCEDURE 16C:
Providing Postmortem Care

PROCEDURE ASSESSMENT

Procedure Steps	Suggested Points	Self Practice	Peer Practice	Peer Testing	Final Testing	Total Earned
PREPROCEDURE						
1. Check that postmortem care should be performed.	3					
2. Check facility policy on how client should be identified.	2					
3. Gather needed equipment.	2					
4. Provide privacy.	3					
5. Raise bed to highest comfortable working position.	4					
• Make sure bed is flat.	3					
6. Wash hands and put on gloves.	4					
PROCEDURE						
7. Position client's body on back.	2					
8. Elevate head and shoulders on a pillow.	2					
9. Close client's eyes.	2					
• If eyes won't stay closed, use moistened cotton ball on eyelids.						
10. Ensure client's dentures or artificial eyes are in place.	2					
11. Close client's mouth.	2					
• If necessary, support jaw, using rolled washcloth or hand towel.						
• Some postmortem kits include a jaw or chin strap.						
12. Remove drainage bags, IVs, bottles, or tubes, if so instructed by supervisor.	2					
13. Use standard precautions whenever there is danger of coming in contact with body fluids.	4					
14. Check facility policy for removal of jewelry.	2					
15. Wear gloves to wash and dry any soiled areas of body.	4					
16. You may need to put protective sheet under client's buttocks.	2					
17. If client has wound dressings, replace them with clean ones.	4					

PROCEDURE 16C: Providing Postmortem Care (continued)

Procedure Steps	Suggested Points	Self Practice	Peer Practice	Peer Testing	Final Testing	Total Earned
18. Complete identification tags and attach them to body, according to facility policy.	2					
• Usually, tags are attached to large toe or ankle.						
19. Cover up body to shoulders if family wishes to view body.	2					
POSTPROCEDURE						
20. Put all client's possessions in bag and label it.	2					
• Check possessions against clothing and valuables list.	1					
21. Remove all equipment and supplies from room.	2					
• Ensure room is clean and neat.	1					
• Turn down lights in room.	1					
22. Let family members into room if they wish to view body.	3					
• Treat them with respect and dignity.						
• Provide emotional support as needed.						
23. Provide family with client's possessions.	3					
24. After family leaves, obtain a stretcher.	2					
25. Check facility policy on how body is to be wrapped.	2					
26. If you use a shroud:	2					
• Position body on top of shroud.	1					
• Bring top down over head.	1					
• Bring bottom up over feet.	1					
• Bring sides in over body and secure them.	1					
27. Put identification tag on shroud according to facility procedure.	2					
28. Move body to stretcher.	4					
• Use same procedure as you would to transfer an unconscious client.						
29. Take body to morgue, if so instructed.	2					
• Make sure doors to other clients' room are closed when body is transferred.	1					
30. Clean stretcher and return it to storage.	2					
31. Straighten client's room:	2					
• Remove all linen and put in proper container.	1					
• Remove all supplies from room.	1					
32. Remove gloves and wash hands.	4					
33. Record procedure in client's record.	2					
34. Report to supervisor that you have done procedure.	3					
• Report any abnormal occurrence.						
TOTAL POSSIBLE POINTS	**100**					

PROCEDURE 16C: Providing Postmortem Care *(continued)*

Comments:

_____

_____

_____

_____

_____

_____

_____

_____

_____

_____

Signatures: _____   **Date:** _____

SCORING   *See Preface for scoring instructions.*

Pharmacy

Reinforcement Activities

Matching

Write the letter of the phrase that best matches each numbered item in the blank provided. Answers can be used more than once.

_____ 1. National Formulary

_____ 2. Anti-neoplastic

_____ 3. Prescription medication

_____ 4. Cytotoxic material

_____ 5. Hazardous drug (HD)

_____ 6. Corrosive

_____ 7. Over the counter (OTC) medications

_____ 8. Franchise

_____ 9. United States Pharmacopeia (USP)

a. Classification of medication used to treat cancer.

b. A pharmacy that is independently operated, yet is owned by a chain or larger company.

c. Substance that is poisonous to cells such as an anti-neoplastic medication.

d. Medications that can have negative health effects when exposed to individuals.

e. A national listing of medications.

f. Medications purchased without a prescription.

g. Medications that are only obtainable if a physician or other licensed practitioner writes an order.

h. A substance that can damage body tissue.

Fill in the Blank

Write the word (or words) that completes the sentence in the blank provided.

10. Three careers in Pharmacy are _____, _____, and _____.

11. The most important responsibility of the pharmacist is to provide the _____ in the _____ to the client.

12. A _____ works as part of a team in developing new medications.

13. The two types of degrees a Pharmacist can earn are _____ and _____.

14. One additional duty of a *hospital* pharmacist is _____.

15. The _____ speeds up drug availability for clients with rare diseases.

16. Tylenol is a _____ and acetaminophen is the _____.

17. Prescription medications are also known as _____.

18. _____ have no accepted medical use in the United States and a high abuse potential.

Name _____   Date _____

True/False

Write "T" in the blank provided if the statement is true. Write "F" if the statement is false.

_____ **19.** A Schedule III drug has a higher potential for abuse than a Schedule I drug.

_____ **20.** Nonchild resistant containers may be used by client request or physician order.

_____ **21.** A pharmacy aide must be certified by the Pharmacy Technician Certification Board.

_____ **22.** The enforcement agency for the Pure Food and Drug Act of 1906 is the FDA.

_____ **23.** OTC medications can have side effects and interfere with other medications.

Name _____ Date _____

Pharmacy

PROCEDURE 17A:
Reviewing Prescriptions and Physician Orders

PROCEDURE ASSESSMENT

Procedure Steps	Suggested Points	Self Practice	Peer Practice	Peer Testing	Final Testing	Total Earned
PREPROCEDURE						
Gain training on how to enter medication from prescription or physician order into system at your place of employment.						
PROCEDURE						
1. Obtain prescription or physician order from client or client's chart.	13					
2. Ensure prescription or order contains all necessary information.	14					
3. Ensure name and identifying information are included and spelled correctly.	14					
4. Verify that medication listed is written legibly.	14					
• Never guess what prescriber meant.						
• If order isn't legible, always notify pharmacist or contact prescribing physician.						
5. Enter complete data into computer system.	13					
• Check your entries carefully.	16					
• If you have questions, ask.						
POSTPROCEDURE						
6. Notify pharmacist that prescription or order has been reviewed, entered, and is ready for filling.	16					
TOTAL POSSIBLE POINTS	100					

Comments: _____

_____

_____

_____

_____

_____

_____

_____

_____

Signatures: _____ Date: _____

SCORING *See Preface for scoring instructions.*

Name _____ Date _____

Pharmacy

PROCEDURE 17B:
Creating a Client Profile and Handling a Prescription

PROCEDURE ASSESSMENT

Procedure Steps	Suggested Points	Self Practice	Peer Practice	Peer Testing	Final Testing	Total Earned
PREPROCEDURE						
1. Become familiar with type of client profile system used.						
• Learn computer system so you can enter profiles independently.	4					
PROCEDURE						
2. Obtain prescription from client.	2					
3. Review name on prescription and retrieve current client profile from computer or hard copy file.	3					
• If you can't find profile, ask client if he/she has visited pharmacy previously.						
• Many chain store pharmacy computer systems will contain profile if client has visited another store of same chain.						
4. If client says he/she has visited pharmacy before, verify his/her complete name and spelling and search again.	3					
• If you still can't find profile, check with pharmacist.						
5. If client says "No," obtain client date for profile, including:	4					
• Name, address, and phone number.	3					
• Date of birth.	3					
• Social security number.	3					
• Allergies.	3					
• Any prescription medications or OTC medications.	3					
• Insurance information.	3					
• Diseases or chronic conditions.	3					
6. Obtain insurance card from client to be viewed and verified by pharmacist.	4					
7. When profile is complete, ask client if he/she will wait for prescription or return.	4					
• If client will wait, tell him/her when prescription will be filled. Estimate time based on number of prescriptions waiting, amount of time it takes pharmacist to fill prescription, and other factors.	3					

PROCEDURE 17B: Creating a Client Profile and Handling a Prescription (continued)

Procedure Steps	Suggested Points	Self Practice	Peer Practice	Peer Testing	Final Testing	Total Earned
8. Prepare prescription for pharmacist to fill medication.	4					
• Check facility policy to see if this is your responsibility.	3					
• Get medication bottle or container from shelf.	3					
• Double-check your medication selection.	3					
• If you are unsure of name, ask pharmacist.	3					
9. Put medication, prescription, and insurance card in proper location for pharmacist to fill.	4					
• In some pharmacies, you will place these items in special container.						
10. In some facilities, you also may be allowed or required to prepare actual prescription.						
• You may count medication after retrieving it.						
• You may select correct container and affix label to it.						
11. Have pharmacist double-check any medication you select and/or prepare.	5					
POSTPROCEDURE						
12. When prescription is ready, call client to counter.	3					
13. Have client sign for prescription.	4					
• Signature documents that client has received medication.						
• In some states, signature documents that client has received counseling and refused child-resistant containers.						
14. Obtain payment for prescription.	4					
• Knowledge of cash register and payment procedures are necessary.	3					
15. Give medication to client.	4					
• Always make sure pharmacist has checked prescription before giving it to client.	6					
16. Thank client.	3					
TOTAL POSSIBLE POINTS	**100**					

PROCEDURE 17B: Creating a Client Profile and Handling a Prescription *(continued)*

Comments: _____
_____
_____
_____
_____
_____
_____
_____
_____
_____

Signatures: _____ **Date:** _____

SCORING   *See Preface for scoring instructions.*

Respiratory Care

Reinforcement Activities

Labeling
In the space provided, write the word(s) that identifies the corresponding part on the diagram.

1. Label the following diagram.

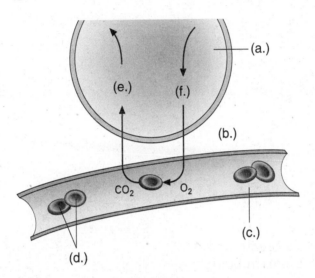

(a.) _____   (d.) _____

(b.) _____   (e.) _____

(c.) _____   (f.) _____

Matching
Write the letter of the phrase that best matches each numbered item in the blank provided.

_____ **2.** Oxygen

_____ **3.** Carbon dioxide

_____ **4.** CRT

_____ **5.** RRT

_____ **6.** Apnea

_____ **7.** Ventilation

_____ **8.** Respiration

a. Gas needed for tissue metabolism.

b. The Advanced Respiratory Therapist credential.

c. Movement of air into and out of the respiratory system.

d. Gaseous waste product of tissue metabolism.

e. Process of gas exchange.

f. The Entry Level Respiratory Therapist credential.

g. Absence of breathing.

True/False
Write "T" in the blank provided if the statement is true. Write "F" if the statement is false.

_____ **9.** A pulse oximetry reading of 99% means the client requires oxygen therapy.

_____ **10.** A nasal cannula delivers the highest percentage of oxygen.

_____ 11. A nasal cannula should be run at less than 6 liters per minute.

_____ 12. Aerosol medications delivered to the lungs can be given at lower doses than oral medications.

Multiple Choice

Circle the letter that best answers the question or completes the statement.

13. What is the size measurement of aerosol particles to be delivered into the lungs?
    a. meters.
    b. microns.
    c. inches.
    d. centimeters.

14. A nasal cannula at 1 liter per minute would deliver approximately what oxygen percentage?
    a. 100%
    b. 20%
    c. 24%
    d. 50%

15. How should the patient taking an MDI be instructed to breathe?
    a. fast and deep
    b. fast and shallow
    c. slow and deep with no breath hold
    d. slow and deep with a breath hold

16. What type of surgical patients are most likely to benefit from incentive spirometry?
    a. nose surgery
    b. chest surgery
    c. eye surgery
    d. mole removal

Fill in the Blank

Write the word (or words) that best completes the sentence in the blank provided.

17. A condition known as _____ exists when there are low levels of oxygen in the blood.

18. The bluish color of the skin due to low oxygen is _____.

19. A device that measures the saturation of oxygen on the hemoglobin is the pulse _____.

20. The medical term for a collapsed lung is _____.

21. The newer gas propellants for MDIs that are ozone layer safe are _____.

Name _____ Date _____

Listing

22. Smoking causes a great many respiratory, cardiac and other diseases. Make a list of reasons why people should *not* smoke.

_____

_____

_____

_____

_____

23. Make a list of techniques people can use to quit smoking.

_____

_____

_____

_____

_____

_____

_____

_____

_____

_____

_____

_____

_____

Respiratory Care

PROCEDURE 18A:
Administering Oxygen

PROCEDURE ASSESSMENT

Procedure Steps	Suggested Points	Self Practice	Peer Practice	Peer Testing	Final Testing	Total Earned
PREPROCEDURE						
1. Verify that doctor's order on client's chart includes prescribed oxygen flow.	4					
• When nasal cannula is used, flow shouldn't exceed 6 liters per minute.						
• With simple mask, flow should be between 5 and 12 liters per minute.						
2. Review client's chart for reason oxygen therapy is being administered.	4					
• Hypoxemia, shortness of breath, or heart conditions are typical reasons.						
3. Gather needed equipment, including:	4					
• Nasal cannula or simple mask.	3					
• Humidifier.	3					
• Oxygen flowmeter.	3					
4. Test equipment to ensure proper functioning.	4					
PROCEDURE						
5. Introduce yourself to client.	4					
6. Identify client by asking his/her full name or checking ID bracelet.	4					
7. Wash hands and observe other standard precautions.	7					
8. Assess client's status:	4					
• Check pulse, respiratory rate, color, and pulse oximetry reading.	3					
9. Explain therapy and ensure client understands.	4					
10. Assemble equipment and ensure it is functioning properly.	4					
11. Adjust flow of oxygen according to doctor's orders.	4					
12. Apply delivery device to client and check to ensure client is comfortable and safe.	3					
13. Explain to client the dangers of smoking or fires or sparks around oxygen device.	4					
• Make sure a "No Smoking" sign is on door.	3					
• Remove flammable items from room.	3					

PROCEDURE 18A: Administering Oxygen *(continued)*

Procedure Steps	Suggested Points	Self Practice	Peer Practice	Peer Testing	Final Testing	Total Earned
14. Monitor client's response to therapy.	4					
• Check color, rate of respiration, pulse, and pulse oximetry reading.	3					
15. Wash your hands when therapy is concluded.	7					
POSTPROCEDURE						
16. Record all necessary information on client's chart, including:	4					
• Delivery device and liter flow.	3					
• Your assessment and results of your monitoring.	3					
17. Report any adverse reactions experienced by client, or therapy suggestions, to appropriate personnel.	4					
TOTAL POSSIBLE POINTS	100					

Comments:

_____

_____

_____

_____

_____

_____

_____

_____

_____

Signatures: _____ **Date:** _____

SCORING *See Preface for scoring instructions.*

Respiratory Care

PROCEDURE 18B:
Delivering an MDI Treatment

PROCEDURE ASSESSMENT

Procedure Steps	Suggested Points	Self Practice	Peer Practice	Peer Testing	Final Testing	Total Earned
PREPROCEDURE						
1. Gather needed equipment.	2					
2. Verify doctor's order.	2					
• Identify medications to be administered.	1					
3. Select and assemble this equipment:	2					
• The appropriate MDI.	1					
• An accessory device, such as a spacer.	1					
4. Test equipment to ensure it is functioning properly.	2					
• Attach and reattach any accessory device to check and ensure proper fit.	1					
PROCEDURE						
5. Introduce yourself to client.	3					
6. Identify client by asking his/her full name and/or checking ID bracelet.	1					
7. Wash hands and observe other standard precautions.	5					
8. Use proper sterile techniques to set up and maintain medicated aerosol devices.	3					
• Sterile conditions are very important.	1					
9. Assess client's premedication status.	3					
• Check breath sounds, pulse, respiratory rate, color, and pulmonary function test.	1					
10. Explain therapy and ensure client understands treatment.	3					
• Tell client you will walk him/her through treatment until he/she masters technique.	1					
11. Make sure client understands which drug is correct for a given situation.	3					
• Antiasthmatic drugs help prevent asthma attacks, but can't help during an attack.						
• Bronchodilators should be used during an attack.						
12. Position client properly.	3					
• Client should be in seated position if able.	1					
13. Warm MDI canister to body temperature by rolling it between palms of hands.	2					
• Shake canister vigorously.	1					
14. Assemble inhaler and uncap mouthpiece.	2					

PROCEDURE 18B: Delivering an MDI Treatment *(continued)*

Procedure Steps	Suggested Points	Self Practice	Peer Practice	Peer Testing	Final Testing	Total Earned
15. Tell client to open mouth.	2					
• Hold MDI device about an inch away.	1					
• If spacer device is used, it should be placed directly in mouth.	1					
16. Tell client to exhale normally.	3					
17. As client slowly begins to inhale through mouth, he/she should depress canister.	2					
18. Tell client to breathe in until lungs are full.	3					
19. Tell client to hold his or her breath for up to 10 seconds if possible.	2					
20. Tell client to breathe out normally.	3					
21. Modify therapy as needed so treatment is effective.	2					
22. Monitor blood pressure of clients receiving these medications.	2					
23. Administer correct number of puffs.	3					
• Usually, 2 or 3 puffs are ordered.	1					
• Wait at least 1 minute between puffs.	1					
24. Disassemble MDI and replace cap.	2					
25. Store equipment properly.	3					
POSTPROCEDURE						
26. Tell client to cough effectively.	2					
27. If steroid is administered, have client rinse mouth with water or mouthwash to prevent thrush.	3					
28. Observe any sputum.	2					
• Record amount, color, and consistency.	1					
29. Monitor client for side effects and drug response.	3					
• Evaluate breath sounds, pulse, respiratory rate, color, and pulmonary function test.	2					
30. Wash your hands.	5					
31. Record data properly in client's chart.	3					
32. Report any adverse reactions experienced by client or therapy suggestions to appropriate personnel.	3					
TOTAL POSSIBLE POINTS	**100**					

PROCEDURE 18B: Delivering an MDI Treatment (continued)

Comments:

_____

_____

_____

_____

_____

_____

_____

_____

_____

_____

Signatures: _____ **Date:** _____

SCORING   *See Preface for scoring instructions.*

Respiratory Care

PROCEDURE 18C:
Administering Incentive Spirometry (IS)

PROCEDURE ASSESSMENT

Procedure Steps	Suggested Points	Self Practice	Peer Practice	Peer Testing	Final Testing	Total Earned
PREPROCEDURE						
1. Verify doctor's order.	4					
• Check client's chart for indications he/she may be at risk of developing lung collapse or already has experienced it.	2					
2. Determine client's appropriate lung volume or goal.	3					
• Use client's lung volume before surgery as goal, obtain calculated goal.	2					
3. Gather needed equipment.	3					
4. Test equipment to ensure it is functioning properly.	3					
PROCEDURE						
5. Introduce yourself to client.	4					
6. Identify client by asking his/her full name or checking ID bracelet.	2					
7. Wash hands and maintain other standard precautions.	6					
8. Assess client's status.	3					
• Check breath sounds, pulse, respiratory rate, and color.	2					
9. Position client properly.	3					
• The best position is sitting upright.	2					
10. Tell client how IS device works.	2					
• Explain what goal is and why you want him/her to use it.	4					
11. Place IS device on flat surface or hold in upright position where client can see it.	2					
12. Have client put lips around mouthpiece.	3					
• Lips should be closed tight around mouthpiece.	2					
• Tongue should be out of the way.	2					
13. Client should exhale normally.	3					
• Ask client to inhale slowly through mouthpiece, raising volume indicator by taking as deep a breath as possible.	2					
14. Tell client to hold his/her breath for 5 to 10 seconds, if possible.	2					
15. Remove mouthpiece and have client exhale normally.	3					

PROCEDURE 18C: Administering Incentive Spirometry (IS) *(continued)*

Procedure Steps	Suggested Points	Self Practice	Peer Practice	Peer Testing	Final Testing	Total Earned
16. Have client relax and breathe normally for a few breaths.	3					
• Then repeat SMI using the IS for a total of 10 to 15 breaths.	2					
POSTPROCEDURE						
17. Tell client to cough effectively.	2					
18. Reassess client's color, heart rate, respiratory rate, and breath sounds.	3					
19. Disassemble and store equipment properly.	3					
20. Wash your hands.	6					
21. Document procedure performed, including:	3					
• Volume goals that were set.	2					
• Volume achieved.	2					
• Breaths per session.	2					
• Ability of client to perform procedure without coaching.	2					
• Cough and breath sounds.	2					
22. Inform appropriate personnel of any adverse reactions client experienced or of any therapy suggestions.	4					
TOTAL POSSIBLE POINTS	**100**					

Comments: _____

_____

_____

_____

_____

_____

_____

_____

_____

_____

_____

Signatures: _____   Date: _____

SCORING   *See Preface for scoring instructions.*

Rehabilitation

Reinforcement Activities

True/False

Write "T" in the blank provided if the statement is true. Write "F" if the statement is false.

_____ **1.** Exercise increases blood flow to the muscles.

_____ **2.** Polio is another name for infantile paralysis.

_____ **3.** Physical therapists never work with children.

_____ **4.** Occupational therapists help clients improve their ability to perform tasks.

_____ **5.** Recreational therapists are baseball coaches that are temporarily out of work.

_____ **6.** Speech and language difficulties can result from a variety of problems.

_____ **7.** A cardiologist uses an audiometer.

Multiple Choice

Circle the letter that best answers the question or completes the statement.

8. When using a cane, walker, or crutches, how should a client move?
   a. Equipment first, strong leg, then weak leg.
   b. Weak leg, strong leg, then equipment.
   c. Strong leg, equipment, then weak leg.
   d. Equipment, weak leg, then strong leg.

9. If a client experiences pain when performing range of motion exercises, you should:
   a. stop the exercises.
   b. continue until the pain becomes greater.
   c. tell the client "no pain, no gain."
   d. report this information to your supervisor.

10. When a client falls, you should
   a. try to catch the client.
   b. cradle the client's head.
   c. push the client away from your body.
   d. hold onto the client's arms.

11. A good walking shoe is one that has
   a. rubber soles.
   b. 2" heels.
   c. low, broad heels, 1½" high.
   d. 1" heels with Velcro closures.

12. Which of the following instruments is used to examine the ears?
   a. otoscope
   b. ophthalmoscope
   c. stethoscope
   d. audiometer

Matching

Write the letter of the term that best matches each numbered item in the blank provided.

_____ **13.** The movement of a body part away from the body.

a. Flexion.

_____ **14.** Turning a body part downward as with the face down or the palm down.

b. Abduction.

_____ **15.** Straightening a body part.

c. Dorsiflexion.

_____ **16.** Bending a body part.

d. Pronation.

_____ **17.** Moving toward the outside.

e. Eversion.

_____ **18.** Excessive straightening.

f. Dressing.

_____ **19.** Bending backward.

g. Extension.

_____ **20.** An activity of daily living. (ADL)

h. Hyperextension.

Rehabilitation

PROCEDURE 19A:
Performing Range-of-Motion Exercises

········ **PROCEDURE ASSESSMENT** ········

Procedure Steps	Suggested Points	Self Practice	Peer Practice	Peer Testing	Final Testing	Total Earned
PREPROCEDURE						
1. Gather equipment:	1					
2. Check orders and obtain authorization from supervisor.	2					
3. Determine what type of range-of-motion exercises are to be performed.	2					
• Determine what joints are involved.						
• Determine if client has any limitations to movement.						
PROCEDURE						
4. Wash your hands.	2					
5. Check client's identification and address client by name.	2					
6. Introduce yourself and explain procedure.	1					
7. Provide for privacy by closing door and/or closing room curtain.	1					
8. Raise bed to comfortable working position.	2					
• Bed should be at waist level or above.						
9. Lower side rail on side of client's body where you will work first.	2					
10. Put client on back and in good body alignment.	2					
• Range-of-motion exercises can be done with client in chair.						
11. Fan-fold top linens down to foot of bed.	1					
12. Use bath blanket or towel to drape client, if necessary.	1					
13. Perform ROM exercises.						
• Exercise client's neck as indicated by supervisor:	1					
a. Move head forward until chin touches chest (flexion).	1					
b. Straighten the head (extension).	1					
c. Move head backward so that chin points upward (hyperextension).	1					
d. Turn head to one side and then other (rotation).	1					
e. Move head to right and then to left (lateral flexion).	1					

PROCEDURE 19A: Performing Range-of-Motion Exercises *(continued)*

Procedure Steps	Suggested Points	Self Practice	Peer Practice	Peer Testing	Final Testing	Total Earned
• Exercise client's shoulder as indicated by supervisor:	1					
a. Hold client's wrist with one hand. Hold the client's elbow with the other.	1					
b. Lower arm down to client's side (abduction).	1					
c. If client is standing or sitting in chair, move client's arm behind his/her body (hyperextention).	1					
d. Move elbow with your other hand.	1					
e. Raise client's arm straight out in front of body and up over head (abduction).	1					
f. Move client's straight arm up and away from side of body (abduction).	1					
g. Move straight arm down to side of body (abduction).	1					
h. Bend client's elbow and position it at shoulder height.	1					
i. Move forearm down and toward body (internal rotation).	1					
j. Move forearm toward head (external rotation).	1					
• Exercise client's elbow as indicated by supervisor:	1					
a. Hold client's wrist with one hand and elbow with other hand.	1					
b. Bend client's forearm so it touches shoulder on same side of body (flexion).	1					
c. Straighten the arm (extension).	1					
• Exercise client's forearm as indicated by supervisor:	1					
a. Turn client's hand so palm faces down.	1					
b. Turn hand so palm faces up (supination).	1					
• Exercise client's wrist as indicated by supervisor:	1					
a. Hold client's wrist with both your hands.	1					
b. Move one hand forward and bend client's hand downward (flexion).	1					
c. Straighten out the hand (extension).	1					
d. Bend the hand back (hyperextension).	1					
e. Turn the wrist and hand toward the thumb (radial flexion).	1					
f. Bend the hand back (hyperextension).	1					
g. Turn the wrist and hand toward the thumb (radial flexion).	1					

Procedure Steps	Suggested Points	Self Practice	Peer Practice	Peer Testing	Final Testing	Total Earned
h. Turn the wrist and hand toward the pinky finger (ulnar flexion).	1					
• Exercise the thumb as indicated by supervisor:	1					
a. With one hand, hold client's hand. With other hand, hold client's thumb.	1					
b. Move thumb away from index finger (abduction).	1					
c. Move thumb toward index finger (abduction).	1					
d. Bend thumb toward palm of hand (flexion).	1					
e. Move thumb out to side of fingers (extension).	1					
f. Move thumb up to touch tip of each finger (opposition).	1					
• Exercise fingers as indicated by supervisor:	1					
a. Spread fingers and thumb apart (abduction).	1					
b. Move fingers and thumb together (abduction).	1					
c. Straighten fingers out (extension).	1					
d. Make a fist (flexion).	1					
• Exercise client's hip as indicated by supervisor:	1					
a. Put one hand under client's knee, and the other under the ankle.	1					
b. Raise the leg (flexion).	1					
c. Straighten the leg (extension).	1					
d. Move leg away from body (abduction).	1					
e. Move leg toward body (abduction).	1					
f. Turn leg inward (internal rotation).	1					
g. Turn leg outward (external rotation).	1					
• Exercise client's knee as indicated by supervisor:	1					
a. Put one hand under client's knee, and the other under the ankle.	1					
b. Bend the leg (flexion).	1					
c. Straighten the leg (extension).	1					
• Exercise client's ankle as indicated by supervisor:	1					
a. Put one hand under client's foot, and the other under the ankle.	1					
b. At same time, pull foot forward and push heel down (dorsiflexion).	1					
c. Point toes forward or turn foot down (plantar flexion).	1					

Procedure Steps	Suggested Points	Self Practice	Peer Practice	Peer Testing	Final Testing	Total Earned
• Exercise client's foot as indicated by supervisor:	1					
a. Turn inside of foot down, and outside of foot up (eversion).	1					
b. Turn outside of foot up, and inside of foot down (inversion).	1					
• Exercise client's toes as indicated by supervisor:	1					
a. Curl the toes (flexion).	1					
b. Straighten the toes (extension).	1					
c. Spread the toes apart (abduction).	1					
d. Pull the toes together (adduction).	1					
14. Raise side rail and move to opposite side of client.	2					
• Lower side rail, if necessary.						
• Repeat the steps to other side of client's body.						
POSTPROCEDURE						
15. Ensure client is comfortable.	2					
• Ensure client's body is properly aligned.						
16. Unfold top linen and cover client. Remove bath blanket and straighten bed linens.	1					
17. Ensure signal light is within client's reach.	1					
18. Raise side rails and lower bed, if necessary.	2					
19. Open curtain and/or door.	1					
20. Wash your hands.	2					
21. Report and record the following information:	1					
• The time of the exercises.						
• The joints exercised and the number of times each joint was exercised.						
TOTAL POSSIBLE POINTS	**100**					

Comments: _____

_____

_____

_____

_____

_____

Signatures: _____   **Date:** _____

SCORING *See Preface for scoring instructions.*

Rehabilitation

PROCEDURE 19B:
Ambulating a Client with a Transfer (Gait) Belt

PROCEDURE ASSESSMENT

Procedure Steps	Suggested Points	Self Practice	Peer Practice	Peer Testing	Final Testing	Total Earned
PREPROCEDURE						
1. Gather needed equipment.	5					
2. Identify client and address client by name.	6					
3. Introduce yourself to client.	6					
4. Explain procedure to client.	7					
5. Wash your hands.	9					
6. Provide for privacy for closing curtain and/or door.	6					
PROCEDURE						
7. Help client move to sitting position using proper body mechanics.	5					
8. Put transfer belt over client's clothes, around waist.	6					
9. Position buckle off center at front or to side.	9					
• Never position buckle at client's back.						
10. Tighten belt snugly around client's waist.	9					
• Don't make belt too tight.						
• Belt shouldn't interfere with breathing or comfort.						
• You should be able to put two fingers comfortably under belt.	5					
11. Transfer client according to supervisor's instructions or physician's order.	6					
POSTPROCEDURE						
12. Wash your hands.	9					
13. Report/record results of transferring.	6					
14. Return transfer belt to proper place.	6					
• Many workers keep belt around own waist so it's handy.						
TOTAL POSSIBLE POINTS	100					

PROCEDURE 19B: Ambulating a Client with a Transfer (Gait) Belt
(continued)

Comments: _____
_____
_____
_____
_____
_____
_____
_____
_____

Signatures: _____   Date: _____

SCORING   *See Preface for scoring instructions.*

Rehabilitation

PROCEDURE 19C:
Ambulating a Client with Crutches

---------- **PROCEDURE ASSESSMENT** ----------

Procedure Steps	Suggested Points	Self Practice	Peer Practice	Peer Testing	Final Testing	Total Earned
PREPROCEDURE						
1. Gather needed equipment.	2					
2. Check orders and obtain authorization from supervisor.	5					
3. Check crutches for safety.	5					
• Rubber tips should be intact.						
• Axillary bars and hand rests should be padded.						
4. Identify client and address client by name.	2					
5. Introduce yourself to client and explain procedure.	2					
6. Wash your hands.	5					
PROCEDURE						
7. Help client put on good walking shoes.	5					
• Shoes should have low, broad heels, 1 to 1½ inches high.						
• Shoes should have nonskid soles.						
8. Put a gait belt on client.	3					
• Use underhanded grasp on belt.	1					
• Assist client to standing position.	1					
• Advise client to bear weight on unaffected leg.	1					
• Position crutches correctly.	1					
9. Check fit of crutches.	2					
10. Position crutches 4 to 6 inches in front of client's feet.	3					
11. Tell client to move crutches 4 to 6 inches to the sides of feet.	2					
12. Ensure there's a 2-inch gap between armpit and axillary bar or rest of crutches.	3					
• If length must be adjusted, check with supervisor.						
13. Ensure each elbow is flexed at 25° to 30° angle.	3					
• If hand rests must be adjusted to achieve this angle, check with supervisor.						
14. Help client with required gait, which depends on client's injury and condition and is determined by therapist.	3					
• Four-point gait: Provides wide base of support and weight bearing on both legs.	2					

Reinforcement Activities and Procedure Assessment   Chapter 19   **A-283**

Procedure Steps	Suggested Points	Self Practice	Peer Practice	Peer Testing	Final Testing	Total Earned
a. Point 1: One crutch moves ahead 4 to 6 inches.	1					
b. Point 2: Opposite foot moves ahead to level of crutch.	1					
c. Point 3: Second crutch moves forward the same distance.	1					
d. Point 4: Second foot moves forward to meet crutch level.	1					
• Two-point gait: Faster than four-point gait, similar to walking.	2					
a. Point 1: Right crutch and left foot move forward at same time.	1					
b. Point 2: Left crutch and right foot move forward at same time.	1					
• Three-point gait: Weight bearing must be on one leg, as with sprain or broken leg.	2					
a. Points 1 and 2: Both crutches and weaker leg move forward.	1					
b. Point 3: Strong leg moves forward to meet other foot.	1					
• Swing to gait: Partial weight bearing on both legs must be allowed.	2					
a. Both crutches move forward at same time.	1					
b. Client swings legs to crutches by lifting body with arms.	1					
• Swing through gait: Similar to swing to but faster-paced.	2					
a. Both crutches move forward at same time.	1					
b. Client swings legs through to other side of crutches, lifting body with arms.	1					
POSTPROCEDURE						
15. Check client's progress and report to therapist or supervisor.	3					
16. When client has finished using crutches, replace all equipment.	3					
17. Help client back to bed or chair.	5					
• Remove gait belt.	2					
• If client is in bed, elevate side rails, lower bed to lowest level, and put call signal within easy reach of client.	2					
18. Leave area neat and clean.	3					
19. Wash your hands.	5					
20. Report/record required information on client's chart or record.	3					
21. Report any problems immediately.	3					
TOTAL POSSIBLE POINTS	100					

PROCEDURE 19C: Ambulating a Client with Crutches *(continued)*

Comments:

_____

_____

_____

_____

_____

_____

_____

_____

_____

_____

Signatures: _____ Date: _____

SCORING *See Preface for scoring instructions.*

Rehabilitation

PROCEDURE 19D:
Ambulating a Client with a Cane

P R O C E D U R E   A S S E S S M E N T

Procedure Steps	Suggested Points	Self Practice	Peer Practice	Peer Testing	Final Testing	Total Earned
PREPROCEDURE						
1. Check orders and obtain authorization from supervisor.	3					
2. Assemble needed equipment.	2					
3. Check cane for safety.	5					
• Ensure bottom has rubber suction tip.	2					
• If client needs extra stability, use tripod or quad cane.						
PROCEDURE						
4. Wash your hands.	5					
5. Introduce yourself.	5					
6. Identify client and explain procedure.	4					
7. Help client put on good walking shoes.	5					
• Shoes should have low, broad heels, 1 to 1½ inches high.						
• Shoes should have nonskid soles.						
8. Have client hold cane on stronger or unaffected side of body.	2					
9. Ensure top of cane is level with top of femur at hip joint.	2					
10. Position bottom tip of cane 6 to 10 inches from side of foot.	3					
11. With cane in client's hand, make sure elbow is flexed.	3					
12. Tell client to balance his/her body weight on strong or unaffected foot and move cane forward.	3					
13. Tell client to move weak or affected foot forward.	3					
14. Help client transfer his/her weight to affected foot and cane.	3					
15. Tell client to move unaffected foot forward.	2					
16. Remain alert at all times.	5					
• Be ready to catch client if he/she falls.						
17. When helping client up and down stairs:	3					
• Always start with good (unaffected) leg.	2					
• Step up with unaffected leg. Bring affected leg up.	2					
• To go down stairs, step down on good leg and follow with cane and weak leg.	2					

PROCEDURE 19D: Ambulating a Client with a Cane (continued)

Procedure Steps	Suggested Points	Self Practice	Peer Practice	Peer Testing	Final Testing	Total Earned
POSTPROCEDURE						
18. Have client take small steps to prevent leaning and loss of balance.	3					
19. Note client's progress.	5					
• Observe/report any problems client experiences.						
20. Help client back to bed or chair.	3					
21. Remove transfer belt.	3					
22. Raise side rails and lower bed to lowest level, if so instructed.	5					
23. Place call signal within easy reach of client.	3					
24. Leave area neat and clean.	3					
25. Wash your hands.	5					
26. Record and report as necessary.	4					
TOTAL POSSIBLE POINTS	100					

Comments: _____

_____

_____

_____

_____

_____

_____

_____

_____

_____

_____

_____

Signatures: _____ Date: _____

SCORING *See Preface for scoring instructions.*

Rehabilitation

PROCEDURE 19E:
Ambulating a Client with a Walker

PROCEDURE ASSESSMENT

Procedure Steps	Suggested Points	Self Practice	Peer Practice	Peer Testing	Final Testing	Total Earned
PREPROCEDURE						
1. Check orders or obtain authorization from supervisor.	2					
2. Gather needed equipment.	2					
3. Check walker for safety.	4					
• Ensure that rubber suction tips are secure on all legs.	2					
4. Check for rough or damaged edges on hand rests.	4					
PROCEDURE						
5. Introduce yourself.	3					
6. Identify client and explain procedure.	4					
7. Wash your hands.	4					
8. Help client put on good walking shoes.	4					
• Shoes should have low, broad heels, 1 to 1½ inches high.						
• Shoes should have nonskid soles.						
9. Put gait belt on client.	3					
• Use underhanded grasp on belt.	2					
• Help client to standing position.	2					
• Position walker correctly.	2					
• Ask client to grasp hand rests securely.	2					
10. Check height of walker for these requirements:	4					
• Hand rests should be level with tops of femurs at hip joints.	2					
• Client's elbows should be flexed at 25° to 30° angle.	2					
• If adjustments need to be made, follow facility policy.	2					
11. Start with walker in position.	3					
• Client should be standing "inside" walker.	2					
12. Have client lift walker and place it forward so back legs of walker are even with client's toes.	4					
• Tell client to avoid sliding the walker; it's dangerous.	1					
13. Tell client to transfer his or her weight forward slightly to walker.	3					
14. Tell client to use walker for support and to walk "into" walker.	4					
• Don't let client shuffle his or her feet.						

Procedure Steps	Suggested Points	Self Practice	Peer Practice	Peer Testing	Final Testing	Total Earned
15. While client is using walker, walk to side and slightly behind client.	4					
• Keep one hand on gait belt.	1					
• Be alert at all times.						
• Be ready to catch client if he or she falls.						
16. Check to ensure client is lifting walker to move it forward.	4					
• Also ensure client is placing walker forward just to his/her toes.	1					
• Ensure client isn't trying to take too large a step.	1					
POSTPROCEDURE						
17. Help client back to bed or chair.	2					
18. Remove gait belt.	2					
19. Ensure client is comfortable.	2					
20. If client is in bed, elevate side rails and lower bed to lowest level, if so instructed.	4					
21. Put call signal within easy reach of client.	4					
22. Replace all equipment and leave area neat and clean.	2					
23. Wash your hands.	4					
24. Report and record all required information.	2					
TOTAL POSSIBLE POINTS	**100**					

Comments: _____
_____
_____
_____
_____
_____
_____
_____
_____
_____
_____

Signatures: _____ Date: _____

SCORING   *See Preface for scoring instructions.*

Rehabilitation

PROCEDURE 19F:
Helping a Client Who Is Falling

PROCEDURE ASSESSMENT

Procedure Steps **PREPROCEDURE**	Suggested Points	Self Practice	Peer Practice	Peer Testing	Final Testing	Total Earned
1. Follow safety measures to reduce and prevent falls:	6					
• Keep floors free of objects that can cause someone to trip.	3					
• Remove equipment when it's no longer needed.	3					
• Keep electrical and extension cords out of the way.	3					
• Provide good lighting in rooms, hallways, and bathrooms. Use night lights.	3					
• Don't use small area rugs unless they have nonskid backing.	3					
• Have clients wear nonskid shoes or slippers.	3					
• Use nonskid bathmats in tubs and showers.	3					
• Clean up any spills immediately.	3					
• Place "Caution" signs when floor is wet from mopping.	3					
PROCEDURE						
2. When fall occurs, position your body so it offers a firm base of support.	3					
• Move your feet a comfortable distance apart.	2					
• Straighten your back.	2					
3. If client is wearing a gait belt, grasp belt.	3					
• If there is no belt, put your arms around client's waist or under arms.	2					
4. Pull client's body toward your body.	2					
5. Position one of your legs as a rest for client's buttocks.	3					
• Let client's buttocks rest on your knee.	2					
6. Gently lower client to floor by letting him/her slide down your leg.	3					
• As you lower client, bend your knees and hips.	2					
7. Stay with client and call for help.						
8. Don't try to stand client up.	6					
• Licensed personnel must examine fallen clients for injuries before they can be moved.	2					

PROCEDURE 19F: Helping a Client Who Is Falling *(continued)*

Procedure Steps	Suggested Points	Self Practice	Peer Practice	Peer Testing	Final Testing	Total Earned
9. Transport client back to bed or chair as directed by license personnel.	2					
• Obtain adequate help.	2					
10. Put signal light within easy reach of client.	6					
POSTPROCEDURE						
11. Check on client frequently after a fall.	6					
• Note unusual behavior or symptoms.	2					
12. Wash your hands after client care.	6					
13. You may be required to complete and/or sign an incident report if you witness or assist a client who is falling.	2					
14. Incident reports should always include:	3					
• Date and time of incident.	2					
• Accurate account of the fall.	2					
• Client's reaction to the fall.	2					
TOTAL POSSIBLE POINTS	**100**					

Comments:

Signatures: _____ Date: _____

SCORING *See Preface for scoring instructions.*

Name _____ Date _____

Rehabilitation

PROCEDURE 19G:
Removing and Inserting a Hearing Aid

PROCEDURE ASSESSMENT

Procedure Steps	Suggested Points	Self Practice	Peer Practice	Peer Testing	Final Testing	Total Earned
PREPROCEDURE						
1. Check batteries before inserting hearing aid.	3					
• Battery case should close easily.						
• If it doesn't, batteries might be wrong size.						
2. Test batteries by turning hearing aid on.	5					
• Turn up volume control.	3					
• When you put hearing aid next to your ear, you should hear a whistle.						
PROCEDURE						
3. Introduce yourself and identify client.	5					
• Address client by name.	3					
• If client doesn't have hearing aid in or it isn't turned on, he/she might not be able to hear you.						
• Look directly at client while speaking.	3					
4. Wash your hands.	7					
5. Tell client you are going to insert and/or remove his/her hearing aid.	4					
6. Provide for privacy by closing curtain or door.	3					
7. Check client's ear for wax buildup or anything unusual.	4					
• Turn hearing aid off.						
8. Insert hearing aid.	4					
• If client is able, let him/her insert hearing aid.	3					
• If you are inserting hearing aid, place aid over client's ear, if appropriate, with ear mold piece hanging free.	3					
• Adjust hearing aid behind ear.	3					
• Pull gently on earlobe and carefully insert ear mold into ear canal. Gently twist ear mold into curve of ear. Push mold up and in.	3					
• Turn hearing aid on and adjust volume to comfortable level.	3					
• If client complains that hearing aid is uncomfortable, it may need to be refitted. Report this to supervisor.	3					

PROCEDURE 19G: Removing and Inserting a Hearing Aid *(continued)*

Procedure Steps	Suggested Points	Self Practice	Peer Practice	Peer Testing	Final Testing	Total Earned
9. Remove hearing aid.	4					
• Turn off hearing aid.	3					
• Gently pull on upper part of ear to loosen outer portion of hearing aid.	3					
• Lift ear mold up and out.	3					
• Remove batteries before storing hearing aid in its case in safe place. Ensure case is labeled with client's name.	3					
POSTPROCEDURE						
10. Make client comfortable and provide for safety.	7					
11. Open curtain or door.	4					
12. Wash your hands.	7					
13. Report any unusual observations to supervisor.	4					
TOTAL POSSIBLE POINTS	**100**					

Comments: _____

_____

_____

_____

_____

_____

_____

_____

_____

_____

_____

Signatures: _____ Date: _____

SCORING *See Preface for scoring instructions.*

Sports Medicine

Reinforcement Activities

Matching

Write the letter of the phrase that best matches each numbered item in the blank provided.

_____ **1.** Strain

_____ **2.** Sprain

_____ **3.** Aerobic

_____ **4.** Anaerobic

_____ **5.** Proprioception

_____ **6.** Fracture

a. Not associated with using oxygen.

b. An injury to a muscle.

c. Body awareness.

d. Involving oxygen.

e. An injury to ligament.

f. An injury to bone.

True/False

Write "T" in the blank provided if the statement is true. Write "F" if the statement is false.

_____ **7.** People who have suffered a heart attack take a VO2 max test to gauge their recovery.

_____ **8.** A client should use a cold whirlpool to treat an acute injury (less than 48 hours old) that has swelling.

_____ **9.** A CPT measures height, weight, and visual acuity on the first visit with a client.

_____ **10.** Athletic trainers only work with athletes on the field.

_____ **11.** A CPT instructs a client to run as fast as possible to elevate heart rate to the maximum amount to burn the most fat.

Multiple Choice

Circle the letter that best answers the question or completes the statement.

11. The formula for body mass index (BMI), where weight is in kg and height is in meters, is
  a. $BMI = kg^2/m^2$.
  b. $BMI = kg/m$.
  c. $BMI = kg^2/m$.
  d. $BMI = kg/m^2$.

12. Which definition of the various parts to a SOAP is incorrect?
  a. S- Subjective
  b. O- Objective
  c. A- Assessment
  d. P- Play

13. ATCs will perform all of the following *except*
   a. control bleeding
   b. taping
   c. CPR
   d. none of the above

14. Sports medicine technicians perform all of the following *except*
   a. filing charts and notes
   b. modifying exercises independently
   c. taking messages from clients
   d. cleaning equipment

15. Heat should *not* be used in which situation?
   a. blood clot
   b. on an injury greater than 48 hours old
   c. tight muscles
   d. elderly clients

16. Which sports medicine worker would *best* be used to rehabilitate an injured athlete?
   a. athletic trainer
   b. strength and conditioning specialist
   c. exercise physiologist
   d. sports physical therapist

Fill in the Blank

Write the word (or words) that best completes the sentence in the blank provided.

17. Before allowing an athlete to return to practice, a sports physical therapist will have him or her perform _____ exercises.

18. When taking skin fold measurements on a male, you will measure the _____, _____, and _____.

19. Strength and conditioning specialists focus on improving _____ _____.

20. An exercise physiologist researches the effects of _____ on the human body.

21. The study of movement of the body is _____.

22. Athletic trainers educate athletes on the _____.

Short Answer

23. What are five skills an athletic trainer must possess?

_____

_____

_____

_____

_____

24. List at least three job duties of a personal trainer.

_____

_____

_____

_____

25. When a sports physical therapist performs an objective evaluation of a client after an injury, what deficits might be found?

_____

_____

_____

_____

_____

_____

Sports Medicine

PROCEDURE 20A:
Applying a Hot Pack

PROCEDURE ASSESSMENT

Procedure Steps	Suggested Points	Self Practice	Peer Practice	Peer Testing	Final Testing	Total Earned
PREPROCEDURE						
1. Gather needed equipment.	3					
2. Test client's sensation to touch by lightly running fingers across area.	6					
• If client reports decreased sensation or hypersensitivity in area, tell licensed supervisor immediately.	4					
3. If sensation is normal, retrieve appropriately sized hot pack from hydrocollator, using tongs.	4					
• If there's a thermometer present, read it.	3					
• Temperature of water should be between 155° and 163°F.	3					
• Temperature shouldn't exceed 165°F.	3					
4. Allow hot pack to drain until water stops streaming off it.	4					
5. Wrap hot pack in 1 to 3 terry cloth covers.	4					
6. Place regular towel on side that will touch client.	4					
PROCEDURE						
7. Help client into a comfortable position.	4					
8. Put hot pack on target area.	4					
• Or, put hot pack in a spot where client can lie on or against it.	3					
9. Set timer for time specified by therapist, usually 15 to 20 minutes.	3					
10. At least every 5 minutes, ask client is he/she is getting too hot.	6					
• If so, immediately help client off hot pack and examine skin.	4					
• If skin is overly red or blistering, stop treatment and tell therapist.	3					
• If skin looks normal, add extra towel or terry cloth cover over those present and help client into position again.	4					
• Tell supervisor about occurrence.	3					
POSTPROCEDURE						
11. When timer rings or time is up, help client off hot pack.	3					
12. Examine skin for adverse effects, such as overly red color or blistering.	6					

PROCEDURE 20A: Applying a Hot Pack *(continued)*

Procedure Steps	Suggested Points	Self Practice	Peer Practice	Peer Testing	Final Testing	Total Earned
13. Hang cover to dry.	4					
• Replace hot pack in hydrocollator.	3					
• Don't splash the water.	3					
• Put used towel in dirty linen bin.	3					
14. Wash your hands.	6					
TOTAL POSSIBLE POINTS	100					

Comments:

_____

_____

_____

_____

_____

_____

_____

_____

_____

_____

Signatures: _____ **Date:** _____

SCORING   *See Preface for scoring instructions.*

Name _____   Date _____

Sports Medicine

PROCEDURE 20B1:
Applying an Ice Pack

PROCEDURE ASSESSMENT

Procedure Steps	Suggested Points	Self Practice	Peer Practice	Peer Testing	Final Testing	Total Earned
PREPROCEDURE						
1. Gather needed equipment.	5					
2. Test client's sensation to touch by lightly running fingers across area.	7					
• If client reports decreased sensation or hypersensitivity in area, tell physical therapist immediately.	5					
3. If sensation is normal, get a plastic bag and put one scoop of crushed ice in it.	4					
4. Compress bag to push all air out.	5					
5. Tie a knot in top of bag, allowing some space to spread ice evenly over affected area.	5					
PROCEDURE						
6. Help client into comfortable position.	4					
7. If client can't tolerate cold put paper or cloth towel between client and ice pack.	4					
8. Put ice bag on affected area and gently push down on it.	4					
• Spread ice evenly, improving contact to target area.	5					
9. Set timer for time specified by therapist, usually 15 to 20 minutes.	5					
10. Periodically check client's skin.	7					
• If you see blistering or client complains of strong burning sensation, immediately help client off ice pack.	5					
• Stop treatment and tell therapist.	6					
POSTPROCEDURE						
11. When timer rings, help client off ice pack.	4					
12. Examine skin for adverse effects.	7					
13. Take ice pack to sink or whirlpool.	3					
14. Tear open bag and discard ice.	4					
15. Throw away empty bag and put used towels in dirty linen bin.	4					
16. Wash your hands.	7					
TOTAL POSSIBLE POINTS	**100**					

Procedure 20B1: Applying an Ice Pack (continued)

Comments: _____
_____
_____
_____
_____
_____
_____
_____

Signatures: _____ Date: _____

SCORING *See Preface for scoring instructions.*

Alternative Medicine

Reinforcement Activities

Multiple Choice

Circle the letter that best answers the question or completes the statement.

1. Which of the following occupations has no national or state system of licensure or certification at present?
   a. chiropractor.
   b. massage therapist.
   c. acupuncturist.
   d. herbalist.

2. When a chiropractor performs an adjustment, the client may hear which of the following sounds?
   a. creaking.
   b. buzzing.
   c. popping.
   d. crackling.

3. Which type of massage is well known and uses five basic strokes to manipulate the soft tissues of the body?
   a. Swedish.
   b. neuromuscular.
   c. shiatsu.
   d. reiki.

4. Most acupuncture treatments last how long?
   a. 5 to 15 minutes.
   b. 20 to 60 minutes.
   c. 60 minutes.
   d. 60 to 90 minutes.

5. Herbal therapy may be contraindicated in which of the following medical conditions?
   a. pregnancy.
   b. hemophilia.
   c. osteoporosis.
   d. cancer.

6. Which of the following is true of herbalists?
   a. they take 2600 hours of training to be certified or licensed.
   b. they prepare herbal medicines ordered by a physician.
   c. they prepare herbal medicines based on their own diagnosis of the client's problems.
   d. they must take college prerequisites, then attend college or university for 4 years.

7. Which of the following is true of chiropractors?
   a. they adjust the spine to realign vertebrae and restore spinal nerve function.
   b. they only treat people who have back pain, neck pain, or headaches.
   c. they take a three-year training program at a chiropractic college.
   d. they prescribe medications to relieve the symptoms of subluxations.

8. Which of the following is true of massage therapists?
   a. they practice a new type of alternative medicine treatment that benefits muscles only.
   b. they may perform a variety of massage types, depending on preference and client problems.
   c. they use lotion to prevent friction, soften the skin, and provide aromatherapy during the massage.
   d. they take 1300 hours of training to become nationally certified.

9. Which of the following is true of acupuncturists?
   a. they must be licensed in traditional Chinese medicine to practice in any state.
   b. they may apply electric current in small amounts through the acupuncture needles.
   c. they can relieve all types of pain if they do the treatment correctly.
   d. they insert needles from 1 to 3 inches under the skin at various points along meridians.

10. Moxibustion is used by which of the following alternative medicine practitioners?
    a. acupuncturist.
    b. chiropractor.
    c. herbalist.
    d. massage therapist.

11. Which of the following alternative medicine practitioners help increase lymph flow which boosts immune function?
    a. acupuncturist.
    b. chiropractor.
    c. herbalist.
    d. massage therapist.

Fill in the Blank
Write the word (or words) that best completes the sentence in the blank provided.

12. _____ is the term for the manual treatments used by chiropractors.

13. The father of chiropractic in America is _____.

14. A chiropractic adjustment is a manual treatment to realign the _____ and restore the function of the spinal nerves.

15. The acupuncturist inserts the needles up to _____ inch(es) in depth.

16. _____ is done by applying a very small amount of electrical current through the acupuncture needles.

17. Moxibustion refers to the application of _____ to the points where the acupuncture needles are inserted.

18. _____ helps the client relax and counteracts the effects of stress.

19. _____ oil is one of the most common and least expensive oils for use in massage therapy.

20. If the client complains of being tickled, the massage therapist may need to apply _____ pressure.

21. _____ determine which individual herbs or herbal combinations to use to treat specific conditions.

True/False

Write "T" in the blank provided if the statement is true. Write "F" if the statement is false.

_____ 22. Chiropractors use drugs or surgery to treat people who are ill or in pain.

_____ 23. Chiropractic care is used to treat respiratory and digestive problems as well as musculoskeletal problems.

_____ 24. During massage therapy, the heart rate and blood pressure are lowered.

_____ 25. Lotion, rather than oil, is preferred to reduce friction on the skin when giving a massage.

_____ 26. The massage therapist should stroke and knead in the direction toward the heart.

_____ 27. Acupressure is a type of acupuncture performed without needles.

_____ 28. The client will feel no sensation as the needles are inserted in acupuncture therapy.

_____ 29. Clients with hemophilia can safely undergo acupressure.

_____ 30. It is normal for the client to feel a sensation similar to a mosquito bite as the acupuncture needles are inserted.

_____ 31. The herbalist recommends individual herbs or combinations to treat specific conditions.

Matching

Write the letter of the phrase that best matches each numbered item in the blank provided.

_____ 32. Acupuncturist

_____ 33. Chiropractor

_____ 34. Herbalist

_____ 35. Massage Therapist

a. Office in a health food store or own a retail store.

b. Work in the client's home or in a spa.

c. Work in pain management center or clinic with other health care professionals.

d. Specialize in sports injuries or occupational health.

Alternative Medicine

PROCEDURE 21A:
Performing a Back Massage

········ P R O C E D U R E   A S S E S S M E N T ········

Procedure Steps PREPROCEDURE	Suggested Points	Self Practice	Peer Practice	Peer Testing	Final Testing	Total Earned
1. Gather needed equipment.	2					
2. Prepare table or bed.	2					
• Cover it with sheet and put large towel or blanket to side.	1					
• Place rolled towel or small blanket under feet.	1					
3. Explain procedure to client.	2					
4. Adjust table or bed height to correct position.	4					
5. Leave room while client removes clothing above waist.	2					
• Tell client to lay on table or bed in prone position.	1					
• If client is unable to undress, help him/her.						
6. Warm oil if needed.	2					
7. Wash your hands.	4					
PROCEDURE						
8. Arrange blanket or towel so only client's back is exposed.	2					
• Ensure any clothing is covered by blanket.	1					
9. Put a quarter-sized amount of oil in your hand.	2					
• Spread oil over your hands and forearms.	1					
• If you notice friction while performing massage, use more oil.	1					
• Always apply oil to your hands and arms, not client's back.	1					
• If you use lotion, apply it to your hands and rub them together to warm them to body temperature before touching client's skin.	1					
10. Stand on left side of table or bed with your feet 18 to 24 inches apart.	4					
• Point your left foot toward client's head.	1					
• Point your right foot toward bed or table.	1					
• Bend slightly at knees and rock from front to back as you do strokes.	1					

Procedure 21A: Performing a Back Massage *(continued)*

Procedure Steps	Suggested Points	Self Practice	Peer Practice	Peer Testing	Final Testing	Total Earned
11. Use flat part of fingers (not just fingertips) to stroke from client's waist to shoulders and from center to outside edge of back.	3					
• Then return to waist.	1					
12. Don't massage over open sores, rashes, or bruises.	4					
13. Repeat strokes, filling in whole back area with oil from your hands.	2					
• Practice to see how much pressure to apply.						
• Client shouldn't feel discomfort.						
• If massage hurts client, you're applying too much pressure.						
• If massage tickles client, you're applying too little pressure.						
14. Put your right forearm on client's back at waist on right side of spine.	3					
• Gently but firmly slide your forearm from waist to shoulder.	1					
• Repeat 3 times.	1					
15. Repeat step 14 with your left forearm on left side of client's spine.	1					
16. Using flat part of fingers, make small circles up each side of spine.	2					
• Start below waist, then up across shoulders, and down edges of back to waist again.	1					
• Repeat until whole of back has been covered in small circles.	1					
17. Make larger circles over low back and upper hip area using your palms and flat part of fingers.	2					
18. Stroke upward to right shoulder area.	3					
• Gently grasp muscle and skin between thumb and curled forefinger, using both hands.	1					
• Work from area where neck and shoulder meet down across trapezius muscle to deltoid muscle.	1					
• This shouldn't hurt client.						
• If it does hurt client, use less pressure.						
19. Continue this grasping stroke down outer edge of back to hip area.	3					
20. Move to right side of table.	4					
• Keep your feet 18 to 24 inches apart.	1					
• Point your right foot toward client's head.	1					
• Point your left foot toward bed or table.	1					
• Bend slightly at knees and rock from front to back as you do strokes.	1					

PROCEDURE 21A: Performing a Back Massage *(continued)*

Procedure Steps	Suggested Points	Self Practice	Peer Practice	Peer Testing	Final Testing	Total Earned
21. Using flat part of fingers, make small circles up each side of spine.	2					
• Start below waist, then up across shoulders, and down edges of back to waist again.	1					
• Repeat until whole of back has been covered in small circles.	1					
22. Stroke from client's waist to shoulders again.	2					
• Use very tips of your fingers with extremely light pressure.	1					
23. Replace blanket or towel over client's back.	2					
POSTPROCEDURE						
24. Tell client you will leave room while he/she gets dressed.	2					
• Tell client to use towel or blanket to wipe off excess oil before dressing.	1					
• Help client dress, if necessary.						
25. Leave room and provide privacy for client.	2					
26. Wash your hands thoroughly to remove oil.	4					
27. Remove used linens from table or bed.	2					
• Put them in dirty linen bin.	1					
28. Clean table using a 1:5 solution of bleach and water.	4					
TOTAL POSSIBLE POINTS	**100**					

Comments:

_____

_____

_____

_____

_____

_____

_____

_____

_____

_____

Signatures: _____   Date: _____

SCORING   *See Preface for scoring instructions.*

Dental Care

Reinforcement Activities

Matching
Write the letter of the phrase that best matches each numbered item in the blank provided.

_____ 1. Cavity
_____ 2. Elastomeric
_____ 3. Amalgamator
_____ 4. Handpiece
_____ 5. Anesthesia
_____ 6. Interdental papilla

a. mechanical mixing device
b. gingiva between adjacent teeth
c. a hole in the tooth
d. rubberlike impression material
e. mechanical device used to shape tooth structure
f. loss of feeling or sensation

True/False
Write "T" in the blank provided if the statement is true. Write "F" if the statement is false.

_____ 7. A model is a negative reproduction of the oral cavity.

_____ 8. The instruments are placed on the tray from left to right in order of use.

_____ 9. All dental cements are mixed the same way.

_____ 10. A high speed handpiece should be sterilized after each use.

Multiple Choice
Circle the letter that best answers the question or completes the statement.

11. Burs with a _____ shank are designed to fit high-speed handpieces
    a. latch
    b. friction-grip
    c. straight

12. A radiograph showing the crowns of both maxillary and mandibular teeth is the
    a. periapical
    b. occlusal
    c. bitewing

13. The dental assistant holds the instrument being transferred _____ to the instrument being returned.
    a. parallel
    b. above
    c. below

14. Charting with _____ indicates work that needs to be done.
    a. red pencil
    b. black pencil
    c. blue pencil

15. Which of the following is not part of the basic instrument setup?
    a. mouth mirror
    b. explorer
    c. burnisher
    d. cotton pliers

16. The _____ side of the film packet is always placed next to the teeth and toward the X-ray tube.
    a. front
    b. back
    c. black
    d. foil

17. What is the dental specialty dealing with diseases of the supporting tissues of the teeth?
    a. prosthodontics
    b. endodontics
    c. periodontics
    d. oral and maxillofacial surgery

Fill in the Blank

Write the word (or words) that best completes the sentence in the blank provided.

18. _____ is the soft tissue that surrounds the neck of the tooth.

19. The tooth is divided into two main sections, the _____ and the _____. The _____ or _____ marks the junction of these two sections.

20. To prevent disease, plaque must be thoroughly removed at least every _____ hours.

21. _____ is the term to describe darker areas on a radiograph. _____ is the term used to describe the lighter areas.

22. _____ is a cement commonly used for temporary fillings and temporary luting.

Matching

Write the letter of the phrase that best matches each numbered item in the blank provided.

_____ 23. explorer
_____ 24. periodontal probe
_____ 25. spoon excavator
_____ 26. discoid-cleoid
_____ 27. scaler

    a. used to remove soft decay
    b. used to remove calculus and cement
    c. used to examine tooth surfaces
    d. used to measure the depth of gingival sulcus
    e. used to remove excess and carve amalgam

Name _____   Date _____

Labeling

28. Label the tooth tissues on the diagram.

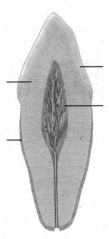

29. On each of the diagrams below of the permanent and primary teeth:
1. Draw the midline.
2. Label the quadrants.
3. Name the teeth of one quadrant. Name teeth in this order: first write the name of the arch (maxillary or mandibular), next write whether the tooth is right or left and then write the full name of the tooth.

(NOTE: When you are looking at the worksheet remember that it is as if you are looking at a person facing you. This means that the teeth on the right of the paper are the left teeth of a person facing you and the teeth on the left side of the paper are the right teeth of a person facing you.)

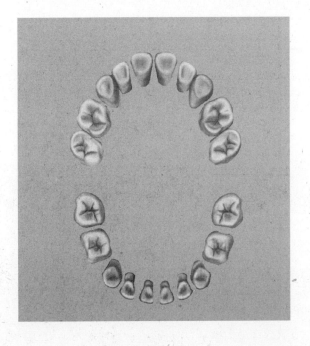   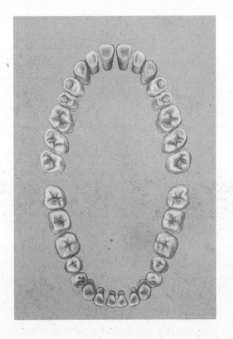

_____   _____
_____   _____
_____   _____
_____   _____
_____   _____

30. Name these teeth identified in the Universal system

#18 _____

#4 _____

#9 _____

#27 _____

#14 _____

b _____

k _____

h _____

p _____

31. Name these teeth identified in the Palmer's system

|3 _____

4| _____

8| _____

|2 _____

|a _____

d| _____

e| _____

|c _____

Name _____   Date _____

Dental Care

PROCEDURE 22A1:
Demonstrating the Bass Toothbrushing Technique

P R O C E D U R E   A S S E S S M E N T

Procedure Steps	Suggested Points	Self Practice	Peer Practice	Peer Testing	Final Testing	Total Earned
PREPROCEDURE						
1. Gather needed equipment.	3					
2. Identify and greet client.	3					
PROCEDURE						
3. Explain relationship of plaque to dental disease.	4					
4. Discuss with client:	4					
• Plaque location.	3					
• Importance of removing plaque.	3					
• Frequency of removing plaque.	3					
5. Advise client on recommended types:	4					
• Toothbrushes.	3					
• Toothpaste.	3					
• Toothbrush replacement.	3					
6. Demonstrate Bass technique beginning with facial of maxillary molars:	4					
• Place toothbrush near gingival margin at a 45° angle to root of tooth.	3					
• With light pressure, vibrate bristles back and forth without dislodging bristle tips.	3					
• Stroke bristles toward occlusal surface.	3					
• Move brush forward and repeat process.	3					
• Continue around maxillary arch.	3					
7. Repeat procedure for facial of mandibular teeth.	4					
8. Use same technique for lingual surfaces of maxillary and mandibular posterior teeth.	3					
9. Clean lingual surfaces of anterior teeth.	4					
• Place head of toothbrush vertically.	3					
• Gently move brush back and forth.	3					
• Stroke bristles toward incisal surface.	3					
10. On all occlusal surfaces:	4					
• Hold bristles flat against surface.	3					
• Brush back and forth or in circular or scrubbing motion.	3					
11. Brush tongue in back-to-front sweeping motion to remove bacteria and food particles.	3					

PROCEDURE 22A1: Demonstrating the Bass Toothbrushing Technique *(continued)*

Procedure Steps	Suggested Points	Self Practice	Peer Practice	Peer Testing	Final Testing	Total Earned
12. Encourage client to ask questions.	3					
13. Have client demonstrate technique on manikin to verify understanding.	3					
POSTPROCEDURE						
14. Dismiss client.	3					
15. Return equipment to storage area.	3					
TOTAL POSSIBLE POINTS	100					

Comments: _____

_____

_____

_____

_____

_____

_____

_____

_____

_____

Signatures: _____ Date: _____

SCORING *See Preface for scoring instructions.*

Name _____   Date _____

Dental Care

PROCEDURE 22A2:
Demonstrating Correct Flossing Technique

.... P R O C E D U R E   A S S E S S M E N T ....

Procedure Steps	Suggested Points	Self Practice	Peer Practice	Peer Testing	Final Testing	Total Earned
PREPROCEDURE						
1. Gather needed equipment.	4					
2. Cut piece of floss approximately 18 inches.	5					
3. Identify and greet client.	6					
PROCEDURE						
4. Explain plaque forms on proximal surfaces of teeth and is not removed by brushing.	4					
5. Demonstrate flossing by using manikin.	5					
6. Wrap floss end around middle finger of right hand.	4					
7. Wrap other end around middle finger leaving 2 to 3 inches of working space.	4					
8. Stretch floss tightly between your fingers.	5					
• Use thumbs or index fingers to guide floss.	4					
• Ease floss through contact area with gentle back-and-forth motion.	4					
9. Curve floss tightly around proximal side of one tooth.	5					
10. Move floss down to sulcus area and back up to contact area repeating several times.	4					
11. Curve floss tightly around proximal side of adjacent tooth.	4					
12. Move floss down to sulcus area and back up to contact area repeating several times.	3					
13. Repeat procedure on each tooth in both arches.	4					
14. After every two or three teeth, unwind clean strip of floss.	5					
15. Always floss distal surface of most posterior tooth in each quadrant.	4					
16. Instruct client to avoid back-and-forth movement of floss once floss is through contact area. Floss can cut gingiva if not used correctly.	3					
17. Inform client when flossing starts, bleeding or soreness of gingival may occur. Client should call office if bleeding continues beyond first week.	5					
18. Encourage client to ask questions.	5					
19. Have client demonstrate technique on manikin to verify understanding.	5					

PROCEDURE 22A2: Demonstrating Correct Flossing Technique *(continued)*

Procedure Steps	Suggested Points	Self Practice	Peer Practice	Peer Testing	Final Testing	Total Earned
POSTPROCEDURE						
20. Dismiss the client.	4					
21. Return equipment to storage area.	4					
TOTAL POSSIBLE POINTS	100					

Comments: _____

_____

_____

_____

_____

_____

_____

_____

_____

Signatures: _____ Date: _____

SCORING   *See Preface for scoring instructions.*

Name _____   Date _____

Dental Care

PROCEDURE 22B:
Maintaining the Dental Treatment Area

PROCEDURE ASSESSMENT

Procedure Steps	Suggested Points	Self Practice	Peer Practice	Peer Testing	Final Testing	Total Earned
PREPROCEDURE						
1. Gather needed equipment.	2					
2. Report to office 15 to 20 minutes before first scheduled client.	2					
3. Change to clinical attire.	2					
PROCEDURE						
Prepare for the First Client of the Day						
4. Switch on air compressor and central vacuum units.	1					
5. Turn on sterilizers.	2					
6. Turn on darkroom safelights and processor.	1					
7. Check daily schedule and review first client's chart.	3					
8. Place current x-rays on view box.	3					
9. Wash hands and put on mask.	4					
10. Switch on units in treatment rooms.	3					
11. If a unit is equipped with an independent water supply, fill water bottles and attach them to the unit.	2					
12. Flush handpiece tubing (without hand piece attached) and air-water syringe for 30 to 60 seconds.	4					
• Flush handpiece and air-water syringe into the suction tubing to reduce airborne microbes.						
13. Discard mask and wash hands.	4					
14. Prepare treatment room for indicated procedure.	2					
15. Select proper tray setup and materials for procedure.	1					
16. Place plastic barriers on:	2					
• Chair.	1					
• Unit.	1					
• Light.	1					
Decontaminate the Treatment Area After a Procedure						
17. While wearing treatment gloves:	2					
• Remove soiled barriers and place on instrument tray.	1					
• Remove saliva ejector tip, oral evacuator tip, air-water syringe tip, and handpieces and place them on the instrument tray.	1					

Reinforcement Activities and Procedure Assessment   Chapter 22   **A-319**

PROCEDURE 22B: Maintaining the Dental Treatment Area *(continued)*

Procedure Steps	Suggested Points	Self Practice	Peer Practice	Peer Testing	Final Testing	Total Earned
• Take contaminated items to contaminated area of sterilization room.	1					
• Remove anesthetic needle and carpule from syringe and place in sharps container.	1					
• Place bloody waste in biohazardous waste container.	1					
• Place soiled instruments, except handpieces, in ultrasonic cleaner.	1					
• Discard waste and treatment gloves.	1					
18. Wash hands and don clean utility gloves.	4					
19. While wearing utility gloves:	2					
• Clean and disinfect instrument tray and towel clips and place in clean area.	1					
• Spray all contaminated surfaces with cleaner or disinfectant.	1					
• Wipe all sprayed surfaces with 4 × 4 gauze pad on paper towels.	1					
• Respray all surfaces with disinfectant and leave wet for 10 minutes.	1					
• Flush hand piece tubing into oral evacuator tubing for 20 to 30 seconds.	1					
20. With gloves on, wash utility gloves then remove gloves and spray with disinfectant.	3					
21. Remove mask and protective eyewear.	2					
22. Wash your hands.	4					
23. Place new barriers on surfaces.	2					
End-of-the Day Routine						
24. Complete steps 17 through 19 to decontaminate treatment room.	4					
25. While wearing utility gloves:	2					
• Check saliva ejector trap and solids collection tank and dispose of filters if debris is present.	1					
• Aspirate sanitizing solution through all suction hoses.	1					
• Clean sinks.	1					
26. Wash, dry, remove and disinfect utility gloves.	2					
27. Remove and empty water bottle and attach dry bottle to unit.	2					
28. Turn off all equipment.	1					
29. Restock consumable supplies.	2					
30. Check next day's appointment schedule and make sure all records and lab work are present.	2					
31. Ensure all lab cases have been or are ready to go to the laboratory.	2					

Procedure Steps	Suggested Points	Self Practice	Peer Practice	Peer Testing	Final Testing	Total Earned
POSTPROCEDURE						
32. Remove clinical attire and place in appropriate container.	4					
33. Wash your hands.	4					
TOTAL POSSIBLE POINTS	100					

Comments: _____

_____

_____

_____

_____

_____

_____

_____

_____

_____

Signatures: _____ **Date:** _____

SCORING *See Preface for scoring instructions.*

Dental Care

PROCEDURE 22C:
Positioning the Client and the Dental Assistant

PROCEDURE ASSESSMENT

Procedure Steps	Suggested Points	Self Practice	Peer Practice	Peer Testing	Final Testing	Total Earned
PREPROCEDURE						
1. Gather needed equipment.	2					
2. Review client's chart.	3					
3. Place current x-rays on view box.	3					
4. Adjust chair height to comfortable entry level for client.	2					
5. Place chair in upright position.	2					
6. Raise chair arm.	2					
7. Clear all equipment so client has clear path to chair.	2					
8. Assemble instrument tray and cover with towel.	2					
PROCEDURE						
9. Greet client in reception area and introduce yourself.	3					
10. Escort client to treatment area.	2					
11. Seat client and lower armrest.	2					
12. Review client's health history and put chart aside.	3					
13. Wash your hands.	5					
14. Drape client.	3					
15. Put on glasses, mask then gloves.	5					
16. If appropriate, have client remove lipstick and retrieve personal items for safekeeping.						
17. Inform client when chair is to be reclined.	3					
18. Lower backrest until client is in supine position.	2					
19. Raise or lower chair to proper working height.	2					
20. If necessary, adjust headrest.						
21. Turn on light and position, moving from client's chest area up, to illuminate field of operation.	3					
22. Position yourself on assistant's stool at side of client:	3					
• Thighs parallel to floor.	2					
• Knees toward head of client's chair.	2					

PROCEDURE 22C: Positioning the Client and the Dental Assistant (continued)

Procedure Steps	Suggested Points	Self Practice	Peer Practice	Peer Testing	Final Testing	Total Earned
• Thigh adjacent to client's shoulder and front edge of chair adjacent to client's mouth.	2					
• Eye level 4 to 6 inches higher than dentist's.	2					
23. Inform client of approximate waiting time.	2					
24. Keep hands away from face and hair.	5					
POSTPROCEDURE						
25. Slowly raise backrest to upright position and lift arm of chair.	2					
26. Check client's face for debris or smudges.	2					
27. Remove drape.	2					
28. Optional: Give client hand mirror or tissue to ensure face is free of debris.						
29. Move equipment out of client's pathway.	2					
30. Remove gloves and mask and wash your hands.	5					
31. Return personal items to client.	2					
32. Assist client in rising from chair if necessary.	2					
33. Escort client to reception desk.	3					
• Communicate client's needs to business assistant.	2					
• Client might make payment or schedule next appointment.						
34. Return to treatment room:	5					
• Put on utility gloves.	2					
• Complete posttreatment aseptic procedures.	2					
TOTAL POSSIBLE POINTS	**100**					

Comments:

_____

_____

_____

_____

_____

_____

_____

Signatures: _____ Date: _____

SCORING *See Preface for scoring instructions.*

Dental Care

PROCEDURE 22D:
Dental Tray Setups

PROCEDURE ASSESSMENT

Procedure Steps	Suggested Points	Self Practice	Peer Practice	Peer Testing	Final Testing	Total Earned
PREPROCEDURE						
1. Gather needed equipment.	3					
2. Wash hands.	5					
PROCEDURE						
Basic or Examination Tray Setup (These are used most often)	3					
• Saliva ejector and/or oral evacuator tip	1					
• Cotton pliers	1					
• Explorer	1					
• Mouth mirror	1					
• Client's chart	1					
• Periodontal probe (optional)	1					
• Client towel	1					
• Towel clips	1					
• 2 × 2 gauze pads	1					
• Air-water syringe tips	1					
Amalgam Tray Setup (Used when a restoration procedure is done)	3					
• Basic setup	1					
• Anesthetic syringe	1					
• Rubber dam setup (optional)	1					
• Handpieces and burs	1					
• Spoon excavator	1					
• Chisel, hatchet, gingival margin trimmer (depends on dentist's preference)	1					
• Matrix band and retainer	1					
• Amalgam carrier	1					
• Amalgam condenser	1					
• Discoid-cleoid	1					
• Hollenback carver	1					
• Burnisher	1					
• Cotton rolls	1					
• Cotton pellets	1					
• Topical anesthetic	1					
• Cotton swab	1					
• Anesthetic carpule	1					
• Anesthetic needle	1					
• Interproximal wedges	1					

Procedure Steps	Suggested Points	Self Practice	Peer Practice	Peer Testing	Final Testing	Total Earned
• Cavity varnish	1					
• Cavity base or liner	1					
• Mixing pad and instrument	1					
• Amalgam capsules	1					
• Amalgamator	1					
• Amalgam well or squeeze cloth	1					
• Articulating paper	1					
Composite Resin Tray Setup (Also used for a restoration procedure)	3					
• Basic	1					
• Anesthetic syringe	1					
• Rubber dam setup (optional)	1					
• Handpieces and burs	1					
• Spoon excavator	1					
• Matrix band and retainer	1					
• Composite placement instrument	1					
• Disposable brush for bonding agent	1					
• Cotton rolls	1					
• Topical anesthetic	1					
• Cotton swab	1					
• Polishing points	1					
• Abrasive strips and discs	1					
• Anesthetic carpule	1					
• Anesthetic needle	1					
• Acid etch	1					
• Bonding agent	1					
• Composite resin compule or syringe	1					
• Curing light	1					
Basic Tooth Extraction Setup	3					
• Mouth mirror	1					
• Cotton pliers	1					
• Anesthetic syringe	1					
• Surgical aspirating tip	1					
• Periosteal elevator	1					
• Root elevator	1					
• Extraction forceps—selected for specific tooth	1					
• Surgical curette	1					
• Hemostat	1					
• Client's chart	1					
• Treatment consent form	1					
• Sterile 2 × 2 gauze pads	1					
• Cotton swab	1					

PROCEDURE 22D: Dental Tray Setups *(continued)*

Procedure Steps	Suggested Points	Self Practice	Peer Practice	Peer Testing	Final Testing	Total Earned
• Topical anesthetic	1					
• Anesthetic needle	1					
• Anesthetic carpules	1					
• Post-treatment instructions	1					
POSTPROCEDURE						
3. Clean and replace equipment.	3					
4. Wash hands.	5					
TOTAL POSSIBLE POINTS	100					

Comments:

_____
_____
_____
_____
_____
_____
_____
_____
_____
_____

Signatures: _____   **Date:** _____

SCORING   *See Preface for scoring instructions.*

Animal Health Care

Reinforcement Activities

Multiple Choice

Circle the letter that best answers the question or completes the statement.

1. Which of the following occupations is considered an entry-level position in animal health care?
   a. veterinarian.
   b. veterinary technician.
   c. veterinary assistant.
   d. animal laboratory technician.

2. Which of the following diagnostic procedures is performed to check for parasites?
   a. fecal examination.
   b. bathing.
   c. urinalysis.
   d. skin testing.

3. The specific gravity is:
   a. the density of the urine.
   b. a small telescopelike device.
   c. a machine to spin and separate the specimen.
   d. a series of tests performed on urine.

4. What must be done to protect the dog's eyes prior to bathing?
   a. place a bland opthalmic ointment in each eye.
   b. tape the eyes shut with hypoallergenic tape.
   c. place antibiotic opthalmic ointment in each eye.
   d. there is no need to protect the dog's eyes.

5. When giving a pill to a dog, in which area of the dog's mouth should the pill be placed?
   a. under the tongue.
   b. front central area.
   c. back central area.
   d. back corner pocket.

Fill in the Blanks

Write the word (or words) that best completes the sentence in the blank provided.

6. A _____ is a medical professional whose primary responsibility is protecting the health and welfare of animals and people.

7. _____ are organisms that live within, upon, or at the expense of another organism without contributing to the organism's survival.

8. A _____ is also called an animal health technician.

9. A _____ is a machine used to determine the specific gravity of the urine.

10. A _____ is a disease that humans may acquire from animals.

Number the Steps

Number the steps of the procedure for giving a pill to a dog in the correct order.

_____ 11. Locate the dog to be medicated.

_____ 12. Close the animal's mouth and gently massage its throat to encourage swallowing.

_____ 13. Position your left hand over the dog's muzzle and use your fingers to manipulate the gums. If you are left-handed, position your right hand over the dog's muzzle.

_____ 14. Check with your supervisor or check the daily treatment sheet to be sure you know which dog needs a pill, and what pill is required.

_____ 15. Return the dog to its cage.

_____ 16. Return the pill bottle to its proper storage place.

_____ 17. Holding the pill in your right hand, use your right index finger to depress the lower jaw enough to allow you to quickly place the pill in the back central area of the mouth. If you are left-handed, use your left hand for this step.

_____ 18. Wash your hands

_____ 19. Find the pill bottle, read the label, and remove the correct number of pills. Double-check the name and amount of medication to be given.

_____ 20. If the dog spits out the pill, repeat the procedure.

_____ 21. With aggressive or large dogs, ask someone to assist you in restraining the dog for this procedure, if necessary.

_____ 22. Indicate in the animal's record which medication was given and cross the procedure off the treatment sheet.

_____ 23. Gently press the upper lips inward over the points of the teeth.

_____ 24. Slightly elevate the dog's head. (Gloves may be worn.)

Name _____   Date _____

Matching

Write the letter of the phrase that best matches each numbered item in the blank provided.

_____ 25. Diagnose and control animal diseases.

_____ 26. Perform experimental surgery.

_____ 27. Collecting blood, urine, tissues, and feces for diagnostic testing.

_____ 28. Cleaning cages.

_____ 29. Performed to remove offensive odors.

_____ 30. Performed to diagnose a urinary infection.

_____ 31. Performed to test for parasites.

_____ 32. Used to give vaccinations.

a. Veterinarian.

b. Veterinary technician.

c. Veterinary assistant.

d. Laboratory animal technician.

e. Subcutaneous injection.

f. Bathing.

g. Urinalysis.

h. Fecal examination.

True/False

Write "T" in the blank provided if the statement is true. Write "F" if the statement is false.

_____ 33. Laboratory animal technicians in biomedical research care for animals in a veterinarian office.

_____ 34. Normal dog stool contains parasites.

_____ 35. When giving a pill to a dog, gently massaging the throat may encourage swallowing.

_____ 36. A hookworm is a parasite.

_____ 37. Medication doses must be double checked prior to administration.

Name _____ Date _____

Animal Health Care

PROCEDURE 23A:
Bathing a Dog

········· **P R O C E D U R E   A S S E S S M E N T** ·········

Procedure Steps	Suggested Points	Self Practice	Peer Practice	Peer Testing	Final Testing	Total Earned
PREPROCEDURE						
1. Gather needed equipment.	5					
2. Identify animal.	6					
3. Ensure you know which products to use and review product instructions.	4					
4. Premix products according to directions, if necessary.	3					
5. You may want to wear a waterproof apron and/or rubber gloves.	3					
6. Remove dog's collar. Ensure it stays with dog throughout process.	4					
PROCEDURE						
7. Carefully put dog in bathtub.	6					
• Two people may be needed to bathe large dogs.						
• Large dogs also can be washed in dog run in warm weather.						
8. Put a bland ophthalmic ointment in dog's eyes to protect from soap.	6					
9. Thoroughly rinse dog with tepid water.	4					
10. Apply soap all over body according to directions.	3					
11. Carefully apply soap around dog's face. Avoid the eyes.	6					
12. Massage soap into dog's coat.	5					
13. Let soap remain on dog's coat for 5 to 15 minutes.	3					
14. Thoroughly rinse soap off dog, from top to bottom.	5					
15. Run your hands through dog's coat and check for suds.	4					
16. Let dog shake off excess water.	3					
17. Use clean towel to dry dog.	4					
• You can dry dog while it's still in tub.						
• Or, you can remove dog from tub and dry it on floor.						
18. Put dog's collar back on.	3					
• Put dry dog in cage.						
• Or, put dog in drying cage or dog run to finish drying.						
19. After dog is dry, brush its coat to remove loose hair.	3					

PROCEDURE 23A: Bathing a Dog (continued)

Procedure Steps POSTPROCEDURE	Suggested Points	Self Practice	Peer Practice	Peer Testing	Final Testing	Total Earned
20. Record bath in dog's medical record.	4					
21. Ensure dog is in correct cage and that it's properly identified.	6					
22. Rinse your gloves and the apron, if worn, and hang them to dry.	4					
23. Wash your hands.	6					
TOTAL POSSIBLE POINTS	100					

Comments: _____
_____
_____
_____
_____
_____
_____
_____
_____
_____

Signatures: _____ Date: _____

SCORING *See Preface for scoring instructions.*

Animal Health Care

PROCEDURE 23B:
Giving a Pill to a Dog

PROCEDURE ASSESSMENT

Procedure Steps	Suggested Points	Self Practice	Peer Practice	Peer Testing	Final Testing	Total Earned
PREPROCEDURE						
1. Gather needed equipment.	6					
2. Identify dog and ensure you know which pill is required for dog.	8					
3. Find pill bottle, read label, remove correct number of pills, and double-check name and amount of medication to be given.	7					
4. Locate dog to be medicated.	4					
5. With large or aggressive dogs, ask someone to help you restrain dog.	5					
PROCEDURE						
6. Slightly elevate dog's head.	5					
7. Put left hand over dog's muzzle and use fingers to manipulate gums. If you're left-handed, use right hand	5					
8. Hold pill in right hand and use right index finger to depress lower jaw.	7					
• Quickly put pill in back central area of mouth.	5					
• If you're left-handed, use left hand for this step.						
9. You may have to gently press upper lips inward over points of teeth so dog doesn't close jaw on your hand.	4					
10. Close dog's mouth and gently massage its throat to encourage swallowing.	6					
11. If dog spits out pill, repeat procedure.	4					
12. Some pills can be mixed with food. If you do this, ensure dog eats pill with the food.	6					
POSTPROCEDURE						
13. Return dog to its cage.	6					
14. Return pill bottle to its proper storage place.	7					
15. Record in dog's medical record which medication was given.	8					
16. Wash your hands.	8					
TOTAL POSSIBLE POINTS	**100**					

PROCEDURE 23B: Giving a Pill to a Dog *(continued)*

Comments: _____
_____
_____
_____
_____
_____
_____
_____
_____

Signatures: _____ **Date:** _____

SCORING   *See Preface for scoring instructions.*

Medical Laboratory   Reinforcement Activities

Matching

Write the letter of the phrase that best matches each numbered item in the blank provided. Answers may be used more than once and more than one answer may be correct.

_____ 1. Proper identification of a blood sample.   **a.** Medical technologist.

_____ 2. Transporting the specimen to the   **b.** Medical laboratory assistant.
designated location.

_____ 3. Maintaining confidentiality.   **c.** Medical laboratory technician.

_____ 4. Examine and analyze body fluids.   **d.** Phlebotomy technician.

_____ 5. Test urine with chemical reagent strips.

_____ 6. Prepare chemical solutions.

_____ 7. Prepare bacteriological smears.

_____ 8. Prepare blood for transfusion.

True/False

Write "T" in the blank provided if the statement is true. Write "F" if the statement is false.

_____ 9. The determination of a client's ABO, or blood type, is never done at a blood bank.

_____ 10. Rh-negative blood agglutinates with anti-D antiserum.

_____ 11. A venous blood sample requires a technique called a phlebotomy.

_____ 12. The normal amounts of hemoglobin never vary.

_____ 13. A hematocrit is a screening test that determines the presence of anemia.

_____ 14. Capillary blood collection is a noninvasive procedure.

_____ 15. The concentration of human chorionic gonadotropin or HCG is highest in the first-morning urine.

_____ 16. Proteinuria is excess protein in the urine.

_____ 17. The copper reduction test measures minerals in the urine.

Matching

Write the letter of the phrase that best matches each numbered item in the blank provided.

_____ 18. Phlebotomy

_____ 19. Venipuncture

_____ 20. Waived tests

_____ 21. Streptococcus pyogenes

_____ 22. Culture

_____ 23. Gram's stain

_____ 24. Point-of-care testing

_____ 25. Bilirubin

_____ 26. Blood

_____ 27. Specific gravity

_____ 28. Supernatant

_____ 29. Hematocrit

_____ 30. Hemoglobin

_____ 31. Agglutination

_____ 32. Protein

a. Helps identify the microorganisms present in specimen.

b. Indicates renal disease if found in urine.

c. Incision or cut into a vein.

d. MLAs can perform these.

e. Clear liquid on top of centrifuged specimen.

f. Measures the amount of solids present in the urine.

g. Puncture into a vein using a special needle.

h. Causes strep throat.

i. Screening test that determines presence of anemia.

j. Testing performed at the client's side; usually done immediately.

k. Indicates infection if found in urine.

l. Confirms the client's blood type.

m. Blood protein that helps transport oxygen.

n. Sign of hepatitis if found in urine.

o. Specimen is placed in a special condition to allow it to grow.

Fill in the Blank

Write the word (or words) that best completes the sentence in the blank provided.

33. _____ is a seaweed extract that is used to grow bacteria and other microorganisms.

34. When you inoculate an agar plate, incubate for _____, then examine.

35. Thick bacterial walls hold the _____ color of Gram's stain and are referred to as being _____.

36. Infectious mononucleosis is an acute disease caused by the _____ virus or _____.

37. As early as 400 B.C.E., physicians checked _____ for clues to illness.

38. _____ in the urine could be a sign of hepatitis, liver disease, or bile duct problems.

39. The _____ confirms the presence of protein in the urine.

40. _____ is an easy way to obtain a small amount of blood.

41. A _____ test determines the oxygen-carrying ability of the red blood cells.

42. The most common site for venipuncture is the _____ of the forearm.

43. A winged infusion set is also known as a _____.

44. _____ is one of the lipids normally found in the blood.

Name _____ Date _____

Medical Laboratory

PROCEDURE 24A:
Preparing Bacteriological Smears

PROCEDURE ASSESSMENT

Procedure Steps	Suggested Points	Self Practice	Peer Practice	Peer Testing	Final Testing	Total Earned
PREPROCEDURE						
1. Wash hands and put on gloves.	9					
2. Gather needed equipment.	6					
3. Label frosted end of slide with client's name.	9					
4. Make a circle on bottom of slide with wax pencil; it is where swab will be placed.	6					
PROCEDURE						
5. Roll specimen swab evenly over smooth part of slide.	6					
6. Dispose of swab in biohazard waste container.	9					
7. Allow smear to air-dry.	6					
8. Heat-fix slide:	7					
• Hold frosted end with forceps.	6					
• Pass clear part of slide, with smear side up, through flame of Bunsen burner 3 or 4 times.	6					
• Let slide cool before staining smear.	6					
POSTPROCEDURE						
9. Return materials to proper locations.	6					
10. Disinfect work area.	9					
11. Remove gloves and wash hands.	9					
TOTAL POSSIBLE POINTS	**100**					

Comments: _____
_____
_____
_____
_____
_____
_____
_____
_____

Signatures: _____ Date: _____

SCORING   *See Preface for scoring instructions.*

Name _____ Date _____

Medical Laboratory

PROCEDURE 24B:
Inoculating an Agar Plate

PROCEDURE ASSESSMENT

Procedure Steps	Suggested Points	Self Practice	Peer Practice	Peer Testing	Final Testing	Total Earned
PREPROCEDURE						
1. Gather needed equipment.	5					
2. Wash hands and put on gloves and face shield.	7					
PROCEDURE						
3. Remove specimen swab from container or use inoculating loop for collected urine.	4					
4. Hold agar plate by bottom (media side) and remove cover. Don't put cover on work area. Hold cover facing down.	4					
5. Roll swab down middle of top half of plate.	5					
• Then use swab to streak the same half of plate.	4					
• If you're using a loop, gently pull loop down middle of top half of plate, then streak the same half of plate.	4					
6. Dispose of swab in biohazard waste container.	7					
7. Sterilize a metal loop by putting it in Bunsen burner or Bacti-cinerator and let it cool.	7					
8. Streak agar to isolate colonies in third or fourth quadrants, using loop. In area of heavy inoculum, use loop to make slices in agar.	4					
9. Sterilize forceps, remove one disk from vial, and put disk on agar between cuts.	4					
10. Label agar side of plate (not lid) with:	7					
• Client's name and date.	4					
• Client's identification number and specimen information.	4					
11. Put plate with agar side of plate on top in incubator.	5					
12. Incubate for 24 hours and then examine. Incubate negative cultures for 24 more hours.	5					

PROCEDURE 24B: Inoculating an Agar Plate (continued)

Procedure Steps POSTPROCEDURE	Suggested Points	Self Practice	Peer Practice	Peer Testing	Final Testing	Total Earned
13. Disinfect work area.	7					
14. Remove gloves and face shield and wash hands.	7					
15. Record test results in client's record or on lab form.	6					
TOTAL POSSIBLE POINTS	**100**					

Comments:

_____

_____

_____

_____

_____

_____

_____

_____

Signatures: _____   **Date:** _____

SCORING   *See Preface for scoring instructions.*

Name _____ Date _____

Medical Laboratory

PROCEDURE 24C:
Staining Culture Smears with Gram's Stain

PROCEDURE ASSESSMENT

Procedure Steps	Suggested Points	Self Practice	Peer Practice	Peer Testing	Final Testing	Total Earned
PREPROCEDURE						
1. Gather needed equipment.	3					
2. Wash hands and put on gloves.	6					
3. Put heat-fixed smear on level staining rack and tray, with smear side up.	4					
PROCEDURE						
4. Completely cover specimen area of slide with crystal violet stain.	5					
5. Let stain sit for 1 minute.	3					
6. Wash slide thoroughly with water from wash bottle.	4					
7. Use forceps to hold slide at frosted end and tilt slide to remove excess water.	5					
8. Put slide flat on rack again and completely cover specimen area with iodine solution.	4					
9. Let iodine remain for 1 minute.	4					
10. Wash slide thoroughly with water.	3					
11. Use forceps to hold and tilt slide to remove excess water.	5					
12. While still tilting slide, apply alcohol or decolorizer drop by drop.	4					
• Do this until no more purple color washes off (usually 10 seconds or less).	3					
• Process usually takes 10 seconds or less.						
13. Wash slide thoroughly with water, using forceps to hold and tip slide to remove excess water.	3					
14. Completely cover specimen with safranin dye.	4					
15. Let safranin remain for 1 minute.	3					
16. Wash slide thoroughly with water.	4					
17. Use forceps to hold stained smear by frosted end and wipe back of slide to remove excess stain.	5					
18. Put smear in vertical position and let it air-dry.	4					
19. If this is a stat procedure, you may carefully blot slide between blotting paper.	4					

PROCEDURE 24C: Staining Culture Smears with Gram's Stain (continued)

Procedure Steps	Suggested Points	Self Practice	Peer Practice	Peer Testing	Final Testing	Total Earned
POSTPROCEDURE						
20. Disinfect work area.	6					
21. Remove gloves and wash hands.	6					
22. Document procedure and note observations.	4					
23. Retain slide for review by your supervisor.	4					
TOTAL POSSIBLE POINTS	100					

Comments:

_____
_____
_____
_____
_____
_____
_____
_____
_____

Signatures: _____ **Date:** _____

SCORING   See Preface for scoring instructions.

Medical Laboratory

PROCEDURE 24D:
Performing a Rapid Strep Test

PROCEDURE ASSESSMENT

Procedure Steps	Suggested Points	Self Practice	Peer Practice	Peer Testing	Final Testing	Total Earned
PREPROCEDURE						
1. Gather needed equipment.	5					
2. Wash hands and put on gloves and face shield.	9					
3. Review request form for proper identification and test procedure to be performed.	6					
4. Label tubes with client's name.	6					
5. Verify that controls for rapid strep test have been run for the day.	7					
• Verify that controls are within correct range.	5					
• Controls should be run daily.						
6. If controls haven't been run, review manufacturer's directions and run controls. Your supervisor may have to check results.	6					
7. Check expiration date of test kit.	5					
PROCEDURE						
8. Position all test reagents in order and follow manufacturer's directions.	6					
9. Be certain to time each reaction accurately.	6					
10. Dispose of all contaminated waste in biohazard waste container.	9					
11. Read test results at end of the timing.	6					
POSTPROCEDURE						
12. Disinfect work area.	9					
13. Remove gloves and face shield and wash hands.	9					
14. Record test results in client's record or on lab form.	6					
TOTAL POSSIBLE POINTS	**100**					

PROCEDURE 24D: Performing a Rapid Strep Test *(continued)*

Comments: _____

_____

_____

_____

_____

_____

_____

_____

Signatures: _____ **Date:** _____

SCORING *See Preface for scoring instructions.*

Name _____ Date _____

Medical Laboratory

PROCEDURE 24E1:
Assessing Urine for Color and Turbidity

PROCEDURE ASSESSMENT

Procedure Steps	Suggested Points	Self Practice	Peer Practice	Peer Testing	Final Testing	Total Earned
PREPROCEDURE						
1. Gather needed equipment.	7					
2. Wash hands and put on gloves. Practice standard precautions while handling specimens.	11					
3. Mix urine by swirling.	8					
4. Label centrifuge tube with client's name.	8					
PROCEDURE						
5. Pour specimen into centrifuge tube.	7					
6. Assess and record color.	8					
7. Assess and record clarity.	8					
8. Assess odor and record abnormalities, if any.	7					
POSTPROCEDURE						
9. Clean work area.	8					
10. Return items to their proper storage location.	8					
11. Remove gloves and wash hands.	11					
12. Record results in client's chart or on lab form.	9					
TOTAL POSSIBLE POINTS	100					

Comments:

_____

_____

_____

_____

_____

_____

_____

_____

Signatures: _____ **Date:** _____

SCORING *See Preface for scoring instructions.*

Name _____   Date _____

Medical Laboratory

PROCEDURE 24E2:
Measuring Specific Gravity Using a Urinometer

P R O C E D U R E   A S S E S S M E N T

Procedure Steps	Suggested Points	Self Practice	Peer Practice	Peer Testing	Final Testing	Total Earned
PREPROCEDURE						
1. Assemble urinometer, cylinder, urine specimen, and distilled water.	6					
2. Wash hands and put on gloves.	8					
3. Put on a face shield.	8					
4. Fill glass cylinder $2/_3$ full with room-temperature distilled water.	6					
5. Read specific gravity of distilled water at lower curve of meniscus. View meniscus at eye level.	6					
6. If urinometer doesn't read 1.000, try a new urinometer or use a correction factor.	5					
PROCEDURE						
7. Mix specimen by swirling.	6					
8. Pour specimen into clean glass cylinder to $2/_3$ to $3/_4$ full.	5					
9. Put cylinder on level surface and gently insert urinometer with a spinning motion.	6					
10. When urinometer stops rotating in specimen, read lower curve of meniscus.	6					
• Read at eye level.	5					
• Normal specific gravity is 1.010 to 1.025.						
POSTPROCEDURE						
11. Clean and dry equipment and return to its proper location.	5					
12. Disinfect work area.	6					
13. Remove face shield and gloves.	8					
14. Wash hands.	8					
15. Record results on client's record or on lab form.	6					
TOTAL POSSIBLE POINTS	100					

PROCEDURE 24E2: Measuring Specific Gravity Using a Urinometer *(continued)*

Comments: _____
_____
_____
_____
_____
_____
_____
_____
_____

Signatures: _____   Date: _____

SCORING   *See Preface for scoring instructions.*

Medical Laboratory

PROCEDURE 24E3:
Testing Urine with Chemical Reagent Strips

PROCEDURE ASSESSMENT

Procedure Steps	Suggested Points	Self Practice	Peer Practice	Peer Testing	Final Testing	Total Earned
PREPROCEDURE						
1. Gather needed equipment.	4					
2. Verify that quality control tests have been performed for the day. If necessary, perform tests as instructed by your supervisor.	5					
3. Review test strip bottle for timing required for each reagent pad. Determine order in which you will view the pads.	4					
4. Prepare client record for recording your results.	5					
5. Wash hands and put on gloves and face shield.	7					
PROCEDURE						
6. Swirl urine specimen to mix it thoroughly.	4					
7. Remove test strip from container and replace cap tightly.	4					
• Exposure to air can destroy reagent pads on test strips.						
• Closing cap immediately is important.						
8. Immerse strip completely in urine and remove it immediately.	5					
9. As you remove strip from urine, pull edge of strip across rim of container, then tap it on side, to remove excess urine.	4					
10. Start timing immediately.	4					
11. Hold dipstick close to, but not touching, container.	5					
• Compare reagent areas to corresponding area on container.	4					
• Record results.	4					
12. Continue process for entire number of reagent pads on dipstick.	4					

PROCEDURE 24E3: Testing Urine with Chemical Reagent Strips *(continued)*

Procedure Steps	Suggested Points	Self Practice	Peer Practice	Peer Testing	Final Testing	Total Earned
POSTPROCEDURE						
13. Dispose of used reagent strips in biohazard waste container.	5					
14. Disinfect work area.	7					
15. Return items to their proper storage location.	5					
16. Remove face shield and gloves.	7					
17. Wash hands.	7					
18. Record results in client's record or on lab form.	6					
TOTAL POSSIBLE POINTS	**100**					

Comments:

_____

_____

_____

_____

_____

_____

_____

_____

_____

_____

Signatures: _____   Date: _____

SCORING   *See Preface for scoring instructions.*

Name _____   Date _____

Medical Laboratory

PROCEDURE 24E4:
Microscopic Urine Analysis

-------- **PROCEDURE ASSESSMENT** --------

Procedure Steps	Suggested Points	Self Practice	Peer Practice	Peer Testing	Final Testing	Total Earned
PREPROCEDURE						
1. Gather needed equipment.	3					
2. Ensure centrifuge has been checked with tachometer for correct rpms. Follow manufacturer's instructions or check with supervisor.	4					
3. Wash hands.	5					
4. Put on gloves and face shield.	5					
PROCEDURE						
5. Mix urine specimen by swirling.	3					
6. Pour urine into labeled centrifuge tube and cap tube.	2					
7. Put tube in centrifuge. If more than one urine specimen is being centrifuged at this time, number each specimen.	2					
8. Balance load by putting another tube containing equal amount of urine or water directly across from specimen.	2					
9. Close lid and centrifuge for time specified for your centrifuge. Review manufacturer's instructions or facility policy.	2					
10. After centrifuge has completely stopped, remove one tube at a time.	3					
11. Pour off supernatant from top of specimen by quickly inverting tube over sink. Make sure to retain sediment in bottom of tube.	2					
12. Grasp tube near top and tap it on countertop until all sediment is resuspended.	3					
13. Aspirate one drop of sediment into disposable pipette and put on clean, labeled slide.	2					
14. Put clean coverslip over drop of sediment and put slide on microscope stage.	2					
15. Remove face shield.	3					
16. Focus under low power and reduce the light.	3					
17. Scan entire coverslip area for abnormal findings.	2					
18. Examine five low-power fields for casts and epithelial cells.	4					
• Always review number of fields specified in lab guidelines.	2					

Procedure Steps	Suggested Points	Self Practice	Peer Practice	Peer Testing	Final Testing	Total Earned
• Count and classify each type of cast you see.	2					
• Indicate if mucus is present.	2					
• If you are new to this analysis, use picture chart or ask supervisor for help.						
19. Switch to high power and adjust the light.	2					
20. Count five high-power fields or the number indicated in lab guidelines. Identify elements viewed.	2					
21. Report the following:	4					
• Red blood cells and white blood cells.	1					
• Epithelial cells and crystals.	1					
• Bacteria, yeast, and parasites.	1					
• Sperm, if so indicated by lab guidelines.	1					
22. Turn off microscope light to avoid drying out specimen.	3					
POSTPROCEDURE						
23. Add elements identified in the five fields, divide by 5 to get average, and report results.	4					
24. Leave slide in microscope so physician can verify results.	3					
25. Return items to proper storage location.	2					
26. Disinfect work area.	5					
27. Remove face shield and gloves.	5					
28. Wash hands.	5					
29. Record verified results on client's chart or on lab form.	3					
TOTAL POSSIBLE POINTS	**100**					

Comments:

_____

_____

_____

_____

_____

_____

_____

_____

_____

Signatures: _____   Date: _____

SCORING   *See Preface for scoring instructions.*

Medical Testing

Reinforcement Activities

Matching

Write the letter of the phrase that best matches each numbered item in the blank provided.

_____ 1. Invasive.

_____ 2. Cardiovascular.

_____ 3. Parkinson's disease.

_____ 4. Electrocardiograph.

_____ 5. Electrocardiogram.

_____ 6. Electroencephalogram.

a. Tracing of the heart's electrical activity.

b. Tracing of the brain's electrical activity.

c. Pertaining to the heart and blood vessels.

d. Instrument used to record the electrical activity of the heart.

e. Entrance into a body cavity.

f. Neuromuscular disorder.

True/False

Write "T" in the blank provided if the statement is true. Write "F" if the statement is false.

_____ 7. It is the ECG technician's responsibility to inform the client of the results of an electrocardiogram.

_____ 8. An electroencephalography technologist only performs electroencephalograms.

_____ 9. During a balloon angioplasty the cardiovascular technologist will monitor the client's heart, blood pressure, and electrocardiogram.

_____ 10. The most likely place you would be employed as an ECG technician is in a hospital.

Multiple Choice

Circle the letter that best answers the question or completes the statement.

11. As an ECG technician which of the following would you most likely be performing?
    a. an electrocardiogram.
    b. an electroencephalogram.
    c. a cardiac catherization.
    d. an balloon angioplasty.

12. After performing an ECG on your client she asks, "Did I pass?" What would be your *best* response to this question?
    a. You will need to discuss this with your doctor who should have the results ready by tomorrow.
    b. Everything looks great, when you return the next week you can talk with the doctor about your results.
    c. I do not know. I am only the ECG technician.
    d. This test is really not a pass/fail.

13. Which of the following *best* describes the duties of a cardiovascular technologist?
    a. performs diagnostic tests on the brain and nervous system.
    b. views and monitors the ECG tracing.
    c. applies electrodes and leads for various diagnostic tests on the heart.
    d. performs a variety of tests on the cardiovascular system.

14. Which of the following diagnostic tests is used to correct coronary artery disease?
    a. cardiac catheterization.
    b. echocardiogram.
    c. balloon angioplasty.
    d. pacemaker.

15. Which of the following is the less likely location for an EEG or END technologist to be employed?
    a. neurologist office.
    b. sleep laboratory.
    c. mobile screening unit.
    d. neurodiagnostic department of a hospital.

16. Which of the following *best* describes an EEG?
    a. A tracing of the electrical activity of the heart used to diagnose disorders.
    b. A tracing of the electrical activity of the brain used to diagnose disorders.
    c. An procedure that evaluates the heart.
    d. A diagnostic test that uses sound waves to evaluate the nervous system.

Fill in the Blank

Write the word (or words) that best completes the sentence in the blank provided.

17. Ask the client to _____ his or her name. For hospitalized clients, check the _____.

18. Move the bed or exam table away from _____.

19. Lead wires should follow the _____ of the body; avoid _____ outside of the body.

20. _____ ECG reports will need to be cut and mounted; _____ ECG reports may need to be attached to a firmer backing.

Labeling

21. Label the parts of the conduction system shown in this figure.

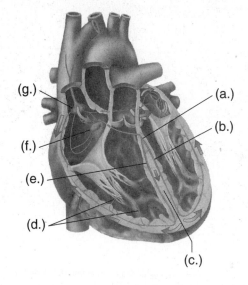

(a.) _____   **(e.)** _____

(b.) _____   **(f.)** _____

(c.) _____   **(g.)** _____

(d.) _____

22. Label the ECG waveform showing the electrical activity of the heart.

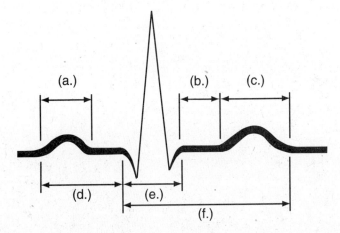

(a.) _____   **(d.)** _____

(b.) _____   **(e.)** _____

(c.) _____   **(f.)** _____

Name _____ Date _____

Medical Testing

PROCEDURE 25A:
Recording an Electrocardiogram

---- P R O C E D U R E   A S S E S S M E N T ----

Procedure Steps	Suggested Points	Self Practice	Peer Practice	Peer Testing	Final Testing	Total Earned
PREPROCEDURE						
1. Receive and validate physician's order and complete requisition form.	2					
2. Ensure machine is working properly.	4					
• Ensure grounding prong is attached to plug.	2					
• Plug in machine securely.	2					
• Check insulation on lead wires for cracks.	2					
3. Gather needed supplies.	1					
4. Read manufacturer's instructions; keep them nearby for reference.	2					
5. Ensure paper supply is adequate.	2					
• Check for a thick red line at base of paper.	1					
• If you see a red line, paper supply may be low.						
6. Change paper as necessary.	2					
7. Enter client data (on completed requisition form) into ECG machine.	2					
PROCEDURE						
8. Identify client.	4					
9. Explain procedure to client.	4					
10. Wash hands and observe standard precautions.	4					
11. Prepare and position client.	2					
• Ask client to remove clothing and jewelry from waist up.	1					
• Place client on back with arms and legs resting on bed or exam table.	1					
12. Provide for client privacy.	2					
• Pull curtain around bed or table or close door.	1					
• Use towel or sheet to drape client's chest.	1					
13. Make sure bed or table isn't touching the wall.	2					
14. Move bed or table away from electrical equipment.	1					
15. Make sure client isn't touching headboard, footboard, or side rails.	2					

PROCEDURE 25A: Recording an Electrocardiogram (continued)

Procedure Steps	Suggested Points	Self Practice	Peer Practice	Peer Testing	Final Testing	Total Earned
16. Clean and prepare skin as necessary.	2					
• Remove lotion or oil from skin with alcohol swab.	1					
• You may have to shave chest hair from small area.						
17. Review manufacturer's instructions, then apply electrodes to chest.	2					
18. Apply electrodes to arms and legs.	2					
• Choose fleshy area with least amount of hair for each electrode.	1					
• Put arm electrodes on wrists or upper arms.	1					
• Put leg electrodes on inside of lower legs.	1					
• If necessary, put leg electrodes on upper legs, close to trunk.						
• Arm and leg electrodes should be at same location on both sides.	1					
19. Attach lead wires.	2					
• Ensure there is no tension on the wires.	1					
• Identify correct cable for each electrode by referring to color and letter abbreviations.	1					
• Lead wire cables should follow the contours of the body.	1					
• Lead wire cables should not form loops.	1					
20. To operate ECG machine.	2					
• For automatic ECG machines, press Run or Auto button.	1					
• Tracing for automatic ECG machine will take 15 to 20 seconds.	1					
• For manual ECG machine, ensure equipment is standardized and set to Lead 1.	1					
• Record each of 12 lead tracings on manual ECG machine by stopping machine and changing lead indicator switch.	1					
• Carefully follow directions in operator's manual.						
21. Observe display for errors.	2					
• Automatic ECG machines will display errors on screen.						
• Correct errors as necessary.						
22. Check tracing for quality and accuracy.	2					

PROCEDURE 25A: Recording an Electrocardiogram *(continued)*

Procedure Steps	Suggested Points	Self Practice	Peer Practice	Peer Testing	Final Testing	Total Earned
23. Troubleshoot any problems. Review pages 818–819 of the textbook before you begin.	1					
24. Turn off and unplug machine.	2					
25. Remove electrodes and clean skin, if necessary.	2					
26. Help client to safe, comfortable position.	2					
• Provide for client privacy.	1					
• Help client dress, if necessary..						
27. Tell client when results will be ready and explain that client needs to talk to physician about results.	2					
28. Practice performing an ECG 3 times, at least, before recording one on a client.	2					
POSTPROCEDURE						
29. Write on tracing any variations in lead placement or reason for poor-quality tracing.	2					
30. Mount and prepare tracing for review.	2					
• For single-channel ECG machine, cut and mount each lead tracing.	1					
• For multichannel ECG machine, you may need to mount tracing on firmer backing.						
31. Give results to physician; if in a "stat" situation, do so immediately.	2					
32. Put completed ECG tracing in a place specified by facility procedure.	1					
33. Ensure client is billed for procedure.	2					
34. Clean lead wires and machine.	1					
• If client is in isolation or has a contagious disease, clean equipment according to facility guidelines.						
• Doing this will help prevent the spread of infection.						
35. Drape lead wires of machine in an orderly fashion.	2					
36. Return machine to designated storage location.	1					
TOTAL POSSIBLE POINTS	**100**					

Comments: _____
_____
_____
_____
_____
_____
_____
_____
_____

Signatures: _____ **Date:** _____

SCORING   *See Preface for scoring instructions.*

Radiology

Reinforcement Activities

Matching

Write the letter of the phrase that best matches each numbered item in the blank provided.

_____ 1. Radiologic technologist.

_____ 2. X ray.

_____ 3. Radiograph.

_____ 4. Radiography.

_____ 5. Fluoroscopy.

_____ 6. Radiologist.

a. An imaging process that projects an image of a client on to an X-ray film.

b. The black and white two-dimensional picture of a client's three-dimensional anatomy that is generated by X rays.

c. The process of projecting an image of a client onto fluorescent screens for real-time viewing.

d. An electromagnetic wave with a shorter wavelength than light that allows for the penetration of objects.

e. A physician who is a specialist in the use of radiant energy to diagnose and treat disease.

f. A person educated and trained to use radiant energy to produce diagnostic images or to administer radiation treatments under supervision.

True/False

Write "T" in the blank provided if the statement is true. Write "F" if the statement is false.

_____ 7. A collimator is a beam restricting device mounted under the X-ray tube housing.

_____ 8. Radiation oncologists conduct the diagnosis of findings for all images produced on clients and generate a written report for the client's attending physician.

_____ 9. Radiologic technologists are physicians.

_____ 10. LINAC stands for Linear Accelerator.

_____ 11. Quality management technology is considered a primary field of radiologic technology.

_____ 12. To remain a registered technologist in good standing with the American Registry of Radiologic Technologists (ARRT), a technologist must obtain a minimum of 24 approved continuing education units within a 24 month period.

_____ 13. Clients who are allergic to peanuts may find it difficult to tolerate iodine-based contrast media used for certain procedures.

_____ 14. A Roentgen ray is the same as an X ray.

_____ 15. An X ray is the same as a radiograph.

_____ **16.** An iodine-based contrast media is swallowed or inserted into the rectum while barium based contrast media is injected into blood vessels.

_____ **17.** X rays were discovered on November 8, 1895, by Dr. Wilhelm Conrad Roentgen.

Multiple Choice

Circle the letter that best answers the question or completes the statement.

18. One of the following is *not* a good radiation protection practice
    a. Perform the procedure correctly the first time.
    b. Collimate to the part being radiographed.
    c. Wear protective aprons when holding clients.
    d. Maintain a safe distance.
    e. Wear a radiation film badge that monitors exposure.

19. One of the following is *not* considered an invasive radiographic procedure
    a. Arteriography.
    b. Cervical Spine.
    c. Venogram.
    d. Myelogram.
    e. Arthrogram.

20. The Mammography Quality Standards Act applies to
    a. Radiographers.
    b. Mammographers.
    c. Magnetic Resonance Technologists.
    d. None of the above.
    e. All of the above.

21. With Picture Archival Communication Systems (PACS), radiologic technologists can do all of the following to images except
    a. Capture images.
    b. Manipulate image quality.
    c. Transmit images.
    d. Archive and retrieve images.
    e. Develop images.

22. The professional association for radiologic technologists is called the
    a. American College of Radiology.
    b. American Board of Radiology.
    c. American Society of Radiologic Technologists.
    d. American Registry of Radiologic Technologists.
    e. American Medical Association.

Name _____ Date _____

Labeling

23. Label the following X-ray production tube and, in the space provided, briefly describe how X rays are produced.

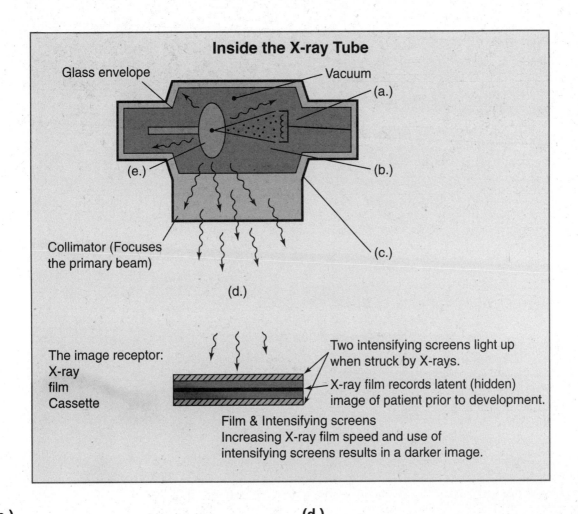

Inside the X-ray Tube

Glass envelope

Vacuum

(a.)

(e.)

(b.)

Collimator (Focuses the primary beam)

(c.)

(d.)

The image receptor:
X-ray
film
Cassette

Two intensifying screens light up when struck by X-rays.

X-ray film records latent (hidden) image of patient prior to development.

Film & Intensifying screens
Increasing X-ray film speed and use of intensifying screens results in a darker image.

(a.) _____   (d.) _____

(b.) _____   (e.) _____

(c.) _____

_____
_____
_____
_____
_____
_____
_____
_____
_____
_____
_____

Radiology

PROCEDURE 26A:
Adult Posterior-Anterior (PA) Chest Radiographic

········ P R O C E D U R E   A S S E S S M E N T ········

Procedure Steps	Suggested Points	Self Practice	Peer Practice	Peer Testing	Final Testing	Total Earned
PREPROCEDURE						
1. Gather needed equipment and wash hands.	5					
2. Ask client to remove all clothing and jewelry from around chest.	4					
• Ask client if he/she has ever had open-heart surgery; if so, chest may contain metal sutures that will block X rays from reaching the film.	3					
• Make a note for the radiologist if client has had open-heart surgery.						
• Ask client to put on gown with straps tied in back and sit down.	3					
3. Select a 14- by 17-inch cassette and put it lengthwise (portrait) in upright chest cassette holder.	3					
• For infants, children, and teenagers, use a 8- by 10-inch, 10- by 12-inch, or 11- by 14-inch cassette.	2					
• Very large clients may require two 14- by 17-inch cassettes, one placed crosswise (landscape) to take top part of chest, and one placed crosswise (landscape) to take bottom part of chest.	2					
4. To affix markers.	3					
• Tape the right "R" lead letter marker in upper right-hand border to coincide with client's right side.	2					
• Or tape the left "L" lead letter marker in upper left-hand side to coincide with client's left side.	2					
• Ensure marker isn't superimposed with client's upper right or left chest lung field or with client's identification field.	2					
5. Direct central ray of X-ray beam (flashlight) horizontal and perpendicular to cassette at distance of 6 feet from tube to cassette.	3					
6. Adjust size of beam to cassette; a good radiation protection measure is ¼ inch just inside the 14- by 17-inch field.	4					
7. Provide lead shielding across posterior pelvis to prevent exposing gonads to direct or scatter radiation.	3					

PROCEDURE 26A: Adult Posterior-Anterior (PA) Chest Radiographic *(continued)*

Procedure Steps	Suggested Points	Self Practice	Peer Practice	Peer Testing	Final Testing	Total Earned
PROCEDURE						
8. Have client stand with front part of chest flush against cassette surface.	4					
9. Adjust median plane of client's body so it is perpendicular to and over center of cassette.	3					
10. Put client's acromion processes (shoulder joint area) 3 inches below upper cassette film border.	4					
11. Adjust central ray of X-ray beam to center of cassette.	3					
12. Immobilize part.	4					
• If client moves during X-ray exposure, image may be blurred and useless for final diagnosis.						
• If necessary, use tape, sand bag, sponge, strap, or handrail to immobilize part.						
• Never should another person immobilize a client during X-ray exposure.						
13. Tell client that soon, you will ask him/her to take a deep breath and blow out several times, then take one final deep breath and hold it.	4					
14. Tell client to take a deep breath, blow it out, and repeat. Then tell client to take a deep breath and hold it.	4					
15. Observe client at height of inhalation.	4					
• Say "Hold it" loudly.	3					
• If client is not breathing or moving, press switch and make exposure.						
POSTPROCEDURE						
16. Give client post-exposure instructions:	3					
• Tell client that he/she may breathe now.	2					
• Tell client that you want him/her to remain unclothed in exam room.	2					
• Tell client that now you will develop radiograph to see if image is good, and then you will come back and tell client to dress.	2					
• Explain that if image quality is poor, you will have to take another radiograph.	2					
17. Remove 14- by 17-inch cassette.	4					
• Put cassette in darkroom pass box with client ID card.	3					
• Have darkroom technician develop the film.	3					
18. Clean area and wash hands.	5					
TOTAL POSSIBLE POINTS	**100**					

PROCEDURE 26A: Adult Posterior-Anterior (PA) Chest Radiographic (continued)

Comments: _____
_____
_____
_____
_____
_____
_____
_____
_____
_____

Signatures: _____ Date: _____

SCORING   See Preface for scoring instructions.

Ophthalmic Care

Reinforcement Activities

Matching

Write the letter of the phrase that best matches each numbered item in the blank provided.

_____ 1. Ishihara color graph

_____ 2. Cornea

_____ 3. Presbyopia

_____ 4. OD, OS

_____ 5. Cataract

_____ 6. LASIK

_____ 7. Retina

a. The inability of the eye lens to focus incoming light.

b. Laser-assisted in situ keratomileusis, a type of corrective eye surgery.

c. Illustrations that contain numbers, lines or symbols that appear as colored dots among other colored dots.

d. Right eye, Left eye.

e. A transparent curved layer of the eye responsible for refracting light.

f. Cloudy or opaque lens in the eye causing blurred vision.

g. The area in the back of the eye where light is focused.

True/False

Write "T" in the blank provided if the statement is true. Write "F" if the statement is false.

_____ 8. One of the duties of the Optometrist may be to prescribe drugs to treat eye disease.

_____ 9. Color deficiency is hereditary, present at birth.

_____ 10. An Optometrist may perform surgery.

_____ 11. Myopia is a condition where near objects are blurry, but far objects are in focus.

_____ 12. Most people develop presbyopia in their 40s.

_____ 13. A far-vision chart should be mounted 20 feet from the client.

Multiple Choice

Circle the letter that best answers the question or completes the statement.

14. All of the following are types of corrective eye surgery *except:*
    a. corneal implants.
    b. strabismus.
    c. radial keratotomy.
    d. PRK.

15. Most clients of orthoptists are:
    a. elderly
    b. men
    c. children
    d. women

16. Which of the following *best* describes glaucoma?
    a. an increase in pressure inside the eyeball
    b. a cloudy area of the eye lens
    c. an itching of the eye area
    d. a muscle weakness of the eye

17. Which of the following is the *best* description for hyperopia?
    a. near and far objects appear blurry
    b. far objects focused, near objects blurry
    c. one eye focused, the other strays
    d. far objects blurry, near objects focused

18. Which of the following interprets the light that is focused on the retina and sends the information to the brain?
    a. cataract
    b. cornea
    c. strabismus
    d. optic nerve

19. The primary function of ophthalmic medical personnel is to:
    a. Teach children and their parents exercises to strengthen the eye muscles.
    b. Examine written prescriptions to determine lens specifications.
    c. Assist the ophthalmologist or optometrist.
    d. Diagnose and treat eye disorders.

Fill in the Blank

Write the word (or words) that best completes the sentence in the blank provided.

20. _____ is the ability of the eye lens to change its shape to focus an image on the retina.

21. The _____ examines the eyes to diagnose vision problems and eye diseases.

22. _____ is blurred vision caused by an irregularly shaped cornea.

23. The shape of the cornea affects the way light focuses onto the retina. Changing its shape _____ and _____ vision.

24. The _____ is a medical doctor who specializes in diseases and disorders of the eye.

25. _____ is a condition in which one eye focuses properly and the other eye strays.

Name _____ Date _____

Labeling

26.

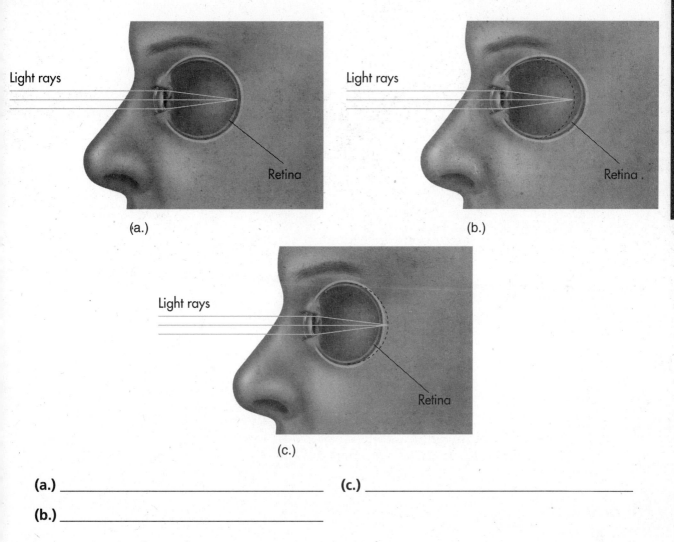

(a.)

(b.)

(c.)

(a.) _____ **(c.)** _____

(b.) _____

Based upon the above pictures answer these questions.

27. Which client would be nearsighted? _____

28. Which client would be farsighted? _____

29. Which client has normal vision? _____

30. What is the retina? _____

_____

Ophthalmic Care

PROCEDURE 27A:
Measuring Visual Acuity

PROCEDURE ASSESSMENT

Procedure Steps	Suggested Points	Self Practice	Peer Practice	Peer Testing	Final Testing	Total Earned
PREPROCEDURE						
1. Assemble equipment.	2					
2. If using reusable eye occluder, clean it.	4					
3. Mount far vision chart 20 feet away.	2					
4. Wash hands.	4					
PROCEDURE						
5. Identify client and explain procedure.	4					
6. If client is a non-reader, use demonstration cards for Snellen E or pictorial chart.	3					
7. Test vision.	3					
a. Test with corrective lenses, then without.	2					
b. Check both eyes.	2					
c. Check each eye separately, right then left.	2					
8. Tell client not to squint, lean forward, or move card.	3					
9. Tell client to keep both eyes open and cover just one eye.	4					
For Far Vision						
• Make sure that client is 20 feet from chart.	3					
• Ask client to read the letters as you point to them at random.	3					
• Note if client is squinting or blinking.	3					
• Ask client to identify all letters on the 20/20 line.	3					
a. If client cannot, note which line he/she can read accurately.	2					
• For children, start at a 40- or 30-foot line, then proceed to 20.	3					
a. Note which line he/she can read with reasonable accuracy.	2					
• Record results with glasses, if worn, and without.	3					
a. Both eyes—O.U. 20/20 cc	2					
b. Right eye—O.D. 20/20 cc	2					
c. Left eye—O.S. 20/20 cc	2					
d. Both eyes without glasses—O.U. 20/20	2					
e. Right eye without glasses—O.D. 20/20	2					
f. Left eye without glasses—O.S. 20/20	2					

Procedure Steps	Suggested Points	Self Practice	Peer Practice	Peer Testing	Final Testing	Total Earned
For Near Vision						
• Have client hold chart 14 to 16 inches from eye.	3					
• Ask client to read letters on chart.	3					
• Note if client is squinting or blinking.	3					
• Note smallest line he/she can read accurately with glasses, if worn, and without.	3					
POSTPROCEDURE						
10. Clean or throw away occluder.	4					
11. If near vision card is laminated, clean it.	4					
12. Dispose of the cleaning supplies properly.	4					
13. Clean area and put away equipment.	3					
14. Wash hands.	4					
TOTAL POSSIBLE POINTS	100					

Comments: _____

_____

_____

_____

_____

_____

_____

_____

_____

Signatures: _____   Date: _____

SCORING   *See Preface for scoring instructions.*

Name _____   Date _____

Ophthalmic Care

PROCEDURE 27B:
Testing Color Vision

········· P R O C E D U R E   A S S E S S M E N T ·········

Procedure Steps	Suggested Points	Self Practice	Peer Practice	Peer Testing	Final Testing	Total Earned
PREPROCEDURE						
1. Have your color vision screened before you perform a color vision test.	5					
2. Gather equipment.	5					
3. Wash hands.	8					
4. Perform test in well-lighted room.	7					
• Avoid direct sunlight and fluorescent lights.	5					
PROCEDURE						
5. Identify client and explain test's purpose.	5					
6. Show client a testing procedure example.	5					
7. Hold chart 14 to 16 inches from client, at a right angle.	6					
8. Record results as client reads number or traces line in each slide.	5					
9. Remain quiet and professional.	5					
10. If you must test each eye separately, use eye occluder or card.	6					
11. Total results and record as "13 correct/1 incorrect."	7					
• Tell doctor which slides were incorrectly identified.	6					
POSTPROCEDURE						
12. If slides are covered with plastic, clean them.	5					
13. Wash hands.	8					
14. Clean area and put away equipment.	7					
• Store slide booklet closed.	5					
TOTAL POSSIBLE POINTS	100					

PROCEDURE 27B: Testing Color Vision *(continued)*

Comments: _____
_____
_____
_____
_____
_____
_____
_____
_____
_____

Signatures: _____ Date: _____

SCORING   See Preface for scoring instructions.

Ophthalmic Care

PROCEDURE 27C:
Caring for Eyeglasses

PROCEDURE ASSESSMENT

Procedure Steps	Suggested Points	Self Practice	Peer Practice	Peer Testing	Final Testing	Total Earned
PREPROCEDURE						
1. Gather equipment.	7					
2. Wash hands.	10					
PROCEDURE						
3. Identify client and explain procedure.	8					
4. Remove glasses, touching only frames.	10					
5. Rinse glasses with mild soap and cool water.	7					
6. Place towel in bottom of sink.	10					
7. If available, rinse with commercial cleaning solution.	7					
8. Dry glasses with lint-free cloth.	8					
9. Give glasses to client.	7					
POSTPROCEDURE						
10. Clean area and put away equipment.	6					
11. Ensure client's safety and comfort.	10					
12. Wash hands.	10					
TOTAL POSSIBLE POINTS	100					

Comments: _____

_____

_____

_____

_____

_____

_____

_____

_____

_____

Signatures: _____   **Date:** _____

SCORING   *See Preface for scoring instructions.*

Medical Office

Reinforcement Activities

Matching

Write the letter of the phrase that best matches each numbered item in the blank provided.

_____ 1. Insured.

_____ 2. Superbill.

_____ 3. Reimbursement.

_____ 4. Form locators.

_____ 5. Delegate.

_____ 6. Co-payment

_____ 7. Subscriber

_____ 8. Fraud

_____ 9. Ethics

_____ 10. Deductible

_____ 11. Benefit

_____ 12. Balance

_____ 13. Tickler report

_____ 14. EOB

_____ 15. Statement

a. Also known as an encounter form.

b. The ability to trust and assign tasks.

c. Payment from an insurance company.

d. Also known as the subscriber.

e. Boxes on the HCFA-1500 form.

f. Misrepresentation of facts with intent to deceive.

g. Written notification of payment from insurance provider.

h. Medical expenses covered and the payable amount owed to a medical provider by the insurance company.

i. A payment usually collected by the front office staff; not a deductible.

j. A written request for payment made to the client.

k. A personal and professional standard of conduct.

l. Helps the billing and insurance specialist keep track of overdue accounts.

m. A payment usually collected by the front office staff; not a co-payment.

n. Amount owed by a client to an office.

o. A client who holds an insurance policy, also known as a policyholder.

True/False

Write "T" in the blank provided if the statement is true. Write "F" if the statement is false.

_____ 16. Computer skills are suggested, but not mandatory for the medical office employee.

_____ 17. When preparing the appointment schedule, the matrix and the buffer are used to schedule clients who may call in for an emergency appointment.

_____ 18. Personal information about a client should be obtained privately.

_____ 19. A medical record can be filed as inactive if the client has not been seen in a certain length of time or no longer needs the services of the physician.

_____ 20. After 90 days the medical office may turn over an account to a collection agency.

Multiple Choice

Circle the letter that best answers the question or completes the statement.

21. The front office employee who greets the client must have a professional appearance including
   a. conservative makeup.
   b. limited jewelry.
   c. wrinkle-free uniform or business dress.
   d. all of the above.

22. A method used by medical office employees answering the phone or greeting clients to determine the urgency for medical care is called
   a. compliance.
   b. triage.
   c. empathy.
   d. professionalism.

23. A spouse or child eligible to receive insurance benefits because of the eligibility of the policyholder is known as a(n)
   a. claim.
   b. resident.
   c. dependent.
   d. subscriber.

24. The medical office employee who is responsible for the efficiency and daily operations of the office is usually the
   a. medical administrative assistant.
   b. insurance specialist.
   c. medical office manager.
   d. billing and collections specialist.

25. A percentage of payment paid by the client upon receiving services is known as a(n)
   a. coinsurance.
   b. deductible.
   c. balance.
   d. copayment.

Fill in the Blank

Write the word (or words) that best completes the sentence in the blank provided.

26. The ability to understand human behavior and use this knowledge positively defines the term _____.

27. The individual record of a client's financial account is kept in the _____.

28. A formal request to an insurance provider for reconsideration of a denied claim is called an _____.

29. Medical office employees who answer the phone should speak clearly and courteously, and _____ client problems efficiently.

30. A reverse _____ record contains the most recent information on top.

Filing Alphabetically

Number the following names in the correct filing order using the alphabetical filing system.

_____ 31. Irene J. MacKay

_____ 32. Samuel L. Jackson

_____ 33. Marsha V. Mason

_____ 34. Beatrice Margaret Jones

_____ 35. Marsha A. Mason

Name _____ Date _____

Medical Office

PROCEDURE 28A:
Using the Telephone

PROCEDURE ASSESSMENT

Procedure Steps	Suggested Points	Self Practice	Peer Practice	Peer Testing	Final Testing	Total Earned
PREPROCEDURE						
1. Gather needed equipment and turn on computer, monitor, and software program used for scheduling, if necessary.	5					
2. Check answering machine or voice mail system for messages.	5					
• Write down information.	4					
• Give messages to appropriate people or handle calls yourself.	4					
PROCEDURE						
3. Answer phone on second ring, if possible, and hold receiver 1 inch from your mouth.	4					
4. Don't answer phone by saying, "Hold, please."	5					
5. Give name of facility and your name; in a pleasant voice, ask how you can help caller.	4					
6. Speak directly into receiver and give caller your full attention.	4					
7. Determine reason for call and urgency of call.	4					
• Ask for caller's name, write it down, and use it while talking to caller.	3					
• Politely ask caller to spell his/her name if you aren't sure of spelling.	3					
8. If call is an emergency, put call through to physician or call 911, depending on office procedure.	7					
9. For all other calls, answer caller's questions if you can. If you can't, take a message. Write down:	5					
• Name of caller.	4					
• General nature of call.	4					
• Date and time of call.	4					
• Return phone number.	4					
10. Restate message and caller's name and phone number; ask caller to confirm accuracy.	5					
11. If you must put caller on hold, first ask permission to do so, and don't leave caller on hold for more than 1 minute.	5					

PROCEDURE 28A: Using the Telephone (continued)

Procedure Steps POSTPROCEDURE	Suggested Points	Self Practice	Peer Practice	Peer Testing	Final Testing	Total Earned
12. Thank caller and let caller hang up first, or transfer call.	4					
13. Send written message to appropriate person.	4					
14. If you handled call, note in client's medical record:	5					
• Date, time, and nature of call.	4					
TOTAL POSSIBLE POINTS	100					

Comments: _____

_____

_____

_____

_____

_____

_____

_____

_____

_____

Signatures: _____   Date: _____

SCORING   See Preface for scoring instructions.

Medical Office

PROCEDURE 28B:
Scheduling Appointments

PROCEDURE ASSESSMENT

Procedure Steps	Suggested Points	Self Practice	Peer Practice	Peer Testing	Final Testing	Total Earned
PREPROCEDURE						
1. Gather needed supplies.	4					
• Check office policy for length of time to schedule appointments.	2					
2. Establish a matrix using a pen. The schedule book is a legal document:	8					
• Record day of week and month, day, and year on top of each page of book.	5					
• Write name of each physician in the practice in top column of daily record, one physician per column.	5					
• Determine what hours office will be closed and when each physician won't be available to see clients.	5					
a. Put large "X" through corresponding times in book.	4					
b. Mark lunch hours and times of physician's personal appointments.	4					
c. Mark "X" through holidays when office will be closed.	4					
PROCEDURE						
3. When a client calls office for appointment:	5					
• Determine nature of call by using telephone triage.	1					
• Get as much information as possible about need for appointment.	1					
4. Determine client's first choice for date and time.	5					
• Check appointment book to determine if that date and time is available.	4					
• Use telephone courtesy.	4					
• Help client find date and time that works for client.	4					
5. When you and client have decided on date and time, write in client's name, phone number, and nature of call in pencil.	3					
• If your facility uses abbreviations for complaints, use them in book.	1					
• List of abbreviations should be placed near book.	1					
• Everyone who writes in book should use same abbreviations.						

Procedure Steps	Suggested Points	Self Practice	Peer Practice	Peer Testing	Final Testing	Total Earned
6. Using pencil, draw downward arrow to block off time for appointment.	5					
• Amount of time necessary is determined by nature of call and office policy.						
• Blocking out time prevents appointment overlaps.						
7. If client makes appointment in person:	5					
• Scheduler should follow above steps.						
• Scheduler also should give reminder appointment card to client.	4					
• Reminder card should contain a place for client's name, date and time of appointment, and name of physician.						
8. Thank client and restate date and time of appointment.	4					
POSTPROCEDURE						
9. At end of day, use pen to write over penciled appointments for day.	8					
• Avoid tampering with or changing information.						
• If client doesn't show up for appointment, note that in appointment book and medical record.						
10. When appointment book is filled, file it in secure location.	4					
• Don't destroy or discard book.						
• State law and office policy determine amount of time book must be kept.						
TOTAL POSSIBLE POINTS	**100**					

Comments: _____

_____

_____

_____

_____

_____

_____

_____

_____

_____

_____

Signatures: _____   **Date:** _____

SCORING *See Preface for scoring instructions.*

Medical Office

PROCEDURE 28C:
Greeting a Client

PROCEDURE ASSESSMENT

Procedure Steps	Suggested Points	Self Practice	Peer Practice	Peer Testing	Final Testing	Total Earned
PREPROCEDURE						
1. At beginning of day, check front desk in reception room for neatness.	7					
• Appointment book should be available.	6					
• Some offices copy page out of schedule book for that day.						
• Daily schedule may be printout from computerized scheduling.						
PROCEDURE						
2. Greet client by name, if possible, and use positive verbal and nonverbal communication.	5					
3. Obtain personal and medical information from client in a discreet manner; no one else should hear your conversation.	6					
4. Demonstrate professionalism and create warm and caring atmosphere.	4					
5. Verify client information (address, phone number, and insurance information). Update medical record.	6					
6. Answer questions truthfully, but don't try to diagnose client.	4					
7. If client is anxious or angry, try to clarify cause while remaining calm and respectful.	7					
• Ease client's anxiety, if possible.	6					
• Offer tissues, water, etc.	6					
• If situation seems urgent, tell clinical staff so client can be taken to another waiting room.						
8. Sign in client on clipboard and daily schedule.	7					
• Ask client to have a seat.	4					
• If physician is running behind schedule, tell client.						
• Indicate approximate length of delay.	6					
• If another client is the cause of delay, don't reveal that fact.						
• Simply tell client that physician had an earlier emergency.	5					
• Offer to reschedule client.	5					
• Always apologize for delay.	6					

PROCEDURE 28C: Greeting a Client (continued)

Procedure Steps	Suggested Points	Self Practice	Peer Practice	Peer Testing	Final Testing	Total Earned
9. Help elderly or disabled clients to their seats, if necessary.	6					
• Help elderly or disabled clients fill out paperwork, if necessary.						
• Remember to be mindful of client confidentiality.						
• Take client into another room to help with paperwork, if necessary.						
POSTPROCEDURE						
10. Note time of client's arrival. If client can't be seen within 15 to 20 minutes after arrival, tell client about delay, give general reason for delay, apologize, and ask client if he/she wants to reschedule.	4					
TOTAL POSSIBLE POINTS	**100**					

Comments:

Signatures: Date:

SCORING   *See Preface for scoring instructions.*

Medical Office

PROCEDURE 28D:
Assembling a Client Record

· · · · · · · · · · · · · · · P R O C E D U R E   A S S E S S M E N T · · · · · · · · · · · · · · ·

Procedure Steps	Suggested Points	Self Practice	Peer Practice	Peer Testing	Final Testing	Total Earned
PREPROCEDURE						
1. Gather needed supplies.	10					
2. Type white file label with client's last name first, followed by first name and middle initial.	11					
PROCEDURE						
3. With file folder in closed position, put typed white label with client's name on tab facing outside. Label should be easily seen when folder is put in file cabinet.	12					
4. Apply a color-coded alphabetic or numerical label on tab above or below white label with client's name.	12					
5. Punch holes in top of blank client data sheet, history and physical form, progress sheet, medication record form, and laboratory or other test result and put them inside record.	12					
• Order of forms is determined by office policy.						
• Often, demographic client data sheet with insurance information is placed on left side of record.						
• Often, information about actual client care is placed on right side of record.						
• Usually, progress or treatment notes and medication forms are on top.						
POSTPROCEDURE						
6. Once record is assembled, put it in area not accessible to unauthorized individuals.	12					
7. To add new pages to record:	11					
• Put empty or blank sheet at top of completed record to create a reverse chronological record of client's care.	10					
• Previous sheets will be directly behind forms containing most current information.	10					
TOTAL POSSIBLE POINTS	**100**					

PROCEDURE 28D: Assembling a Client Record *(continued)*

Comments: _____
_____
_____
_____
_____
_____
_____
_____
_____
_____

Signatures: _____ **Date:** _____

SCORING   *See Preface for scoring instructions.*

Name _____ Date _____

Medical Office

PROCEDURE 28E:
Filing Medical Records

P R O C E D U R E   A S S E S S M E N T

Procedure Steps	Suggested Points	Self Practice	Peer Practice	Peer Testing	Final Testing	Total Earned
PREPROCEDURE						
1. Gather all records in one area.	5					
2. Quickly check each record for loose papers, illegible labels, or misfiled documents; if you find problems, fix them before continuing.	5					
3. Put files on cart or table for easy access.	5					
4. Assemble records in order in which they will be filed.	6					
5. If you're using vertical files, use a stable stepladder to file; never stand on chairs or other furniture.	8					
6. If you're using a filing cabinet with drawers, open only one drawer at a time to prevent cabinet tipping over.	8					
PROCEDURE						
7. Remove medical record to be filed from stack of records.	5					
8. Open file drawer on filing cabinet or locate proper vertical file.	5					
9. Locate general area where file will be placed.	6					
• Some offices place an "out guide" folder where the record has been kept.						
• Look for "out guide" folder (which is often red).						
• Before you remove "out guide" folder, ensure it's in the right place; often, more than one "out guide" is in the file.	5					
10. When you find correct location, insert file with alphabetic tab facing outward.	6					
• Use letters of client's last name and then first name to file.	5					
• Consider a hyphenated name as one unit.	5					
• Alphabetize a last name with a prefix (Mc, Mac, Van) as if prefix is part of last name.	5					
• If more than one client has same last name, use letters of first name to determine where to place file. Use middle initial when two or more clients have same first and last name.	5					
11. Continue until you correctly file all records.	6					

PROCEDURE 28E: Filing Medical Records (continued)

Procedure Steps	Suggested Points	Self Practice	Peer Practice	Peer Testing	Final Testing	Total Earned
POSTPROCEDURE						
12. Return filing supplies to proper location.	5					
13. Put away stepladders, etc.	5					
TOTAL POSSIBLE POINTS	100					

Comments: _____

_____

_____

_____

_____

_____

_____

_____

_____

Signatures: _____   **Date:** _____

SCORING   *See Preface for scoring instructions.*

Medical Office

PROCEDURE 28F:
Using the *Physicians' Desk Reference*

········ **PROCEDURE ASSESSMENT** ········

Procedure Steps	Suggested Points	Self Practice	Peer Practice	Peer Testing	Final Testing	Total Earned
PREPROCEDURE						
1. Obtain *Physicians' Desk Reference* and any available supplements.	10					
2. Have paper, pencil, or pen available to note information.	9					
3. Determine which index or section of PDR will be useful in looking up specific medication.	10					
PROCEDURE						
4. If using drug category to locate a drug, turn to drug category section in front of PDR and locate general category or classification of drug.	11					
5. If using generic category of drug, turn to that section of PDR and locate generic name of drug. Drugs are listed alphabetically.	11					
6. If trade or brand name of drug is known, turn to that section and locate trade or brand name of medication.	10					
7. When medication is located, turn to listed page number in larger section of book (white pages).	10					
8. Once correct page is located, find specific medication and make note of spelling and any other relevant information.	10					
POSTPROCEDURE						
9. Provide information to appropriate person.	10					
10. Return PDR to original location.	9					
TOTAL POSSIBLE POINTS	100					

Comments: _____

_____

_____

_____

_____

Signatures: _____   **Date:** _____

SCORING   *See Preface for scoring instructions.*

Health Information

Reinforcement Activities

Multiple Choice

Circle the letter that best answers the question or completes the statement.

1. Which of the following occupations would be more likely to provide an opportunity for an independent private practice?
    a. health care receptionist.
    b. medical coder.
    c. privacy officer.
    d. medical transcriptionist.

2. Which of the following actions best protects patient confidentiality?
    a. talking about the patient in the elevator.
    b. discussing the patient while having lunch in the cafeteria.
    c. turning the computer screen away from the view of the public.
    d. leaving the patient notes on the counter.

3. Which volume of the ICD-9-CM would be used to find the correct code for a cardiac catheterization procedure?
    a. volume 1.
    b. volume 2.
    c. volume 3.
    d. volume 4.

4. Two-digit modifiers can be assigned to the five-digit code for
    a. procedures.
    b. primary diagnoses.
    c. secondary diagnoses.
    d. medical diagnoses.

5. Which of the following actions will help prevent repetitive motion injuries to health information professionals?
    a. placing papers flat on the desk while working on the computer.
    b. position the monitor above eye level.
    c. alternate keyboarding with noncomputer activities.
    d. keep feet slightly raised off the floor.

Fill in the Blank

Write the word (or words) that best completes the sentence in the blank provided.

6. An _____ is a client whose services require at least an overnight stay in the hospital.

7. _____ work to keep their facilities in compliance with the laws about confidentiality.

8. Clients' diagnoses are assigned codes from the **International Classification of Diseases, Ninth Revision, Clinical Modification,** called the _____.

9. _____ is a type of repetitive motion injury to the wrist that commonly occurs in those who use the keyboard often in their job.

10. One of the first forms you are likely to sign as a health information professional will be a _____ statement.

Matching

Write the letter of the phrase that best matches each numbered item in the blank provided.

_____ 11. Prepares bills to send to clients.

_____ 12. Collects insurance co-payments and gives receipts.

_____ 13. Types dictation from physicians into a word processing program.

_____ 14. Assigns codes to inpatient and outpatient records.

_____ 15. Makes sure the hospital record is complete and correct.

a. Medical biller

b. Health care receptionist

c. Medical coder

d. Medical transcriptionist

e. Health information technician

True/False

Write "T" in the blank provided if the statement is true. Write "F" if the statement is false.

_____ 16. Client information must remain strictly confidential.

_____ 17. Clients own their own health record.

_____ 18. Health care information professionals are responsible for organizing and maintaining clients' health records.

_____ 19. Mistakes in the health record can be covered with correction fluid and written over.

_____ 20. The healthcare receptionist is responsible for sending the bill to the client.

_____ 21. No part of a record should be otherwise altered or removed, deleted, or destroyed.

_____ 22. To avoid repetitive motion injuries, you should vary your work duties by alternating keyboarding with noncomputer tasks.

_____ 23. Medicare is the medical insurance program for people under the age of 65.

_____ 24. HIPAA is a federal law that provides rules for the use of client health information.

_____ 25. Each entry in the health record must be signed.

Health Information

PROCEDURE 29A:
Diagnostic Coding Practice

-------- P R O C E D U R E   A S S E S S M E N T --------

Procedure Steps	Suggested Points	Self Practice	Peer Practice	Peer Testing	Final Testing	Total Earned
PREPROCEDURE						
1. Review diagnostic coding steps, particularly guidelines for selecting main term.	4					
2. Review contents of Tabular List.	3					
PROCEDURE						
3. Determine main term in each of the following diagnoses.	5					
• Abdominal pain	4					
• Acute cerebrovascular disease	4					
• Postoperative fibrillation	4					
• Night sweats	4					
• Singer's nodule	4					
• Carpal tunnel syndrome	4					
• Popliteal fat pad hernia	4					
• Harvest itch	4					
• Urinary incontinence without sensory awareness	4					
• Little's disease, congenital	4					
4. Using Table 29-2 in your textbook, determine range of codes which you expect to be able to locate correct code for following diagnosis.	5					
• Muscle spasms	4					
• Attention deficit disorder	4					
• Detached retina	4					
• Tuberculosis	4					
• Skin cancer	4					
• Disorder of thyroid	4					
• Gastric ulcer	4					
• Acute tonsillitis	4					
• Cesarean delivery	4					
• First-degree burn	4					
POSTPROCEDURE						
5. Compare answers with those provided in the Teacher Resource Guide.	3					
TOTAL POSSIBLE POINTS	**100**					

PROCEDURE 29A: Diagnostic Coding Practice *(continued)*

Comments:

_____

_____

_____

_____

_____

_____

_____

_____

_____

Signatures: _____ **Date:** _____

SCORING   *See Preface for scoring instructions.*

Name _____ Date _____

Health Information

PROCEDURE 29B:
Procedural Coding Practice

··········· **PROCEDURE ASSESSMENT** ···········

Procedure Steps	Suggested Points	Self Practice	Peer Practice	Peer Testing	Final Testing	Total Earned
PREPROCEDURE						
1. Review procedural coding steps.	6					
2. Review CPT in Table 29-3 in your textbook.	6					
PROCEDURE						
3. Locate codes for procedures:	6					
• Primary adenoidectomy.	5					
• Excision of tonsil tags.	5					
• Secondary adenoidectomy.	5					
• Tonsillectomy and adenoidectomy.	5					
4. Using Table 29-3, list code range:	6					
• ECG.	5					
• Anesthesia for delivery.	5					
• Glucose tolerance test.	5					
• Physician and psychiatrist medical conference.	5					
• Physical examination of infant.	5					
• Appendectomy.	5					
• Permanent pacemaker insertion.	5					
• Intensive care observation.	5					
• Dialysis.	5					
• White blood cell count.	5					
POSTPROCEDURE						
5. Compare code numbers and ranges with the Teacher Resource Guide.	6					
TOTAL POSSIBLE POINTS	**100**					

Comments: _____
_____
_____
_____
_____
_____
_____
_____
_____
_____

Signatures: **Date:**

SCORING   *See Preface for scoring instructions.*

Biomedical Technology | Reinforcement Activities

Matching

Write the letter of the phrase that best matches each numbered item in the blank provided.

_____ **1.** Macroshock

_____ **2.** PET

_____ **3.** Electrically Sensitive Patient Locations (ESPL)

_____ **4.** Medical Treatment Facility (MTF)

_____ **5.** Teleradiology

_____ **6.** Ampere

_____ **7.** Microshock

_____ **8.** Leakage current

_____ **9.** Calibration

_____ **10.** Asset management

_____ **11.** Thermocouple

a. Unit of electrical current.

b. Insuring the instrument is operating at its intended settings.

c. A large value electrical current that passes arm to arm.

d. Areas of the hospital where clients are connected via an intravenous line of electrical conduction to the heart.

e. Undesired current.

f. A small value electrical current that passes directly through the heart.

g. Energy generated by heat.

h. Communications between radiologists of different medical treatment facilities or research centers.

i. Managing the life cycle of the equipment.

j. Places where medical treatment or health care is provided.

k. Positron emission tomography.

Fill in the Blank

Write the word (or words) that best completes the sentence in the blank provided.

12. Students planning biomedical careers frequently train in _____ and _____.

13. CBET stands for _____.

14. AAMI stands for _____.

15. _____ is a primary concern of the biomedical technician.

16. Electrical safety principles can be referenced in five words: Keep _____ in its place.

17. Electrical wires, plugs, and outlets in a medical treatment facility are color-coded and marked _____.

18. Electrical currents continuing for more than one heart cycle may cause _____.

19. Class A equipment is used in _____ areas.

20. _____ promote occupational health and safety within organizations.

Labeling

21. Label the parts of the following piece of equipment and explain what it is used for in the space provided.

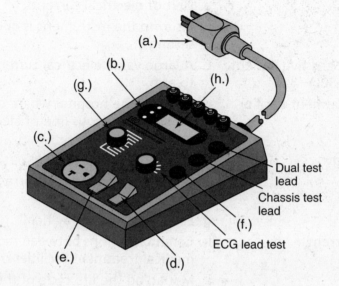

Dual test
lead

Chassis test
lead

ECG lead test

(a.) _____   (e.) _____

(b.) _____   (f.) _____

(c.) _____   (g.) _____

(d.) _____   (h.) _____

_____

_____

_____

_____

Biomedical Technology

PROCEDURE 30A:
Performing an Electrical Safety Test

PROCEDURE ASSESSMENT

Procedure Steps	Suggested Points	Self Practice	Peer Practice	Peer Testing	Final Testing	Total Earned
PREPROCEDURE						
1. Gather needed equipment.	5					
2. Calibrate safety analyzer if necessary. Do this at least annually.	6					
PROCEDURE						
3. Plug equipment into electrical safety analyzer. Equipment being tested shouldn't be in use on a client.	9					
4. Turn on the analyzer.	7					
5. Place the cable with a clamp clip from the safety analyzer on the unpainted metal case of the piece of equipment.	6					
6. Read leakage current if it's detected on meter or digital readout of safety analyzer.	7					
7. Test equipment in both "on" and "off" positions.	6					
8. Using reverse polarity buttons on safety analyzer, check for correct wiring of electrical plug, cord, and machine under test.	7					
9. When reverse polarity test is performed, readings on analyzer shouldn't change.	7					
• If readings change, or if meter readings are high, it usually means that plug, electrical cable, or machine is wired incorrectly.						
• Immediately remove equipment from use and report problem.	7					
POSTPROCEDURE						
10. Record all readings on proper forms.	6					
11. If leakage current for type of equipment is within limits, certify it safe for continued use.	6					
12. If equipment is beyond electric current leakage limits:	7					
• Remove it immediately from use.	7					
• Report the malfunction.	7					
TOTAL POSSIBLE POINTS	**100**					

PROCEDURE 30A: Performing an Electrical Safety Test *(continued)*

Comments: _____

_____

_____

_____

_____

_____

_____

_____

_____

Signatures: _____ Date: _____

Central Supply/ Processing

Reinforcement Activities

Matching

Write the letter of the phrase that best matches each numbered item in the blank provided.

_____ 1. Ethylene oxide

_____ 2. Chemical sterilant

_____ 3. Surgical asepsis

_____ 4. Spores

_____ 5. Ultrasonic cleaner

_____ 6. Autoclave

_____ 7. Sterilization

_____ 8. Medical asepsis

a. Instrument used to sterilize with steam under pressure.

b. Microorganisms in an inactive state that allow them to survive extreme living conditions until more favorable conditions exist.

c. Gas used for sterilization.

d. The process of destroying all microorganisms and spores.

e. Special chemical used during immersion to sterilize; must be registered with environmental protection agency.

f. Practices used at all times to maintain areas and individuals free from gross contamination and most microorganisms.

g. A container filled with a cleansing solution that vibrates to loosen contamination and clean instruments and equipment.

h. Sterilization of items to be used during sterile technique.

Fill in the Blank

Write the word (or words) that best completes the sentence in the blank provided.

9. The Central Supply is also known as the _____.

10. Soiled items are brought to _____ from client care areas for sorting and first stage cleaning.

11. _____ make inventory of supplies much easier and quicker.

12. A _____ is an area free of microorganisms.

13. Sterile gloves are used for _____ procedures that are done on parts of the body that are considered _____.

14. As a Central Supply technician, you may be expected to collect and/or receive _____, _____, _____, _____, and other supplies in the daily operation of a health care facility.

15. _____ is when an instrument is autoclaved unwrapped for a shorter period of time.

16. Linen and/or supplies are stored in _____.

17. In decontamination, PPE must be worn, including _____, _____, _____, _____, _____, and _____ at all times.

Multiple Choice
Circle the letter that best answers the question or completes the statement.

18. _____ is used on items that steam will not penetrate.
   a. Chemical sterilant
   b. Auto claving
   c. Dry heat sterilization
   d. Ethylene oxide

19. The time required for cold chemical sterilization is about _____, but depends on the chemical and manufacturer's directions.
   a. 6 hours
   b. 10 hours
   c. 4 hours
   d. 12 hours

20. This career choice requires 2 years of community college and/or experience in inventory management or business administration.
   a. Central Supply technician
   b. Central Supply assistant
   c. Supply Supervisor/coordinator
   d. Central Supply aide

Fill in the Blank and Ordering
Write the word (or words) that best completes the sentence in the blank provided.

21. Contaminated instruments just arrived at the Central Supply/Processing department and must be processed and returned. Number the following steps of the journey the instruments will take through the department and identify where each step in the process will occur.

   _____ All microscopic organisms and spores are removed in _____.

   _____ Ultrasonic cleaning occurs in _____.

   _____ Brought via a closed cart to _____.

   _____ Instruments are wrapped and packaged in _____.

   _____ Instruments returned to floors from the _____.

Name _____ Date _____

Labeling

22. The following pictures identify the steps of wrapping for sterilization. Number the pictures in the correct order of how you would perform this procedure. Describe each step on the lines provided.

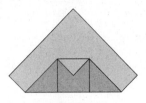 _____   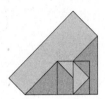 _____   _____

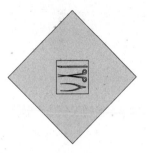 _____   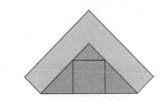 _____   _____

 _____

1. _____

2. _____

3. _____

4. _____

5. _____

6. _____

7. _____

Central Supply/ Processing

PROCEDURE 31A:
Performing Decontamination Cleaning

PROCEDURE ASSESSMENT

Procedure Steps	Suggested Points	Self Practice	Peer Practice	Peer Testing	Final Testing	Total Earned
PREPROCEDURE						
1. Gather needed equipment and wash hands.	7					
2. Put on personal protective equipment (PPE).	7					
PROCEDURE						
3. Determine proper cleaning substance for items to be washed.	4					
• Soaps or solutions may need to be diluted.						
• Check directions to ensure correct mixture.						
4. Separate items for cleaning.	5					
• Put items into automatic washer baskets and put in washer.	4					
• Apply correct amount of cleaning substance.	4					
• Operate dishwasher according to manufacturer's instructions.	4					
5. Wipe surfaces of items that can't be put in washer with cleaning substance, according to manufacturer's directions and facility policy.	5					
6. Clean instruments according to policy; some items may need hand cleaning before being put in washer.	5					
7. Items with serrated edges or hinges and heavily soiled items may need ultrasonic cleaning.	5					
• Measure detergent and add water to machine. Check manufacturer's directions.	4					
• Put items in basket; don't overload.	4					
• Turn machine on for correct amount of time.	4					
• Rinse items in tap water.	4					
• Rinse items in distilled or demineralized water as policy dictates.	4					
• Thoroughly dry each item.	4					

PROCEDURE 31A: Performing Decontamination Cleaning *(continued)*

Procedure Steps POSTPROCEDURE	Suggested Points	Self Practice	Peer Practice	Peer Testing	Final Testing	Total Earned
8. Pass clean items to the preparation and packing area or other clean area.	5					
9. Clean and replace equipment.	7					
10. Remove and discard protective equipment correctly outside of contaminated area.	7					
11. Wash hands.	7					
TOTAL POSSIBLE POINTS	**100**					

Comments: _____

_____

_____

_____

_____

_____

_____

_____

_____

_____

Signatures: _____ Date: _____

SCORING *See Preface for scoring instructions.*

Central Supply/ Processing

PROCEDURE 31B:
Cleaning Instruments

PROCEDURE ASSESSMENT

Procedure Steps	Suggested Points	Self Practice	Peer Practice	Peer Testing	Final Testing	Total Earned
PREPROCEDURE						
1. Wash hands.	8					
2. Gather needed equipment.	5					
3. Apply gloves; you may wear two pairs of gloves or thicker gloves if you're handling instruments contaminated with blood or body fluids.	8					
PROCEDURE						
4. Unclamp, open, or take apart all instruments.	4					
5. Put items in solutions to loosen dried substances.	5					
6. Remove contaminating materials from instruments by rinsing them under cold running water.	6					
7. Clean instruments with warm soapy water.	4					
• Scrub instruments with brush if heavily soiled.	1					
• Use ultrasonic or sonic cleaner if required.	1					
8. Rinse again with tap water, then with distilled or demineralized water.	4					
9. Wipe large items with disinfectant and leave to air dry.	5					
10. Dry instruments with clean cloth or put in hot-air oven.	4					
11. Oil instruments with special oils if required by manufacturer's instructions.	4					
12. Arrange instruments on trays for storage and/or packing for sterilization; trays are prepared depending on instruments' use.	6					
13. Put trays and/or packages in designated area.	6					
POSTPROCEDURE						
14. Dispose of soiled water and replace equipment.	8					
15. Clean area using specified procedure.	5					
16. Remove gloves.	8					
17. Wash hands.	8					
TOTAL POSSIBLE POINTS	**100**					

PROCEDURE 31B: Cleaning Instruments *(continued)*

Comments:

_____
_____
_____
_____
_____
_____
_____
_____

Signatures: _____   Date: _____

SCORING   *See Preface for scoring instructions.*

Central Supply/ Processing

PROCEDURE 31C:
Packaging for Sterilization

PROCEDURE ASSESSMENT

Procedure Steps	Suggested Points	Self Practice	Peer Practice	Peer Testing	Final Testing	Total Earned
PREPROCEDURE						
1. Gather needed equipment.	5					
2. Wash hands.	6					
3. Put on gloves.	6					
PROCEDURE						
4. Separate articles to be packaged.	5					
• You may be wrapping linens, instruments, or other equipment.						
• Instruments are left open and sometimes grouped on trays for various procedures.	2					
• Inspect linen prior to wrapping if necessary.	1					
• Check policy at your facility.	3					
5. When using prepared packages:	5					
• Insert instruments and/or article into package.	3					
• Include appropriate autoclave indicator. Check indicator for damage.	3					
• Seal according to manufacturer's directions.	3					
6. When using a wrapping muslin or permeable material:	5					
• Select the correct size square of wrapping material. The wrap is usually 3 times longer from corner to corner than the item to be wrapped.	3					
• Place instrument, tray of instruments, or linens diagonally across center of wrapping materials. Put hinged instruments in pack in open position. Ensure items don't touch inside pack.	3					
• Put an indicator device beside items. Indicator tape on outside of package doesn't mean inner contents are sterilized.	3					
• Fold bottom corner of material across items until completely covered. Fold corner back.	3					
• Fold right corner in to center. Fold back small portion of point, making a flap.	3					
• Fold left corner in to center. Make a flap. Package should resemble an open envelope.	3					

PROCEDURE 31C: Packaging for Sterilization (continued)

Procedure Steps	Suggested Points	Self Practice	Peer Practice	Peer Testing	Final Testing	Total Earned
g. Fold top corner down. Grasp package to make sure it's snug but not too tight. Bring last corner around package and make a small flap.	3					
7. Secure with autoclave indicator tape. Folding tape back upon itself can make a quick-opening tab with the tape.	5					
8. Label package or tape with date and time of sterilization, contents, and your initials.	5					
9. Put items in appropriate locations for sterilization.	5					
POSTPROCEDURE						
10. Clean area and replace equipment used.	5					
11. Remove gloves.	6					
12. Wash hands.	6					
TOTAL POSSIBLE POINTS	**100**					

Comments: _____

_____

_____

_____

_____

_____

_____

_____

_____

Signatures: _____ Date: _____

SCORING *See Preface for scoring instructions.*

Central Supply/ Processing

PROCEDURE 31D:
Sterilization

PROCEDURE ASSESSMENT

Procedure Steps	Suggested Points	Self Practice	Peer Practice	Peer Testing	Final Testing	Total Earned
PREPROCEDURE						
1. Gather needed equipment.	3					
2. Wash hands and put on gloves.	5					
3. Check distilled water reservoir and add water, if necessary.	3					
PROCEDURE						
4. Load autoclave.	4					
a. Rest packages on their edges.	3					
b. Put jar and containers on their sides.	3					
c. Don't let large packages block steam flow to smaller ones.	3					
d. Ensure items don't touch sides, top, or door of autoclave.	3					
e. If load is mixed, put unwrapped items below wrapped ones.	3					
5. Double check load and fill chamber. Check manufacturer's instructions for starting and stopping fill cycle.	4					
6. Close and lock door.	3					
7. Start autoclave.	3					
8. Set timer when indicator shows correct temperature and pressure amounts.	4					
• Check manufacturer's instructions or facility policy.	3					
• Maintain items at a constant temperature and pressure for recommended length of time.	3					
• Check temperature and pressure gauges at intervals to ensure temperature and pressure is maintained throughout time period.	3					
9. When specified time has elapsed, turn autoclave to vent or dry.	4					
• When all steam has escaped and pressure gauge is at zero, open autoclave door to 1/4 inch for items to dry.	3					
• Wear safety goggles when opening autoclave.	5					

PROCEDURE 31D: Sterilization *(continued)*

Procedure Steps	Suggested Points	Self Practice	Peer Practice	Peer Testing	Final Testing	Total Earned
10. Unload items when drying is complete.	4					
• Don't touch items that aren't thoroughly dry.	3					
• Use a cloth or oven mitt to remove items.	5					
• Use sterile transfer forceps for items that aren't wrapped.	3					
11. Check each package. Items must be resterilized if indicator is underexposed, there are tears in the packages, or the packages have any moisture.	4					
POSTPROCEDURE						
12. Put each package in proper location for storage or use.	3					
13. Clean area.	3					
14. Remove gloves.	5					
15. Wash hands.	5					
TOTAL POSSIBLE POINTS	**100**					

Comments: _____

_____

_____

_____

_____

_____

_____

_____

_____

_____

Signatures: _____   Date: _____

SCORING   *See Preface for scoring instructions.*

Name _____   Date _____

Central Supply/ Processing

PROCEDURE 31E:
Handling and Preparing Linens

PROCEDURE ASSESSMENT

Procedure Steps	Suggested Points	Self Practice	Peer Practice	Peer Testing	Final Testing	Total Earned
PREPROCEDURE						
1. Gather needed equipment.	7					
2. Wash hands.	9					
PROCEDURE						
3. Inspect linens by placing them over well-lit table. Look for holes, tears, or other defects.	7					
4. Circle defects with pencil or other linen marker and send for repair.	8					
5. Prepare linens for sterilization by folding according to policy.	7					
6. Sort and stack linens according to use.	7					
7. Package linens by placing last item to be used on bottom and first item to be used on top.	8					
• Alternate layers of linens.	7					
• Place gauze in center of package.	7					
8. Wrap packages according to facility policy.	4					
• Use Procedure 31c for folding method.	2					
• Maintain size and weight limit for each complete package.	2					
• One standard for linen packages is 12 by 12 by 20 inches and not greater than 20 pounds.						
9. Sterilize linens according to Procedure 31d.	8					
POSTPROCEDURE						
10. Clean area and put equipment away.	8					
11. Wash hands.	9					
TOTAL POSSIBLE POINTS	100					

PROCEDURE 31E: Handling and Preparing Linens (continued)

Comments: _____
_____
_____
_____
_____
_____
_____
_____

Signatures: _____ Date: _____

SCORING *See Preface for scoring instructions.*

Name _____   Date _____

Central Supply/ Processing

PROCEDURE 31F:
Performing a Surgical Scrub

PROCEDURE ASSESSMENT

Procedure Steps	Suggested Points	Self Practice	Peer Practice	Peer Testing	Final Testing	Total Earned
PREPROCEDURE						
1. Gather needed equipment.	5					
2. Remove all your jewelry and roll up your sleeves.	5					
PROCEDURE						
3. Turn on water and adjust it to comfortable warm temperature.	2					
• Use a foot or knee pedal for adjusting the temperature.	2					
• If there is no foot or knee pedal, use a clean dry paper towel to turn sink handle.	2					
4. Wet hands from fingertips to elbows. Keep hands higher than elbows so water doesn't run down arms and contaminate washed areas.	5					
5. Use surgical soap from dispenser to scrub.	6					
• Scrub fingers, between fingers, palms and backs of hands, wrists and forearms.	4					
• Scrub should take at least 2 minutes.	4					
6. Rinse hands and forearms with hands higher than elbows.	6					
7. Use orange wood stick to clean under each fingernail.	5					
8. Rinse hands again.	5					
9. Apply more soap.	6					
• Repeat washing process with surgical brush.	4					
• Use firm circular motion for up to 3 minutes.	4					
10. Rinse hands again with hands above elbows.	5					
11. Thoroughly pat dry your hands and forearms with sterile towels, working from hands to elbows.	6					
12. Turn off faucet. If it's a hand faucet, use a clean dry towel.	5					

PROCEDURE 31F: Performing a Surgical Scrub (continued)

Procedure Steps POSTPROCEDURE	Suggested Points	Self Practice	Peer Practice	Peer Testing	Final Testing	Total Earned
13. To avoid contamination:	6					
• Don't touch anything with your hands.	4					
• Keep hands in front of you, between your shoulders and your waist.	4					
14. Apply sterile surgical gloves immediately if required.	5					
TOTAL POSSIBLE POINTS	100					

Comments: _____
_____
_____
_____
_____
_____
_____
_____
_____

Signatures: _____ Date: _____

SCORING See Preface for scoring instructions.

Dietetics

Reinforcement Activities

Matching

Write the letter of the phrase that best matches each numbered item in the blank provided.

_____ 1. Medical nutrition therapy

_____ 2. Bacteria

_____ 3. Sanitation

_____ 4. Aspiration

_____ 5. Low-fat, low-cholesterol diet

_____ 6. Food-borne illness

a. a therapeutic diet used to treat heart disease

b. using nutrition to treat illness or other conditions

c. a type of microorganism that may cause food-borne illness

d. sickness that results from eating food that is not safe

e. when food or liquid enters the airway

f. preventing illness through cleanliness

True/False

Write "T" in the blank provided if the statement is true. Write "F" if the statement is false.

_____ 7. A CDM may be employed in a clinical setting or may be part of a management team that supervises a foodservice operation.

_____ 8. A dietetic aide must complete an approved training program and pass a national examination.

_____ 9. A registered dietitian may work in variety of settings, including a hospital, school, fitness center, food company, public health office, university, research center, and more.

_____ 10. Many people are becoming interested in using nutrition and dietary supplements to improve the way they feel, how they look, and their overall well-being, which means increased opportunities for RDs.

Multiple Choice

Circle the letter that best answers the question or completes the statement.

11. As a DTR, which of the following responsibilities might you have?
    a. Performing basic nutrition counseling
    b. Developing specialized nutrition care plans
    c. Passing menus to clients
    d. Checking the temperatures of foods on a tray line

12. An RD may use medical nutrition therapy to treat which disease or condition?
    a. Flu
    b. Ear infection
    c. Heart disease
    d. Pneumonia

13. Which microorganism is the most common cause of foodborne illness?
    a. viruses
    b. parasites
    c. spores
    d. bacteria

14. Which is **not** a common symptom of foodborne illness?
    a. diarrhea
    b. fever
    c. sore throat
    d. vomiting

15. Which diet is recommended as a preventive measure and as part of the treatment for osteoporosis?
    a. Low-sodium diet
    b. Diabetic diet
    c. Calcium-rich diet
    d. Pureed diet

16. Which of the following BEST describes a diet history?
    a. Assessing whether a client's diet is nutritionally adequate
    b. Collecting information about a client's usual diet
    c. Understanding the history of therapeutic diets
    d. Teaching a client about a special diet

Fill in the Blank

Write the word (or words) that best completes the sentence in the blank provided.

17. If juices from raw meat touch cooked or ready-to-eat foods, _____ can occur.

18. Correct _____ is important before a client begins to eat to prevent choking and _____.

19. The best way to be sure that foods are cooked enough is to use a _____ to measure the internal _____ of meat, poultry, casseroles, and other cooked foods.

20. A _____ is recommended for people with high blood pressure; a _____ is recommended for people with digestive problems, such as constipation.

21. Describe the hand-over-hand assistance technique for feeding a client.

_____

Name _____ Date _____

22. Fill in the blank. Complete the table below related to therapeutic diets.

TYPE OF DIET	DESCRIPTION	SAMPLE FOODS INCLUDED
Low-fat, low cholesterol		
	Reduces blood pressure.	
		Variety of foods spaced evenly over the day—sugary foods and sweets are avoided
High-fiber		
Calcium rich		
		Chopped or pureed meats, mashed fruits and vegetables, Most raw fruits and fried foods are excluded
Liquid		

Reinforcement Activities and Procedure Assessment   Chapter 32   **A-423**

Labeling

24. Mark the danger zone for bacterial growth in food.

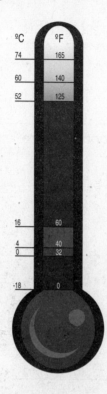

Dietetics

PROCEDURE 32A:
Cleaning and Sanitizing Surfaces, Utensils, and Other Items

PROCEDURE ASSESSMENT

Procedure Steps	Suggested Points	Self Practice	Peer Practice	Peer Testing	Final Testing	Total Earned
PREPROCEDURE						
1. Prepare sanitizing solutions for different types of surfaces, utensils, etc.	4					
• When you mix solutions, wear plastic gloves and stay away from food preparation areas.	3					
• Store each solution in a plastic gallon container with a tight lid.	3					
• Label each container with the type of solution.	3					
For hard, nonporous surfaces:	2					
1 tablespoon liquid bleach						
1 gallon water						
For porous surfaces (like wooden cutting boards):	2					
3 tablespoons liquid bleach						
1 gallon water						
Disinfecting solution:	2					
¾ cup liquid bleach						
1 gallon water						
2. Follow contact time guidelines shown below to allow enough time to kill microorganisms.	4					
PROCEDURE						
3. For wooden and plastic cutting boards:	4					
• Wash board with hot sudsy water and rinse thoroughly.	3					
• For porous surfaces, spray on sanitizing solution.	3					
• Keep surface wet for 2 minutes.	3					
• Rinse and let surface air-dry. Don't dry with towel.	3					
4. For dinnerware, plastic, and glassware:	4					
• Wash with soap and water and rinse thoroughly.	3					
• Use sanitizing solution for hard surfaces. Soak items in solution for 2 minutes. Don't use on aluminum, metal, or silverware.	3					
• Allow to air-dry.	3					
Note: These items also can be cleaned and sanitized in a dishwasher.						

Procedure Steps	Suggested Points	Self Practice	Peer Practice	Peer Testing	Final Testing	Total Earned
5. For dishcloths and sponges:	3					
• Soak dishcloths and/or sponges in disinfecting solution in a sink for 2 minutes.	3					
• Rinse sink and cloth or sponge in clean water.	3					
• Squeeze out excess water and allow to air-dry.	3					
6. For countertops and surfaces:	3					
• Remove any loose food or dirt.	3					
• Wash with hot, sudsy water and rinse.	3					
• Use sanitizing solution for hard surfaces. Apply solution to surface for 2 minutes.	3					
• Rinse and let air-dry or wipe with clean paper towel.	3					
7. For frequency of cleaning and sanitizing surfaces, utensils, and equipment:	3					
• Tableware must be washed, rinsed, and sanitized after each use.	3					
• Kitchenware and equipment must be washed, rinsed, and sanitized after each use.	3					
• Food preparation utensils and equipment being used continuously must be washed, rinsed, and sanitized at regularly scheduled intervals.	3					
• Grills, griddles, microwave ovens, and other cooking devices must be cleaned at least once a day. Other chemical solutions also may be used in food service departments.	3					
POSTPROCEDURE						
8. Discard any sanitizing solution left at end of day.	2					
9. Store cleaned and sanitized cutting boards, utensils, and dishware in drawers and cupboards that are cleaned and sanitized regularly.	2					
10. Discard cracked or chipped containers, utensils, cooking pots, cups, and dishes.	2					
TOTAL POSSIBLE POINTS	**100**					

PROCEDURE 32A: Cleaning and Sanitizing Surfaces, Utensils, and Other Items *(continued)*

Comments: _____

_____

_____

_____

_____

_____

_____

_____

_____

Signatures: _____   **Date:** _____

SCORING   *See Preface for scoring instructions.*

Dietetics

PROCEDURE 32B:
Assisting the Client to Eat

PROCEDURE ASSESSMENT

Procedure Steps	Suggested Points	Self Practice	Peer Practice	Peer Testing	Final Testing	Total Earned
PREPROCEDURE						
1. Gather equipment.	4					
2. Wash your hands and help client wash hands, if necessary.	6					
3. Ensure that correct food tray was delivered.	4					
• Client's name and specific diet type should be marked on tag.	3					
• If you question any foods on tray, immediately notify supervisor.	3					
4. Ensure client isn't scheduled for any tests; if tests are scheduled, sometimes tray should be withheld.	4					
5. If client was able to make food selections, ensure these foods are on tray.	5					
6. Ensure that fork tines aren't bent, spoon edges are smooth, and plastic coatings are unbroken.	4					
7. Help client get into comfortable, upright position.	4					
8. Provide napkin or apron.	3					
9. Ensure environment is free from distractions (i.e. TV).	3					
PROCEDURE						
10. Arrange place setting so client can reach foods and utensils.	4					
11. Let client decide what foods to eat first, next, and so on.	5					
12. Help client cut foods into small bites. Suggest that client use spoon to eat, as it is easier than fork.	4					
13. If client has trouble using utensils, cut foods into pieces that can be picked up easily or use hand over hand assistance technique.	3					
14. Offer a drink between bites to soften foods. Use a straw, if necessary.	4					
15. Sit at same level as client and share pleasant conversation.	5					
16. Keep napkin handy to clean any spills immediately.	4					
17. Relax, be patient, and don't rush meal.	4					
18. Respect client's needs and desires. Ask client when he/she is done.	5					

PROCEDURE 32B: Assisting the Client to Eat *(continued)*

Procedure Steps POSTPROCEDURE	Suggested Points	Self Practice	Peer Practice	Peer Testing	Final Testing	Total Earned
19. Clear away finished tray of food.	4					
20. If needed, help client clean hands and mouth, and clean any spills on client's clothing.	5					
21. Record how much client ate and drank or report it to supervisor.	5					
22. If client is on Intake and Output, note exact amount of fluids on Intake and Output record. Review this section in Chapter 14, if necessary.	5					
TOTAL POSSIBLE POINTS	100					

Comments: _____
_____
_____
_____
_____
_____
_____
_____
_____
_____

Signatures: _____   **Date:** _____

SCORING   *See Preface for scoring instructions.*

Dietetics

PROCEDURE 32C:
Feeding a Helpless Client

PROCEDURE ASSESSMENT

Procedure Steps	Suggested Points	Self Practice	Peer Practice	Peer Testing	Final Testing	Total Earned
PREPROCEDURE						
1. Gather equipment.	3					
2. Wash hands thoroughly before feeding. If necessary, tie your hair back.	5					
3. Prepare client by offering oral hygiene, toileting and washing hands.	5					
4. Wear clean clothes. Don't smoke, drink, eat, or chew gum during feeding.	4					
5. Don't feed a client if you have open sores on exposed areas of your body.	3					
6. Wear gloves during feeding if your hands will touch client's mouth.	2					
7. Ensure correct food tray was delivered.	3					
• Client's name and specific diet type should be marked on tag.	2					
• If you question any foods on tray, immediately notify supervisor.	2					
8. Ensure client isn't scheduled for any tests; if tests are scheduled, sometimes tray should be withheld.	3					
9. Ensure that fork tines aren't bent, spoon edges are smooth, and plastic coatings are unbroken.	2					
10. Ensure environment is free from distractions (i.e. TV).	3					
11. Help client get into comfortable, upright position.	3					
12. Provide a napkin or apron.	3					
PROCEDURE						
13. Sit at same level as client and share pleasant conversation.	3					
14. Ask client what foods he/she would like to eat first. If client can't respond, offer foods in normal sequence.	3					
15. Test hot liquids and foods on inside of your wrist before serving.	2					
16. Touch only handles of utensils. Pick up glasses by base, not rim.	3					
17. If you touch client's mouth or eating end of utensil, wash hands before assisting another client.	2					

PROCEDURE 32C: Feeding a Helpless Client *(continued)*

Procedure Steps	Suggested Points	Self Practice	Peer Practice	Peer Testing	Final Testing	Total Earned
18. Present a small amount of food at a time.	4					
• You may need to prompt client to open mouth.	2					
• Tell client what food you're offering.	2					
• Tell client when you're switching to another food.	2					
• Be sure client has swallowed before offering next bite.	2					
19. Offer a drink between bites to soften foods. Use a straw, if necessary.	3					
20. Keep napkin handy to clean any spills immediately.	3					
21. Relax, be patient, and don't rush meal.	3					
22. Ask client when he/she has had enough. If client doesn't speak, look for cues that client is done:	3					
• Refusal to open mouth.	2					
• Turning away when food is presented.	2					
POSTPROCEDURE						
23. Clear away finished tray of food.	3					
24. Wipe client's face and mouth with moistened napkin.	3					
25. Clean off any food spills.	3					
26. Record how much client ate and drank or report it to supervisor.	3					
27. If client is on Intake and Output, note exact amount of fluids on Intake and Output record. Review this section in Chapter 14, if necessary.	4					
TOTAL POSSIBLE POINTS	**100**					

Comments: _____
_____
_____
_____
_____
_____
_____
_____
_____
_____

Signatures: _____   Date: _____

SCORING   *See Preface for scoring instructions.*

PART B

Additional Career Skills

Procedure LM4-1 | Amputation

Amputations occur when the body is subjected to forces that tear away body parts or sever them from the body. Amputations occur in industrial and home settings. Machines, saws, and lawn mowers can cause them. When assisting a client with an amputation, whether it is a toe or a finger, it is important to remember that the first priority is to provide first aid to the client. Retrieval and first aid for the amputated part is second. Figure LM4-1 shows some steps to take when you provide first aid for an amputation.

Tourniquet

A tourniquet is used as a last resort, when all other bleeding control methods have failed. Tourniquets close off the entire blood supply to and from the bleeding extremity. When applied, a tourniquet may control life-threatening bleeding, but it is likely to cause extensive damage to the blood vessels, nerves, and muscle tissue of the bleeding extremity. Tourniquets are most likely to be used in cases of partial or rough-edged extremity amputations.

When you provide first aid for amputations, refer to the step-by-step guide in the following sections.

Equipment and Supplies

Latex or vinyl gloves • client • sterile gauze dressing

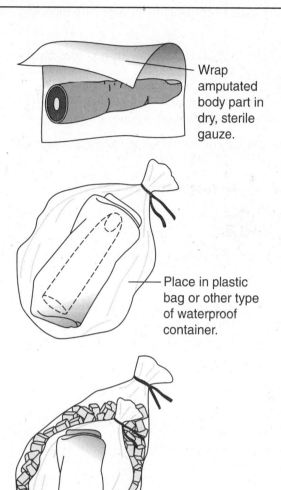

Wrap amputated body part in dry, sterile gauze.

Place in plastic bag or other type of waterproof container.

Place on bed of ice: do *not* bury it.

Figure LM4-1. Why is it necessary to place an amputated body part on ice?

PREPROCEDURE

1. Before you begin, gather needed equipment.
2. Make sure that the scene is safe. If it is safe, observe standard precautions by wearing latex or vinyl gloves.
3. Call EMS.
4. Check the client's level of responsiveness and ABCs. Carry out first aid measures to restore ABCs if required.

PROCEDURE

Keep the following points in mind when you provide first aid for an amputation.

5. If possible, retrieve amputated part with your gloved hand.
6. Control all major external bleeding.
7. Treat the client for shock. See textbook Procedure 4H, "Shock."

Procedure LM4-1: Amputation (continued)

8. Provide first aid to the part that remains. Apply a tourniquet to control life-threatening bleeding only.

9. Wrap the amputated part with a sterile gauze dressing or other clean cloth.

10. Place the amputated part in a waterproof plastic bag or other waterproof container.

11. Place the bag or container containing the part on ice.

12. Keep the part cool but do not freeze it.

13. Comfort and reassure client while waiting the arrival of EMS.

14. Send amputated part with client to hospital.

POSTPROCEDURE

Once you have provided first aid for an amputation remove your gloves and wash your hands with soap and water.

PRACTICE LM4-1

Using Procedure Assessment Sheet LM4-1 in your Lab Activity Manual, practice first aid for amputation. Review the step-by-step procedure until you have mastered the skill. Follow your teacher's guidelines for completion of hands-on testing.

Procedure LM13-1A Preparing an Oxygen Cylinder

Equipment and Supplies

Medical grade oxygen cylinder (indicated by the letters USP)

Figure LM13-1 shows the preparation of the oxygen delivery system.

PREPROCEDURE

1. Gather needed equipment.
2. Place the cylinder in an upright position and stand it to one side.

PROCEDURE

3. Remove the protective seal from the valve of the cylinder.
4. Keep the plastic valve.

Figure LM13-1.
Preparation.
(a.) Select appropriate cylinder.
(b.) Place cylinder in upright position.
(c.) Remove plastic protecting cylinder outlet.
(d.) Keep plastic valve.
(e.) Crack valve for one second.
(f.) Place gasket on oxygen regulator.
(g.) Place regulator on cylinder and align pins.
(h.) Tighten the T-screw.
(i.) Turn on oxygen and assess for leaks.
(j.) Attach delivery device.
(k.) Adjust Oxygen flow rate.
(l.) Place device on client.

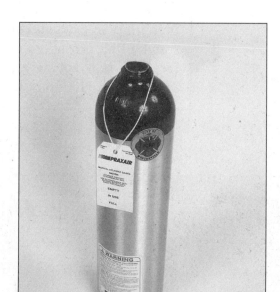

Steps (a.) and (b.)

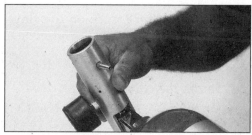

Step (g.)

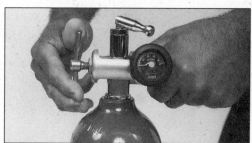

Step (h.)

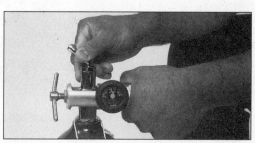

Step (e.)

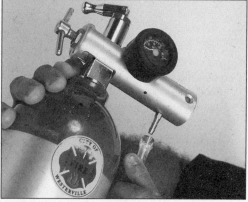

Step (j.)

5. Open the cylinder's valve for one second.

6. Select the appropriate flow meter.

7. Place the cylinder's nylon O ring on the regulator's oxygen port.

8. Align the regulator's pins with the cylinder's valve inlets.

9. Tighten the "T-screw."

10. Open the cylinder's main valve all the way, and then close it a half turn.

11. Check for leaks. If there is a leak, turn off the valve and bleed oxygen from the regulator by turning it on. Once it is bled, remove the regulator and repeat steps starting at step 7.

12. If there is no leak, attach oxygen tubing and the delivery device, turn on the flow meter, and adjust flow to prescribed rate.

13. Apply the delivery device to the client.

14. Secure the cylinder or lay it down.

POSTPROCEDURE

Figure LM13-2 shows the procedure for discontinuing oxygen.

15. Remove the delivery device from the client.

16. Turn off oxygen's main valve.

17. Disconnect the flow device from the regulator.

18. Turn on the flow meter and bleed, or discharge, residual oxygen from the regulator.

PRACTICE LM13-1A

Using Procedure Assessment Sheet LM13-1A in your Lab Activity Manual, practice preparing an oxygen cylinder. Review the step-by-step procedure until you have mastered the skill. Follow your teacher's guidelines for completion of hands-on testing.

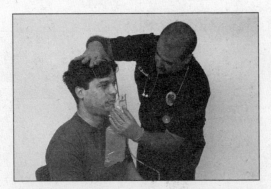
Step (a.)

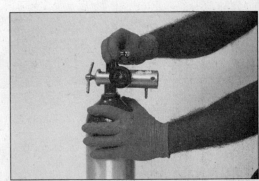
Step (b.)

Figure LM13-2.
Discontinuing oxygen.
(a.) Remove delivery device from client.
(b.) Close Main valve
(c.) Remove oxygen tubing
(d.) Bleed regulator. What does it mean to "bleed" the regulator?

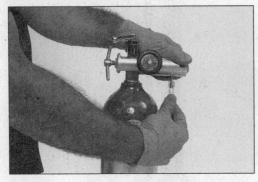
Step (c.)

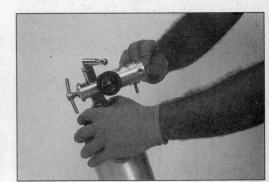
Step (d.)

Procedure LM13-1B Providing Oxygen

Equipment and Supplies

Gloves • goggles or a face shield • other appropriate protective equipment • nonrebreather mask • oxygen cylinder • nasal cannula

PREPROCEDURE

1. Gather needed equipment.
2. Determine the need for oxygen use based upon your assessment findings of the client and the probable condition of the client. The client must have spontaneous adequate air exchange to safely use this device.
3. (CAUTION) Follow appropriate infection control practices while providing oxygen.

PROCEDURE

Procedure for Nonrebreather Mask

Figure LM13-3 shows a nonrebreather mask.

- Remove the nonrebreather mask and tubing from packaging.
- Uncoil tubing and the reservoir bag and tubing.
- Connect the female connector of tubing to the nipple of oxygen source flow meter.
- Turn on the oxygen cylinder valve and adjust flow meter to between 12 to 15 liters per minute.

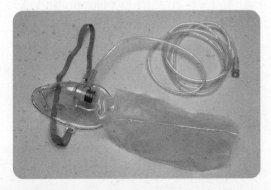

Figure LM13-3. A nonbreather mask. Set oxygen concentration percentages and flow rates.

- Place your thumb over the one-way inlet valve between the mask and the reservoir bag, until the bag becomes fully inflated.
- Remove your thumb from the valve.
- Explain to the client that you are going to place him or her on oxygen.
- Place the mask over the client's nose and mouth and slip the elastic strap over the client's head so that the strap is placed between each ear and the back of the client's head.
- Tighten the elastic strap as needed.
- Squeeze the pliable metal strip across the portion that is covering the nose so that a better seal is achieved. If a tight seal has been achieved, the reservoir bag will remain partly inflated when the client breathes in.
- If the bag completely flattens, increase the flow of oxygen.
- Monitor the client's status.

Procedure for Nasal Cannula

- Remove the nasal cannula from packaging.
- Uncoil the tubing.
- Connect the female connector of tubing to the nipple of the oxygen source flow meter.
- (CAUTION) Turn on the oxygen cylinder valve and adjust the flow meter to between 2 to 6 liters per minute. Never exceed the 6 liters per minute flow rate with a cannula. Exceeding this flow rate will not increase the oxygen concentration and it may cause severe drying and potential injury to the client's nasal passages.
- Check that the oxygen properly flows from the cannula's prongs.
- Explain to the client that you are going to place him or her on oxygen.
- Hold the loop part of the cannula in front of the client's face so that the prongs are oriented on the upper side of the loop.

PROCEDURE LM13-1B: Providing Oxygen (continued)

- Orient the curvature of the prongs so that the tips face upward.

- Point the tips of the prongs toward each nostril and advance them into each nostril until they are fully inserted.

- Hold the loop at the nose to keep the prongs inserted. With the other hand, carefully pass one side of the loop over and behind the ear on one side of the client's head.

- Continue to hold the inserted prongs in the nostrils, and pass the other loop over and behind the ear on the other side of the client's head.

- Once the loop is over each ear, grasp the loop at the neck and advance the plastic slide fastener up under the client's chin until the bottom of the loop is held firmly in place.

- Recheck the loop. Make sure it is firmly in place to hold the prongs securely in the nostrils, but it should not be so tight that it is uncomfortable or places undue pressure on the client's trachea.

POSTPROCEDURE

4. Carefully remove the oxygen delivery device from the client.

5. Turn off oxygen at the flow meter and cylinder valve.

6. Bleed flow meter dry.

7. Replace the cylinder if pressure is 500 psi or below.

PRACTICE LM13-1B

Using Procedure Assessment Sheet LM13-1B in your Lab Activity Manual, practice providing oxygen with a nonrebreather mask and nasal cannula. Review the step-by-step procedure until you have mastered the skill. Follow your teacher's guidelines for completion of hands-on testing.

Procedure LM13-2A Manual Stabilization of the Head and Neck

The object of this procedure is to maintain the client's head and neck motionless in a neutral, inline position as shown in Figure LM13-4. In this position, the head is facing forward, not turned to either side, nor tilted forward or backward. Applying manual stabilization prevents further movement of the head and neck and is used for possible head or neck injury.

client is completely immobilized on a long spine board.

PROCEDURE

Depending upon the client's position provide stabilization as follows:

- Client is sitting up.
    a. Position yourself behind the client's head.
    b. Grasp the sides of the client's head with both hands, spread your fingers and thumb over each side of the head.
    c. Hold the head motionless. Do not allow the client to move his or her head.

- Client is supine, lying on his or her back, face up.
    a. Kneel behind the client's head.

Equipment and Supplies
No equipment needed.

PREPROCEDURE

1. (CAUTION) Identify that the client requires head and neck stabilization by assessment and observation of signs and symptom. Once applied, manual stabilization cannot be released until the

PROCEDURE LM13-2A: Manual Stabilization of the Head and Neck

(continued)

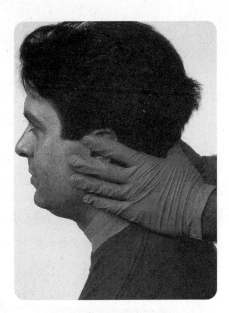

Figure LM13-4. The inline position. Name the situations that require manual stabilization of the head and neck.

b. Grasp the sides of the client's head with both hands, spread your fingers and thumb over each side of the head.
c. Hold the head motionless. Do not allow the client to move his or her head.

- If the client is in another position, for example, on his or her side, adapt the above procedure so that the head can remain motionless, in a neutral position.

POSTPROCEDURE

2. Maintain stabilization until the client is completely immobilized on a long spine board.

PRACTICE LM13-2A

Using Procedure Assessment Sheet LM13-2A in your Lab Activity Manual, practice manual stabilization of the head and neck. Review the step-by-step procedure until you have mastered the skill. Follow your teacher's guidelines for completion of hands-on testing.

Procedure LM13-2B Applying Cervical Collars

Cervical collars are rigid collars applied to protect the cervical spine of victims of head and neck trauma. They must be appropriately sized and applied after taking care of life-threatening problems and only after assessing the front and back of the client's head and neck. Varieties of cervical immobilization collars are found on the market. Regardless of the collar's construction, make sure the collar is the right size for the client. The correct size of the collar depends on the length of the client's neck. The front height of the collar should fit between the point of the chin and the U-shaped dip where the sternum and clavicles meet. The collar should rest on the clavicles and support the lower jaw. A properly fitted collar will not stretch or lift the chin or hyperextend the neck, nor will it allow the chin to drop too low, and it will not constrict the neck too tightly. The general steps for sizing and applying a cervical collar on the neck of a client with a suspected spinal injury are shown in Figure LM13-5.

PROCEDURE LM13-2B: Applying Cervical Collars *(continued)*

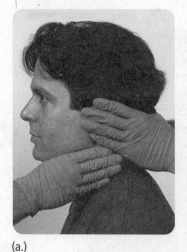 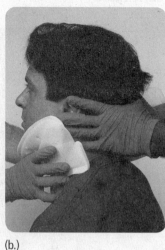

Figure LM13-5.
(a.) Measure client's neck.
(b.) Measure the collar. What are the characteristics of a properly fitted collar?

(a.)   (b.)

Equipment and Supplies

Correct size cervical collar

PREPROCEDURE

1. Gather needed equipment.

2. Ensure that the scene is safe and secure. Advise the client not to move his or her head or neck.

3. Have a partner position himself or herself behind the client's head and apply manual stabilization to the head and neck. Continue manual stabilization without interruption.

4. Perform initial assessment:
   - Without moving the client's neck or with assistance from another, obtain a general impression of the client's condition and injuries.
   - Evaluate airway, breathing, signs of circulation, and level of responsiveness.
   - Assess motor and sensory abilities in all four extremities.

5. Examine the head and neck for signs of injury.

6. Measure the correct size of the cervical collar. Collar size is best determined by measuring the height between the top of the shoulder and the tip of the chin when the head is in the neutral, inline position. To perform a quick size check,

use your fingers to measure the shoulder to chin distance. Make sure that the chin piece will not lift the client's chin and hyperextend the neck. Make sure that the collar is not too small or too tight.

PROCEDURE

Depending upon the client's position, apply the cervical collar as follows and as shown in Figure LM13-6:

- If the client is sitting:
   a. Your partner maintains manual inline stabilization of the head and neck. See Figure LM13-4.
   b. You properly angle the collar for placement.
   c. You then position the collar bottom under chin and lower jaw.
   d. Set the collar in place around the neck.
   e. Secure Velcro straps on collar.
   f. Have your partner spread fingers and maintain manual support for the head and neck until the client is completely immobilized on the appropriate spinal immobilization device.

- If the client is lying:
   a. Your partner kneels at the client's head and neck and applies manual stabilization to the head and neck. Manual stabilization should be continued without interruption.

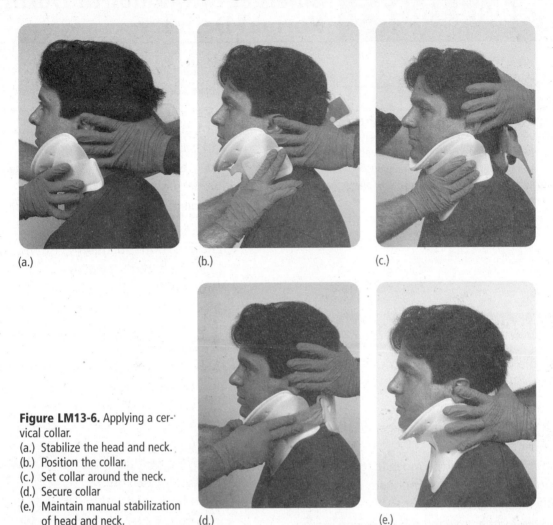

(a.)   (b.)   (c.)

Figure LM13-6. Applying a cervical collar.
(a.) Stabilize the head and neck.
(b.) Position the collar.
(c.) Set collar around the neck.
(d.) Secure collar
(e.) Maintain manual stabilization of head and neck.

(d.)   (e.)

b. You position the collar in place.
c. Position the collar bottom under the chin and lower jaw.
d. Set the collar around the neck.
e. Secure Velcro straps on collar.
f. Have your partner spread fingers and maintain manual support for the head and neck until client is completely immobilized on a suitable spinal immobilization device.

PRACTICE LM13-2B

Using Procedure Assessment Sheet LM13-2B in your Lab Activity Manual, practice applying a cervical collar. Review the step-by-step procedure until you have mastered the skill. Follow your teacher's guidelines for completion of hands-on testing.

POSTPROCEDURE

7. Monitor client until he or she is safely transported to a medical facility.

Procedure LM13-3 — Emergency Childbirth During a Normal Delivery

Equipment and Supplies

OB kit • impervious gown or apron and face shield • two or more pairs of sterile gloves • towels or sheets • one rubber bulb syringe • gauze pads or clean towels • cord clamps, umbilical tape or hemostats • individually wrapped sanitary napkins • clean sheets or blankets • plastic bag for the placenta • sterile knife

PREPROCEDURE

1. Assemble or obtain an obstetrics (OB) kit with the items listed above.

2. Evaluate the expectant mother.
   - Ask the mother her name, age, and expected due date.
   - Labor for a first-born is much longer, whereas labor for a second or subsequent birth is typically much shorter.
   - Ask the mother how long she has been in labor and how often she is having pains. When contractions last 30 seconds to 1 minute and are 2 to 3 minutes apart, delivery of the baby is imminent.
   - Ask the mother if she has experienced any bleeding or discharge of mucus.
   - Ask the mother if her amniotic sac (bag of water) has ruptured.
   - Ask, "Do you feel the need to move your bowels?" If the answer to this question is yes, this usually means that the baby has moved into the birth canal. Do not allow the mother to use the bathroom.
   - Check the mother to see if she is crowning. The presence of crowning means the birth is imminent.
   - During a contraction, feel the abdomen of the mother. Is it hard? A very hard abdomen means delivery of the infant is underway.
   - Take vital signs.

3. Observe for signs of imminent delivery.
   - Crowning is present.
   - Contractions are closer than 2 minutes apart and last from 30 to 90 seconds.
   - The client feels the child's head moving down the birth canal.
   - The client's abdomen is very hard.

4. Prepare the mother.
   - (CAUTION) Put on gloves, gown, and face shield. Childbirth involves a lot of blood and amniotic fluid. First Responders and EMTs should follow strict standard precaution guidelines to protect themselves from an exposure.
   - Place the mother on a bed or on the floor. Elevate the buttocks with blankets or pillows and have the mother lie with knees drawn up and legs and thighs spread apart. If possible, raise up her back.
   - Remove the mother's clothing below the waist and her underpants.
   - Drape both legs and knees with clean sheets or towels. Cover the abdomen with another clean sheet.
   - Position someone at the head of the mother to assist you.
   - Position all OB supplies near you and within easy reach.

PROCEDURE

5. Deliver the baby.
   - Position yourself so that you have a clear view of the vaginal opening.
   - Calmly speak to the mother throughout the delivery.
   - Have the person at the head monitor the mother for vomiting. This person can also take vital signs.
   - Position your gloved hand at the opening of the vagina when the infant's head begins to appear.

Procedure LM13-3: Emergency Childbirth During a Normal Delivery

(continued)

- As the head delivers, place one gloved hand over the baby's head. Spread your fingers evenly over the bony part of the skull. Avoid the soft areas.
- Continue to support the head but do not allow it to pop out. As the head is delivering, have suction available.
- With a towel in the other hand, support the tissue between the mother's vagina and anus. Supporting this tissue may help to prevent tearing, as the baby's head delivers.
- If the amniotic sac has not ruptured by the time the head has delivered, tear it using your fingers. Pull the membrane away from the mouth and nose of the baby.
- Once the head has delivered, check to see if the umbilical cord is wrapped around the baby's neck. If you determine that the cord is around the infant's neck, use your fingers to slip it over the head. If this is not possible, carefully clamp the cord in two places and cut between the clamps.
- Suction the baby's airway with the bulb syringe as soon as the head delivers. Compress the bulb before placing it in the baby's mouth. Always suction the mouth first, then the nostrils. Continue to support the head with one hand as you suction the airway.
- Help deliver the first shoulder by exerting gentle downward pressure on the head.
- Help deliver the second shoulder by gently guiding the head upwards.
- As the torso and full body are born, support the newborn with both hands. Be sure to grasp the feet as they are born. Remember, a newborn is very slippery.

- After delivery, immediately clean and dry the newborn's head, face, and torso.
- Wrap the baby in a warm, dry, clean blanket or sheet and position the infant on his or her side with the head slightly lower than the body. It may be necessary to periodically suction the infant's airway.
- Record the date and time of the baby's birth.

POSTPROCEDURE

6. Assign your partner to monitor and complete the assessment of the infant.
7. Observe the mother for delivery of the placenta.
8. After the placenta delivers, wrap the delivered placenta in a towel and place in a plastic bag.
9. After the delivery of the placenta, place two sanitary napkins over the vaginal opening.
10. Have the client lower her legs and massage the uterus.
11. Transport mother and baby to a hospital for evaluation.

PRACTICE LM13-3

Using Procedure Assessment Sheet LM13-3 in your Lab Activity Manual, practice emergency childbirth of a normal delivery. Review the step-by-step procedure until you have mastered the skill. Follow your teacher's guidelines for completion of hands-on testing.

Procedure LM15-1 | Measuring Blood Glucose Using a Glucometer

When you measure blood glucose using a glucometer, refer to the step-by-step guide given in the following sections.

Equipment and Supplies

Gloves • sterile gauze or tissue • glucometer machine • sterile-lancet or automatic device • capillary testing sticks • antiseptic wipe • biohazard sharps container

PREPROCEDURE

Before you measure blood glucose with a glucometer, review these steps.

1. Gather needed equipment.
2. **(CAUTION)** Wash your hands.
3. Review the glucometer operator's manual or user's guide if necessary.
4. Perform a quality control check on the glucometer according to the manufacturer's instructions and use a test strip and/or control solution.
5. **(CAUTION)** Note the expiration date on the testing strips. Do not use the strips if the expiration date has passed.
6. Review the request form to verify the test ordered.

PROCEDURE

Keep the following points in mind when you measure blood glucose using a glucometer.

7. **(CAUTION)** Identify the client by asking his or her full name.
8. Explain the procedure to the client.
9. **(CAUTION)** Put on examination gloves and choose one of the client's fingers for the capillary stick. The finger should be free of bruises, scars, calluses, cuts, or sores.

10. Clean the finger with the antiseptic wipe. With a sterile lancet or capillary puncture device, quickly puncture the site at a 90° angle. See Figure LM15-1.
11. **(CAUTION)** Properly dispose of the lancet by placing it into a biohazard sharps container.
12. Remove the first drop of blood with a piece of clean gauze or tissue.
13. Gently squeeze a second drop of blood onto the testing strip and place the strip into the glucometer at the appropriate time according to the manufacturer's instructions. You may be required to remove the first drop of blood prior to inserting the testing strip into the glucometer. You may use a small pipette to obtain the blood from the finger and place on the strip. Check the manufacturer's instructions.
14. When the glucometer is finished processing the blood specimen on the testing strip, you will hear a "beeping" sound or see a flash.
15. Note the number that appears in the digital display window. This is the blood glucose amount. If the display is less than 20 or greater than 300, or if something other than a number appears, repeat the test. Review the Procedure Troubleshooting box on the next page for more guidelines on measuring blood glucose.

POSTPROCEDURE

Once you have completed measuring blood glucose, do the following.

16. **(CAUTION)** Place the used gauze or tissue and the testing strip in the appropriate biohazard container.
17. Turn off the glucometer and replace it in the storage cabinet.
18. **(CAUTION)** Remove gloves and wash your hands.
19. Document the procedure and the blood glucose result in the client's record.

PROCEDURE LM15-1: Measuring Blood Glucose Using a Glucometer

(continued)

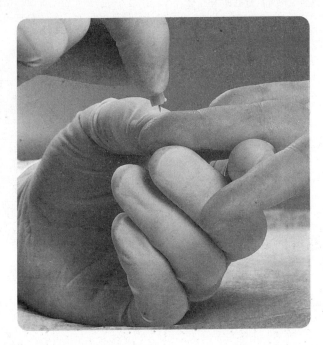

Figure LM15-1. Hold the lancet, or puncture device, at a right angle to the clients' finger.

PROCEDURE TROUBLESHOOTING

Using a Glucometer

The expected reading for a fasting blood sugar (glucose) is 74 to 120 mg/dL. If your client has had nothing to eat or drink for 8 hours, this reading is considered normal. If your client has had food or drink during the last 8 hours, the blood sugar could be higher.

When an error message is displayed before repeating the test, review the following points to make sure that your results will be accurate.

- Check the reagent strips to make sure they are not out of date. Do not touch the reagent pads or leave the container of strips open for longer than necessary.
- Check the glucometer to be sure that it is clean. Dust, dirt, or other residue can cause an inaccurate reading. The lens of the glucometer is usually cleaned with lens paper or a special cleaning solution. The lens is usually not cleaned with alcohol. Check the manufacturer's instructions.
- Be sure that you have the correct amount of blood on the reagent pad. Many machines require you to blot the drop of blood after you have placed it on the pad. Be careful not to wipe too much blood off the pad. Some machines do not use a reagent pad; a full drop of blood is placed in a small container that is inserted into the machine. Review the manufacturer's directions.
- The reagent pad or container must be inserted into the glucometer correctly. Double-check that the pad or container is facing in the right direction and is firmly in place. Make sure that you wait the appropriate amount of time before reading the machine.

Procedure LM15-2 | Assisting with Minor Office Surgery

Many physicians perform minor surgical procedures in the office setting. Although the physician is responsible for explaining the procedure to the client, the office staff is responsible for setting up the treatment area and surgical tray for the physician. See Figure LM15-2. The office assistant is also responsible for preparing the client for the procedure and making sure that the consent form for treatment has been signed. During the procedure, the assistant reassures the client and assists the physician as needed. After the procedure, the client is given specific instructions for wound care as determined by the physician.

When you assist with minor office surgery, follow the step-by-step guide in the following sections.

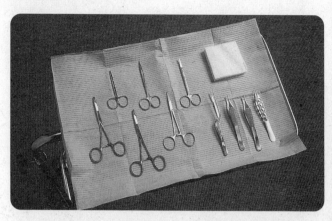

Figure LM15-2. It may be the responsibility of the MA to set up the sterile tray with all sterile items before the minor office procedure. What are the assistant's other responsibilities related to these procedures?

Equipment and Supplies

Sterile gauze pads of an appropriate size for the procedure • two sterile drapes • suture material, which is wire or thread for surgically closing a wound; and local anesthetic • syringe and needle: 1 or 3 cc, 1/2 to 1 inch, 22 to 26 gauge • disposable scalpel, a sharp instrument used for cutting and disecting tissue; (this instrument may also be nondisposable) • individually wrapped and sterilized surgical instruments, determined by the procedure • sterile gloves for the physician • container for collecting contaminated instruments and supplies • biohazard sharps container • biohazard waste container • sterile dressing and tape • specimen container and preservative, if appropriate • laboratory request for any specimens collected • examination light • mayo stand

PREPROCEDURE

Before you assist with minor office surgery, do the following. Also refer to Figures LM15-3 and LM15-4.

1. (CAUTION) Wash your hands and assemble the equipment:

2. Check the client's medical record for a signed consent form.

3. Identify the client by asking for his or her full name.

4. Prepare the client by instructing him or her on clothing removal, gown, and draping.

5. If instructed by the physician, prepare the surgical area by shaving unwanted hair from the area and/or cleaning the area with an antiseptic solution.

PROCEDURE

Keep the following points in mind when you assist with minor office surgery.

6. Take all equipment and supplies to the treatment area or examination room.

7. Carefully open one sterile drape and place it on the mayo stand, from the back of the tray to the front of the tray. Refer to Figure LM15-5.

8. Do not allow the top of the sterile drape to touch any items while you place the sterile drape over the Mayo stand, and do not allow your arms to pass over the sterile field.

9. (CAUTION) A one-inch border around the sterile drape is considered nonsterile. Do not, however, touch any other area of the drape without wearing sterile gloves.

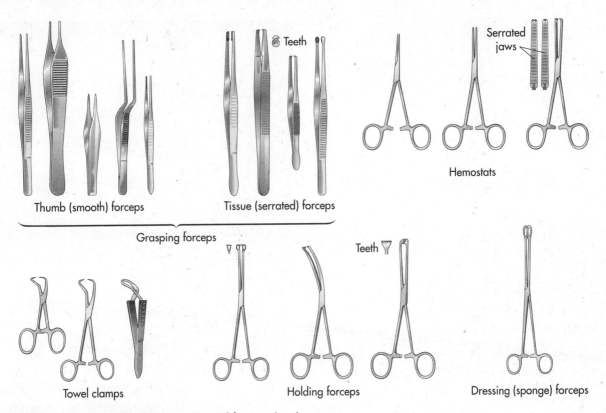

Figure LM15-3. These are surgical instruments used for grasping tissue.

10. (CAUTION) Do not talk or cough over the sterile drape or while applying articles.

11. Add various articles to the sterile field by gently flipping open items in peel-apart packages onto the drape. Items that may be gently flipped onto the field include the gauze, sterile instruments, suture, needle, syringe, and scalpel.

12. Leave non-sterile items and other items such as the anesthetic, additional gauze pads, the physician's unopened sterile gloves, a biohazard container, a specimen container, the laboratory request, and a roll of bandage tape on a side table for easy access. See Figures LM15-6 and LM15-7.

13. Put on sterile gloves and straighten the items on the sterile field or use sterile transfer forceps shown in Figure LM15-8.

14. Remove the sterile gloves and discard them.

15. Open the second sterile drape and place it over the sterile field, from the front of the field to the back of the setup. Avoid touching any non-sterile surfaces with the drape while placing the drape over the sterile tray setup.

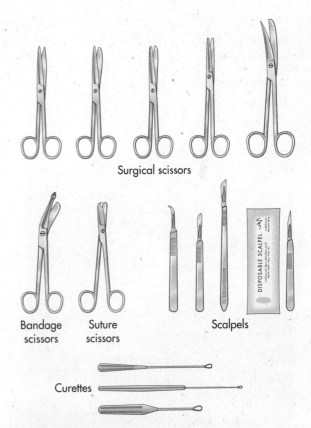

Figure LM15-4. Scalpels, scissors, and currettes are several types of instruments used for cutting and dissecting during surgical procedures.

PROCEDURE LM15-2: Assisting with Minor Office Surgery *(continued)*

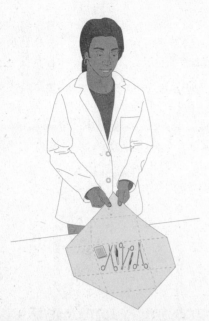

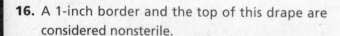

Figure LM15-5. Once the sterilized pack is opened, the inside wrapper of the sterilized pack can become the sterile field. Otherwise, a sterile drape must be applied to the Mayo stand and sterile supplies added.

16. A 1-inch border and the top of this drape are considered nonsterile.

17. Once the tray setup is covered, push the tray to the side by grasping the Mayo stand on the bottom; avoid touching the sterile drapes.

18. Notify the physician that the client and supplies are ready.

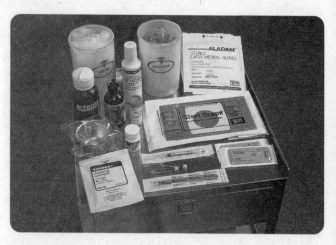

Figure LM15-7. The items that cannot be placed on the sterile field are shown assembled on a side table or countertop.

19. Assist the physician during the procedure by holding a basin or bowl for used instruments or a specimen container, opening sterile items for the physician, or placing additional items on the sterile field as needed. See Figure LM15-9.

20. Reassure the client during the procedure as needed.

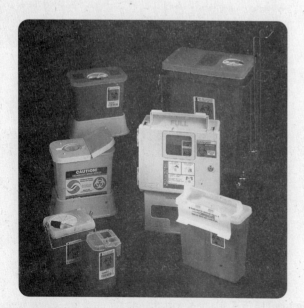

Figure LM15-6. All biohazard sharps containers should be puncture resistant. Why is this an important feature?

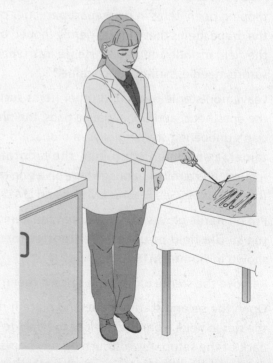

Figure LM15-8. Sterile items can be placed on the sterile field by using sterile transfer forceps.

PROCEDURE LM15-2: Assisting with Minor Office Surgery *(continued)*

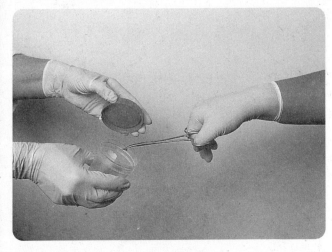

Figure LM15-9. Hold the specimen container so that the physician can place the tissue in it without touching the rim on the outside of the container with the tissue.

POSTPROCEDURE

Once the surgery is completed, do the following.

21. Apply antibiotic ointment, a sterile dressing, and tape to the surgical area if ordered to do by the physician.

22. Help the client get dressed if necessary.

23. Instruct the client on how to care for the surgical area and when to return for suture removal or additional wound care.

24. (CAUTION) Put on clean examination gloves and clean the examination or treatment room by discarding any disposable items in the appropriate containers, sanitizing and disinfecting the work surfaces and tables, and putting away any unused items.

25. Take nondisposable instruments to the utility room and sanitize, disinfect, and prepare them for the sterilization procedure.

26. (CAUTION) Remove gloves and wash your hands.

PRACTICE LM15-2

Using Procedure Assessment Sheet LM15-2 in your Lab Activity Manual, practice assisting with minor office surgery. Review the step-by-step procedure until you have mastered the skill. Follow your teacher's guidelines for completion of hands-on testing.

Procedure LM15-3   Removing Sutures

When you remove sutures, refer to the step-by-step guide in the following sections.

Equipment and Supplies

Clean examination gloves • a disposable or nondisposable suture removal kit consisting of: suture scissors • 2 × 2 inch gauze • sterile thumb forceps, an instrument used to hold or grasp tissue • antiseptic and sterile gauze

PREPROCEDURE

Before you begin removing sutures, review the following steps.

1. (CAUTION) Gather needed equipment and wash your hands.

PROCEDURE

Keep the following points in mind when you remove sutures.

2. (CAUTION) Identify the client by asking for his or her full name.

3. Explain the procedure to the client.

4. (CAUTION) Using clean examination gloves, remove any dressings and discard them in a biohazard waste container.

PROCEDURE LM15-3: Removing Sutures (continued)

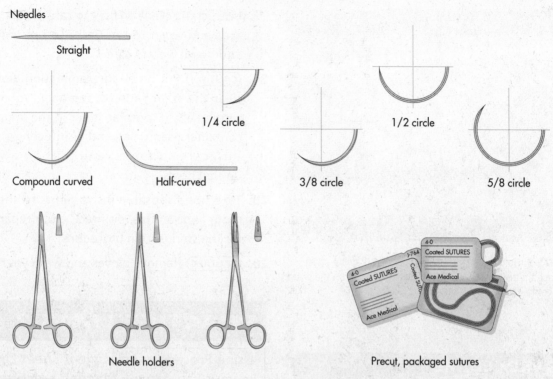

Figure LM15-10. The items shown here will be needed for suturing open wounds. Would these supplies need to be sterile?

5. Inspect the wound for redness, swelling, drainage, and **approximation**, or how close together the edges of the wound have become. If you observe any problems, report them to the physician before you remove the sutures.

6. If the wound appears well healed, determine the number of sutures to be removed.

7. Clean the wound with antiseptic solution and sterile gauze.

8. Pick up the thumb forceps in your nondominant hand and place the suture scissors in your dominant hand. See Figures LM15-3 and LM15-4.

9. Using the thumb forceps, carefully lift one suture by the knot. Slip the curved end of the suture scissors under the suture material closest to the skin and cut it while holding the forceps in place as shown in Figure LM15-11.

10. Pull the suture with the thumb forceps until it is completely removed from the skin.

11. Place the suture onto the 2 × 2-inch gauze pad.

12. Continue this procedure until all the sutures have been removed.

13. (CAUTION) When all the sutures have been removed, count the sutures on the gauze pad and discard the gauze pad in a biohazard waste container.

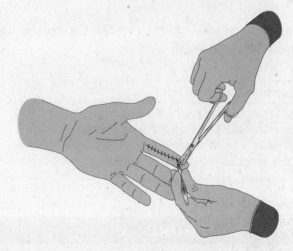

Figure LM15-11. When you remove sutures, be sure to lift the knot away from the skin and cut the suture material as close as possible to the skin.

PROCEDURE LM15-3: Removing Sutures *(continued)*

POSTPROCEDURE

Once you have removed the sutures, do the following.

14. **(CAUTION)** Discard disposable items and or sanitize and disinfect nondisposable items.

15. **(CAUTION)** Remove gloves and wash your hands.

16. Record the procedure, including the number of sutures removed, in the client's record. Also, note the condition of the wound.

PRACTICE LM15-3

Using Procedure Assessment Sheet LM15-3 in your Lab Activity Manual, practice removing sutures. Review the step-by-step procedure until you have mastered the skill. Follow your teacher's guidelines for completion of hands-on testing.

Procedure LM15-4 | Opening Medication Vials and Ampules

When you open medication vials and ampules, refer to the step-by-step guide in the following sections.

Equipment and Supplies

Vial or ampule • 2 X 2 gauze and glove for ampule • PDR or other medication reference book

PREPROCEDURE

Before you open medication vials or ampules, review these steps.

1. **(CAUTION)** Gather needed supplies and wash your hands.

2. Using a drug reference book, look up the drug and note the normal dosages and route of administration. Also refer to textbook Procedure 28F using a PDR for this procedure. Note any contraindications and alert the physician about any questions or concerns before you prepare or administer the medication.

3. Obtain the correct medication from the storage area. Medication containers are shown in Figure LM15-12.

4. **(CAUTION)** Check the medication label carefully against the physician's order.

PROCEDURE

Keep the following points in mind when you open medication vials or ampules.

- To open a medication vial:
    a. Take the medication vial to a well-lit, clean area.
    b. Remove the plastic cap on the top of the bottle by snapping it off with your fingers.
    c. Under the plastic cap, the vial will have a special rubber diaphragm that can be punctured more than once without producing permanent holes. This feature is useful if the vial contains more than one dose. (A vial

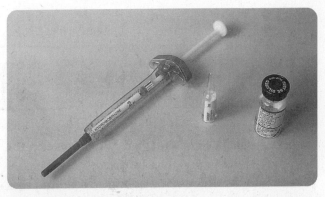

Figure LM15-12. Injectible drugs come prepared in a cartridge (left), an ampule (center), and a vial (right).

containing more than one dose is known as a multiple-dose vial.) Some vials contain only one dose and are therefore called single-dose vials.

- To open a medication ampule:
  a. Take the medication ampule and a 2- × 2-inch gauze pad to a clean, well-lit area.
  b. **(CAUTION)** Put on clean examination gloves.
  c. Holding the ampule by the base, or bottom, gently tap the top, or stem, to remove any medication that may be trapped inside the ampule.
  d. When all medication has been moved to the base, hold the base of the ampule with your nondominant hand and, using your dominant hand, place the gauze around the neck of the ampule.
  e. Gently but firmly break the ampule at the scored area on the neck of the ampule where the stem and the base meet. See Figure LM15-13.

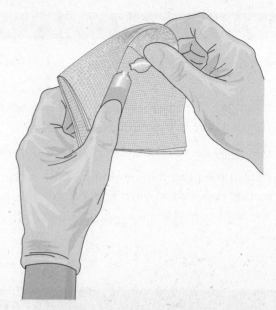

Figure LM15-13. Use a piece of gauze over the neck of the ampule before breaking the glass. What other safety measures should you take?

POSTPROCEDURE

Once you have opened the vial or ampule, do the following.

5. **(CAUTION)** Discard the glass stem of the ampule in a biohazard sharps container.

6. Prepare the medication for withdrawing and administration. See Procedures LM15-5 and LM15-6.

PRACTICE LM15-4

Using Procedure Assessment Sheet LM15-4 in your Lab Activity Manual, practice opening medication vials and ampules. Review the step-by-step procedure until you have mastered the skill. Follow your teacher's guidelines for completion of hands-on testing.

Procedure LM15-5 | Aspirating Medication from Vials and Ampules

Medications packaged in vials and ampules must be removed by suction, or **aspirated**, from the containers into a syringe to be administered. Ampules cannot be used more than once and are usually supplied as single doses.

Regardless of the packaging, the medical office employee must calculate the correct amount to be aspirated into the syringe based upon the dosage ordered by the physician. Review Chapter 17 regarding calculation of dosages. Any unused medication

PROCEDURE LM15-5: Aspirating Medication from Vials and Ampules

(continued)

in the single-dose vial or the ampule must be discarded according to the policy of the physician's office and the procedure manual.

When you aspirate medication from vials or ampules, refer to the step-by-step guide in the following sections.

Equipment and Supplies

Appropriate size needle and syringe (See Procedure LM15-7)
• vial or ampule • alcohol or antiseptic wipe • gloves •
2 x 2 gauze pad

PREPROCEDURE

Before you aspirate medication from vials or ampules, review these steps.

1. **(CAUTION)** Gather needed equipment and wash your hands.

2. **(CAUTION)** Calculate the dosage ordered. Check your calculation at least two times. If you are uncertain, ask someone else to check your calculation.

3. Assemble the needle and syringe without contaminating them.

4. Refer to Procedure LM15-4 for opening the vial or ampule.

PROCEDURE

Keep the following points in mind when you aspirate medication from vials or ampules.

- To aspirate medication from a vial:
  a. Clean the top of the vial with an alcohol, antiseptic wipe.
  b. Carefully remove the needle cap and place it on a clean counter.
  c. Pull back on the plunger of the syringe until an amount of air equal to the amount of medication to be withdrawn is obtained. Figure LM15-15 shows the parts of the syringe.
  d. Inject this air into the vial through the rubber stopper. See Figure LM15-16(a.).
  e. Lift the vial so that it is upside down with the needle inside the vial.
  f. Use your dominant hand to pull back on the plunger of the syringe, keeping the bevel of the needle under the fluid of the medication at all times. See Figure LM15-16(b.).
  g. Pull back on the plunger until more than the correct amount of medication has been drawn into the syringe.
  h. Avoid bubbles if possible, but if any bubbles appear in the syringe, firmly tap the outside of the syringe to move them to the top, near the hub of the needle. See Figure LM15-15.

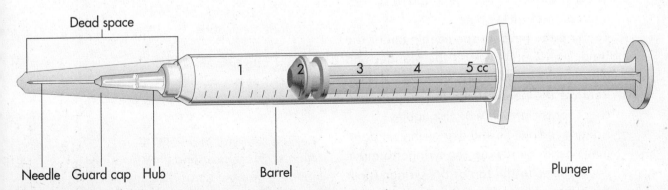

Figure LM15-15. Note the plunger, hub, and barrel on this syringe and needle. What areas of the syringe and needle should be kept sterile?

PROCEDURE LM15-5: Aspirating Medication from Vials and Ampules
(continued)

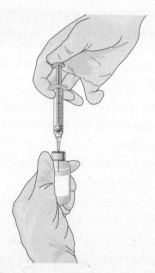

Figure LM15-16(a.). Injecting air into the vial creates an increase in the pressure on the inside of the vial, making it easier to withdraw the medication.

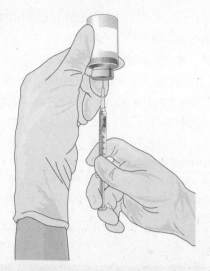

Figure LM15-16(b.). Keep the level of the needle below the level of the medication to avoid aspirating air. What should you do if you aspirate air?

i. Gently push any extra medication and air bubbles out of the syringe and into the vial until the correct dosage is obtained in the syringe.

j. **CAUTION** Remove the needle from the vial and recap the vial by scooping the needle cap onto the needle, or use a needle guard. Do not use two hands to recap the needle. You may accidentally stick yourself with the needle.

- To aspirate medication from an ampule:
  a. Open the ampule according to the steps in Procedure LM15-4 on page B-21.
  b. Carefully remove the filtered needle cap and place it on a clean counter.
  c. Pick up the ampule with one hand and quickly invert it.
  d. Insert the needle into the ampule. Do not inject air into the ampule.
  e. Keeping the bevel of the needle under the fluid, slowly pull back on the plunger and withdraw the medication.
  f. Remove the needle from the ampule and check for the presence of air bubbles.
  g. Holding the needle and syringe in your dominant hand, gently tap the syringe to move any bubbles to the top of the syringe (near the hub) and carefully push excess medication and air out of the syringe.

h. **CAUTION** Recap the needle by scooping the needle cap onto the needle, or use a needle guard. Do not use two hands to recap the needle. You may accidentally stick yourself with the needle.

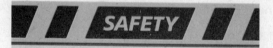

SAFETY

Medical Administration
Medication errors can cause serious or even fatal effects. When preparing and administering medications, you must practice extreme caution and check the following "Five Rights" at least three times prior to administering the medication to the client.
1. Right medication
2. Right client
3. Right dose or amount
4. Right time
5. Right route, for example, oral, subcutaneous, or intramuscular

Be sure that you know the "Five Rights" of medication administration before you prepare or give any medication.

PROCEDURE LM15-5: Aspirating Medication from Vials and Ampules
(continued)

POSTPROCEDURE

Once you have aspirated the medication from the vial or ampule, do the following.

5. **(CAUTION)** Check the label on the vial or ampule for accuracy at least three times: First, when you obtain the medication from the storage area; second, before you withdraw the medication from the ampule or vial: and third, after you aspirate the medication.

6. Discard single-dose vials in the appropriate waste container or replace multiple-dose vials in the proper storage area.

7. **(CAUTION)** Carefully discard the stem and the base of ampules in the biohazard sharps container.

PRACTICE LM15-5

Using Procedure Assessment Sheet LM15-5 in your Lab Activity Manual, practice aspiring medication from vials and ampules. Review the step-by-step procedure until you have mastered the skill. Follow your teacher's guidelines for completion of hands-on testing.

Procedure LM15-6 — Reconstituting Powder Medication for Injection

Some medications come packaged in the powder form and must be mixed with a sterile solution—a liquid agent called a **diluent**—before being injected. Many manufacturers provide the sterile diluents. Other manufacturers suggest using sterile water for injection. In either case, the diluent and the powder medication are packaged in separate vials. Several extra steps must be taken before the medication can be withdrawn and injected into the client.

When you reconstitute powder medication, refer to the step-by-step guide in the following sections.

Equipment and Supplies

The diluent (if it is not packaged with the medication) • two sterile needle and syringe units • alcohol or antiseptic wipes

PREPROCEDURE

Before you begin reconstituting powder medication, review the following steps.

1. Gather needed supplies.

2. **(CAUTION)** Obtain the correct medication from the storage area. Verify the medication against the physician's order and refer to a drug reference book as needed.

3. Determine the amount of diluent to be used according to the medication information insert supplied with the medication or stated in the drug reference book.

4. **(CAUTION)** Wash your hands.

PROCEDURE

Keep the following points in mind when you reconstitute powder medication.

5. Open the vials containing the medication and the diluent. Refer to Procedure LM15-4.

6. Wipe the tops of the vials with alcohol or antiseptic wipe.

PROCEDURE LM15-6: Reconstituting Powder Medication for Injection
(continued)

7. Assemble the needle and syringe without contaminating them.

8. Remove the needle cap and place it on a clean counter.

9. Pull back on the plunger of the syringe until the amount of air is equal to the amount of diluent to be used.

10. Insert the needle into the vial of diluent and invert the vial using your nondominant hand.

11. Push the plunger so that the air in the syringe is inserted into the vial.

12. Remove the appropriate amount of diluent by pulling back on the plunger. Carefully remove any air bubbles if necessary and withdraw the needle from the diluent vial.

13. Insert the needle and syringe containing the diluent into the medication vial.

14. Inject the diluent into the vial containing the powder.

15. (CAUTION) Without aspirating any medication, remove the syringe and needle and discard them in the biohazard sharps container.

16. Gently roll the vial between your hands to mix the powder completely with the diluent.

POSTPROCEDURE

When you have finished reconstituting powder medication, do the following.

17. (CAUTION) Calculate the correct amount to be aspirated and injected using the newly reconstituted mixture.

18. Always use a new syringe and needle to aspirate reconstituted medication before administering the medication to the client.

19. (CAUTION) Discard the used vials in the appropriate waste containers.

PRACTICE LM15-6

Using Procedure Assessment Sheet LM15-6 in your Lab Activity Manual, practice reconstituting powder medication for injection. Review the step-by-step procedure until you have mastered the skill. Follow your teacher's guidelines for completion of hands-on testing.

Procedure LM15-7 | Performing Injections

When you perform **intramuscular (IM)**, **intradermal (ID)**, and **subcutaneous (SC)** injections, refer to the step-by-step guide in the following sections.

Equipment and Supplies

Syringe and needle (the size is determined by injection method) • alcohol antiseptic wipes • band-aid • 2- by 2-inch gauze pad • biohazard sharps container • gloves

PREPROCEDURE

Before you perform injections, review the following steps.

1. (CAUTION) Check the physician's order and obtain the correct medication.

2. (CAUTION) Refer to the drug reference book to note correct dosages, route of administration,

PROCEDURE LM15-7: Performing Injections *(continued)*

contraindications, and special administration instructions.

3. (**CAUTION**) Compare the medication label on the vial or ampule with the physician's order.

4. (**CAUTION**) Wash your hands and assemble the supplies.

5. (**CAUTION**) Calculate the dosage according to the amount ordered by the physician and how the medication is supplied. Reconstitute powder medications if necessary.

6. (**CAUTION**) Always check the medication label three times for accuracy: once when obtaining the medication, again before withdrawing, and a third time before discarding the used vial or ampule.

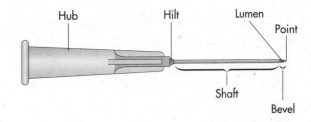

Figure LM15-17. It is important to understand the parts of a needle so that you can use it accurately.

PROCEDURE

Keep the following points in mind when you perform injections.

7. Assemble the syringe and needle.
   Intramuscular
   - Assemble a 3-mL syringe and a needle size ranging from 18 to 23 **gauge**, with a shaft of 1 to 3 inches in length. The term gauge describes the diameter of the lumen of the needle. See Figure LM15-17 for an illustration of the parts of a needle. The gauge and length of the needle are determined by the viscosity, or thickness, of the medication and the location of the muscle to be injected. Typically, a 22- or 23-gauge needle is used. Of course, the size of the client should also be taken into consideration. Refer to the following guide when you determine the needle length:
   - Deltoid muscle—1-inch needle
   - Dorsogluteal muscle—1½-inch needle
   - Vastus lateralis muscle—1½-inch needle

   Subcutaneous
   - 3-milliliter syringe and a needle size ranging from 23- to 27-gauge, ½ to ¾ inch in length.
   Intradermal
   - 1-milliliter syringe and a needle size ranging from 25- to 26-gauge, ⅜ to ½ inch in length.

8. Using the proper technique, aspirate the correct amount of medication from the vial or the ampule. Refer to Procedure LM15-5.

9. Place the syringe and needle filled with the correct amount of medication, an antiseptic wipe, a small gauze pad, clean examination gloves, and an adhesive bandage on a small tray to carry to the examination room. (**CAUTION**) In addition, a biohazard sharps container should be available to discard the used needle and syringe.

10. (**CAUTION**) Identify the client by asking for his or her full name.

11. (**CAUTION**) Check the client's medical record for documentation of any **allergy**, that is, a hypersensitive reaction to a substance that normally does not cause a reaction. Also ask the client about medication allergies if these are not documented. Chart NKA if "no known allergies" are noted. If the injection is for an Intradermal tuberculin test, ask the client about previous tests and results.

12. If the client is not allergic to the medication to be given, instruct the client on clothing removal and positioning.

PROCEDURE LM15-7: Performing Injections (continued)

13. **(CAUTION)** Put on clean examination gloves.

14. Find the correct site:

   Intramuscular
   • Use appropriate landmarks on the body. Refer to Figure LM15-18.

   Subcutaneous
   • Refer to Figure LM15-19.

Intradermal
• Refer to Figure LM15-20. Usually the anterior forearm is used for tuberculin screening tests.

15. Clean the chosen site with an antiseptic wipe, starting in the center and moving in a circular and outward motion.

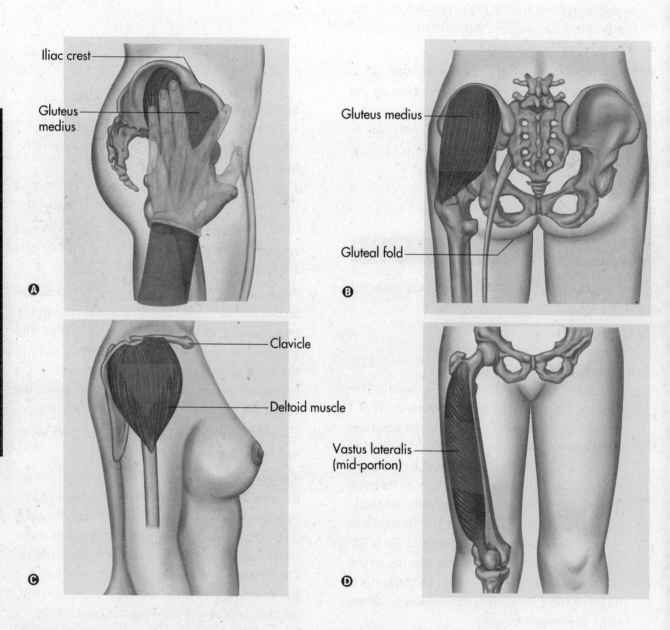

Figure LM15-18. Three common sites for administering intramuscular injections are shown: the gluteus medius (shown in A and B), the deltoid, and the vastus lateralis. Note the bony landmarks that must be palpated to accurately locate the muscle.

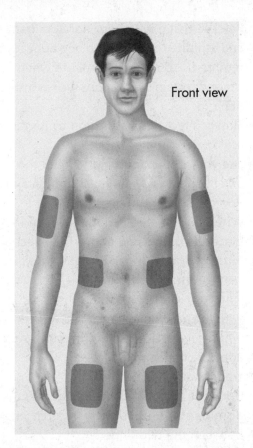
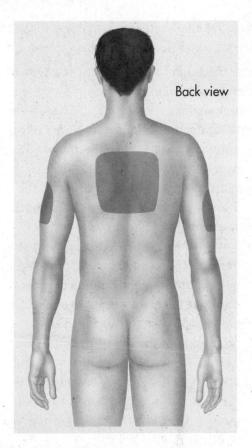

Figure LM15-19. The shaded areas shown on the anterior of this body are suitable for subcutaneous injections.

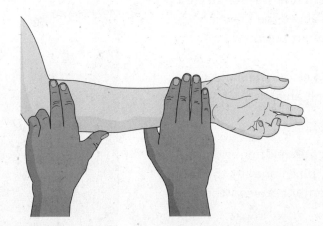

Figure LM15-20. Using the anterior forearm, the space shown between the physician office employee's finger is adequate for the intradermal injection.

PROCEDURE LM15-7: Performing Injections (continued)

16. Remove the needle cap, making sure that the sharps container is within easy access.

17. Use the proper technique for the type of injection to be given.

Intramuscular

- Using the thumb and index finger of your nondominant hand, hold the muscle firmly between the two fingers.
- With the needle at a 90° angle to the muscle, insert the needle quickly and smoothly with your dominant hand.
- **(CAUTION)** Release the muscle with your nondominant hand and aspirate, or create suction, by pulling back gently on the plunger to make sure that the needle is not in a blood vessel. If blood appears in the hub of the needle, do not proceed with the injection and withdraw the needle. Begin the procedure over again after obtaining a new syringe and needle. However, if no blood is produced in the hub of the needle after aspirating, continue with the injection.
- Slowly inject the medication into the muscle by gently pressing on the plunger.
- Use your dominant hand to keep the syringe and needle steady during aspiration and injection of the medication.
- When all the medication has been injected, place the gauze pad above the injection site with your nondominant hand and quickly remove the needle.
- Gently massage the injection site, unless contra indicated, and apply an adhesive bandage if necessary.

Subcutaneous

- Using the thumb and index finger of your nondominant hand, pinch and lift the subcutaneous tissue gently between the two fingers.
- With the needle at a 45° angle to the skin, insert the needle quickly and smoothly with the dominant hand with the bevel of the needle up. See Figure LM15-21. Use a 90° angle for abdominal SC injections for heavier clients.

- Release tissue with your nondominant hand and aspirate to check for blood appearance (if required). You do NOT aspirate when administering certain medications such as insulin and heparin.
- Slowly inject the medication by gently pressing on the plunger.
- Use your dominant hand to keep the syringe and needle steady during aspiration and injection of the medication.
- When all the medication has been injected, place the gauze pad above the injection site with your nondominant hand and quickly remove the needle.
- **(CAUTION)** Gently massage the injection site with the gauze pad if required. Never message when giving a heparin injection. Apply an adhesive bandage if necessary.

Intradermal

- Using the thumb and index finger of your nondominant hand, tightly stretch the skin between the two fingers.
- **(CAUTION)** With the needle at a 10° to 15° angle to the skin, insert the needle smoothly, with the bevel of the needle up. Insert the needle only until the bevel is completely under the skin. Do not aspirate for this injection. See Figure LM15-21.

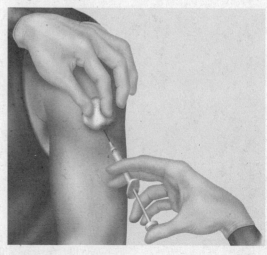

Figure LM15-21. During a subcutaneous injection, keep the needle at a 45° angle so that the medication is administered into the fatty tissue. What is the danger of a needle wrongly placed or placed at a different angle?

PROCEDURE LM15-7: Performing Injections *(continued)*

- Release the skin with your nondominant hand and slowly inject the medication by gently pressing on the plunger. A small wheal, or bubble, on the skin will be produced. It indicates that the medication has been injected correctly. See Figure LM15-22.
- Use your dominant hand to keep the syringe and needle steady during the injection of the medication.
- (CAUTION) When all the medication has been injected, gently remove the needle. Do not massage the injection site and do not apply an adhesive bandage.

18. (CAUTION) Place the needle and syringe into a biohazard sharps container.

19. (CAUTION) Remove your gloves and wash your hands.

20. Instruct the client in the procedure for reporting the results if necessary.

POSTPROCEDURE

Once you have performed the injection, do the following.

21. Document the injection by recording the date, time, name, and dose of the medication, route and site of administration, and your name in the client's record.

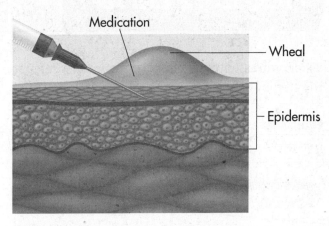

Figure LM15-22. Medication injected into the dermal layer of the skin correctly will produce a wheal.

22. Observe and report any reactions to the medication immediately to the physician.

PRACTICE LM15-7

Using Procedure Assessment Sheet LM15-7 in your Lab Activity Manual, practice performing intramuscular, intradermal, and subcutaneous injections. Review the step-by-step procedure until you have mastered the skill. Follow your teacher's guidelines for completion of hands-on testing.

Procedure LM16-1 | Administering Chemical Restraints

When you administer chemical restraints, refer to the step-by-step guide in the following sections.

Equipment and Supplies

Medication • glass of water

PREPROCEDURE

Before you begin, review these steps.

1. Check to make sure there is a written order for the chemical restraint or medication. The order should be in the plan of care of the supervising nurse or other licensed practitioner.

2. (CAUTION) The licensed practitioner must have instructed you on the medication that is to be given.

3. (CAUTION) Wash your hands.

4. (CAUTION) Identify the client.

5. Introduce yourself to the client if necessary.

6. Provide for privacy for the client.

7. Explain the procedure to the client.

8. Make sure that the client is in a comfortable position.

9. Have on hand a glass of water so that the client can take the medication.

PROCEDURE

Keep the following points in mind when you administer chemical restraints.

10. Help the client to sit up.

11. Hand the medication to the client.

12. Help the client put the medication in his or her mouth if necessary.

13. Hand the glass of water to the client so that he or she can swallow the medication. If the client has difficulty swallowing the medication, you may suggest that he or she take a drink of water before taking the medication.

14. (CAUTION) Make sure that the client has put the medication in his or her mouth and has swallowed it.

15. (CAUTION) Make sure that the client can reach the signal bell.

16. (CAUTION) Make sure that the client is comfortable.

17. (CAUTION) Wash your hands.

18. Record the procedure in the client's record.

19. Report to your supervisor that you have done the procedure and any abnormal occurrence.

POSTPROCEDURE

When you have administered a chemical restraint, do the following.

20. (CAUTION) Check on the client frequently to make sure that he or she is safe. Offer fluids as necessary. Check to see whether the client needs to use the bathroom.

21. Report any adverse findings to your supervisor immediately.

PRACTICE LM16-1

Using Procedure Assessment Sheet LM16-1 in your Lab Activity Manual, practice administering chemical restraints. Review the step-by-step procedure until you have mastered the skill. Follow your teacher's guidelines for completion of hands-on testing.

Procedure LM19-1 — Assisting with an Examination of the Ear

When you assist with an examination of the ear, refer to the step-by-step guide in the following sections.

Equipment and Supplies

Otoscope • disposable speculum • disposable gloves • pen or pencil.

PREPROCEDURE

Before you begin, do the following.

1. Gather needed equipment.
2. Identify the client and introduce yourself.
3. Explain the procedure.
4. Ask the client to remove glasses and hearing aides if the client is wearing these items.

PROCEDURE

Keep the following points in mind when you assist with an examination of the ear.

5. Pass the lighted otoscope to the doctor or nurse.
6. Help the client sit in the correct position for examination. The client should tip his or her head slightly toward the shoulder so that the ear to be examined is pointing up. The doctor or nurse may hold the ear lobe as the speculum is inserted into the ear. The client may need to adjust her position so that the doctor can get a better view

of the ear canal and eardrum. Both ears are usually examined, even if there seems to be a problem with just one ear.

POSTPROCEDURE

When you have completed assisting with an examination of the ear, do the following.

7. When the examination is complete, help the client put on glasses, hearing aid(s), and other articles as necessary.
8. (CAUTION) Provide for the client's safety and comfort. If you are in an inpatient facility, place the signal light within easy reach of the client.
9. Clean and replace all equipment. Dispose of the cone-shaped plastic tip to prevent cross-contamination.
10. (CAUTION) Wash your hands.
11. Record all required information.

PRACTICE LM19-1

Using Procedure Assessment Sheet LM19-1 in your Lab Activity Manual, practice assisting with an examination of the ear. Review the step-by-step procedure until you have mastered the skill. Follow your teacher's guidelines for completion of hands-on testing.

Procedure LM20-1 | Using a Cold Whirlpool

Equipment and Supplies

Whirlpool • ice scoop or bucket • thermometer • disinfectant • timer • towel(s)

PREPROCEDURE

1. Gather needed equipment.

2. (CAUTION) Test the client's sensation to touch by lightly running your hand or fingers across the area. If the client reports decreased sensation or hypersensitivity in the area, tell your licensed supervisor immediately.

3. If sensation is normal, fill the whirlpool in the following manner.
   - Close the drain to the whirlpool.
   - Turn on the faucet to facilitate filling.
   - Use scoops or buckets of ice from a nearby ice maker to regulate the temperature of the water. The temperature should be between 50° and 60°F.
   - Add the appropriate amount of disinfectant to the water, such as Chlorazene®, and turn on the turbine to mix it.
   - (CAUTION) Be sure the water is deep enough to cover the lower 2/3 of the turbine. If not, damage can occur to the engine.
   - Run the turbine for approximately 5 minutes to ensure proper disinfecting.

PROCEDURE

4. Help the client place the affected extremity in the whirlpool.

5. Turn the turbine on.

6. Aim the jet of the turbine at the affected limb.

7. Adjust the force of the output of the turbine by opening or closing the outflow valve.

8. Set a timer for the time specified by the therapist.

9. (CAUTION) Periodically check the client's condition. Some clients may not tolerate cold well. On rare occasions, a client may have an adverse affect to the treatment. If the client reports feeling dizzy, lightheaded, or looks pale, immediately assist the client out of the whirlpool. Stop the treatment and tell your supervisor.

POSTPROCEDURE

10. When the timer rings, help the client out of the whirlpool.

11. (CAUTION) Examine the skin for any adverse effects such as blistering or extreme redness.

12. Assist the client in drying the extremity with a towel.

13. You may need to help the client put on his or her clothes or walk initially, depending on what extremity is treated. Altered sensation may result in decreased balance or a hazardous condition.

PRACTICE LM20-1

Using Procedure Assessment Sheet LM20-1 in your Lab Activity Manual, practice using a cold whirlpool. Review the step-by-step procedure until you have mastered the skill. Follow your teacher's guidelines for completion of hands-on testing.

Procedure LM20-2 | Calculating Body Fat

Equipment and Supplies

Caliper • paper and pen or pencil

PREPROCEDURE

1. Gather needed equipment.

2. If the client is male, have him take off his shirt and put on short pants; if female, have her put on short pants and a short-sleeved shirt.

3. Adjust the age and sex settings on the caliper to make them appropriate for the client.

4. Have the client stand for the measurements.

5. Take measurements on the right side of the body.

6. Do not take measurements immediately after exercise or if the skin is wet. This can lead to inaccurate readings.

PROCEDURE

Male

7. Hold the body fat caliper in one hand.

8. With the other hand, pinch the chest with your thumb and forefinger vertically approximately 2 inches above and lateral to the nipple. Try to pinch only skin and fat, not the underlying muscle. It may help to lift the skin away from the muscle.

9. Open the caliper by squeezing the trigger and allow it to close over the skin being held in your opposite hand.

10. Click the switch on the side of the caliper to lock in the measurement.

11. Repeat steps 7 to 10 for the abdominal region just lateral to the umbilicus and mid-thigh.

12. The caliper will calculate the percent body fat for the client and show it on the display.

Female

Repeat steps 7 to 12, but the measurements are taken on the back of the arm (mid-tricep with the arm relaxed by the side), abdominal region just above the iliac crest, and at mid-thigh. Note: Some calipers use measurements taken just inferior to the scapula. Read the directions accompanying the caliper you use to determine the suggested sites.

POSTPROCEDURE

13. Instruct the client to put on his or her clothes.

14. Interpret and discuss the findings with the client.

PRACTICE LM20-2

Using Procedure Assessment Sheet LM20-2 in your Lab Activity Manual practice measuring body fat percentages. Review the step-by-step procedure until you have mastered the skill. Follow your teacher's guidelines for completion of hands-on testing.

PROCEDURE LM20-2: Calculating Body Fat *(continued)*

PROCEDURE TROUBLESHOOTING

Measuring Body Fat Percentages

Techniques for calculating body fat percentage have their drawbacks. Hydrostatic testing is very expensive and accounting for the volume of air in the lungs can be difficult to determine. The air in the lungs affects the buoyancy and thus can affect the results. Electrical impedance can be affected by a client's hydration level at the time of the test. If a client has just exercised and lacks body fluid, or has an excess of body fluid, this can affect the test results. When using the skin fold caliper for measurements, reliability among testers can be a problem. Each tester may take a different amount of skin or apply a different amount of pressure. Even the same tester could apply different amounts of force. Using different amounts of force when pinching the test sites can result in varying body fat calculations. Take all body fat measurement consistently and follow the manufacturer's directions for accuracy.

Many people enjoy having their feet massaged. Even people who have ticklish feet can enjoy massage when the correct amount of pressure is used. Reflexology is a type of foot massage. It is based on the theory that zones in the feet and hands correspond to all glands, organs, parts, and systems of the body. Pressure is applied to the zones using the thumbs and fingers to help improve the overall condition of the body. The foot massage you will learn is not based on reflexology. It is massage of the foot to relieve tension in the muscles and improve circulation. It would be included in a total body massage.

When you provide a foot massage, follow the step-by-step guide given in the following sections.

Equipment and Supplies

Table or bed • large towel or blanket • rolled towel or small blanket • massage oil or lotion

PREPROCEDURE

Before you begin a foot massage, review the following steps.

1. Gather needed equipment.

2. Prepare the table or bed. Cover it with a sheet and place a large towel or blanket to the side for the client to use as cover. Use a rolled towel or small blanket placed under the foot to keep the toes from pressing against the bed or table.

3. Explain what you will do and what the client is to do.

4. (CAUTION) Adjust table or bed height to the correct position.

5. Leave the room while the client removes shoes, socks, and any clothing on the lower leg and then positions himself or herself on the table or bed in a prone position. Assist the client if necessary.

6. Warm the oil if needed.

7. (CAUTION) Wash your hands.

PROCEDURE

Follow these steps when you do the foot massage.

8. Arrange the blanket or towel so that only the client's lower leg and foot are exposed and any clothing is covered.

9. Put a quarter-size amount of oil in the palm of your hands and spread it over your hands and forearms. As you perform the massage, use more oil if you notice friction during the strokes. Always apply the oil to your hands and arms, not to the client.

10. (CAUTION) Do not massage over open sores or rashes. Do not massage the calf of the leg if there is a warm, red, tender area. This could indicate a blood clot.

11. (CAUTION) Stand on the left side of the table or bed with your feet about 18 to 24 inches apart. Point your left foot toward the client's head and point your right foot toward the bed or table. Bend slightly at the knees and rock from front to back as you do the strokes.

12. Spread the oil on the client's left foot and lower leg, using the flat part of your fingers. Stroke from the foot toward the knee and back down to the foot.

13. (CAUTION) Shift your weight and turn your body so that you are facing the foot of the bed or table. Point your right foot straight and your left foot toward the bed or table. Bend slightly at the knees.

14. Gently lift the client's leg, bending it at the knee. Support the leg in this position during the foot massage.

15. Use the palm of your left hand to cup the client's heel. Rotate your palm over the heel, massaging it firmly.

16. Use the sides of your thumbs to gently but firmly massage the sole and ball of the foot and the lower side of each toe.

PROCEDURE LM21-1: Performing a Foot Massage *(continued)*

17. **(CAUTION)** Shift your weight and turn your body so that you are facing the head of the bed or table again. Point your left foot straight and your right foot toward the bed or table. Bend slightly at the knees.

18. Massage the client's arch by firmly stroking it with the lateral portion of your left forearm. Rotate your arm, using the lateral side on the upstroke, and the medial side on the down stroke. Repeat three to five times.

19. Use the sides of your thumbs to gently but firmly massage the top of the foot, covering all areas with thumb strokes.

20. Massage the tops of each toe using thumb strokes. Pull gently on each toe.

21. Massage around the inner and outer ankle bones using thumb strokes.

22. Gently lower the leg and foot to table or bed.

23. Using thumb strokes, massage from the ankle up the calf to the back of the knee. Do not massage the popliteal area (behind the knee).

24. **(CAUTION)** Massage the entire calf with thumb strokes, working from the ankle toward the back of the knee. This helps increase circulation from the legs to the heart. Remember to use the sides of the thumbs, not the tip of the thumb. With some clients, the calves may be tender. Massage with lighter pressure if the client complains of discomfort. Do not massage the calves of clients who have a history of blood clots.

25. Massage the calf from the ankle to the knee and back to the ankle using the flat part of your fingers. Lighten your touch as you do this stroke.

26. Stroke from the client's leg to knee again, using the very tips of your fingers with extremely light pressure.

27. Cover the client's leg and foot with the blanket or towel.

28. Move to the right side of the table. Repeat steps 8 through 27 on the client's right leg. Reverse your foot position in steps 11, 13, and 17 when you are on the right side of the table.

POSTPROCEDURE

Once you have completed the foot massage, do the following.

29. Tell the client that you will leave the room while he or she gets dressed. Instruct the client to use the towel or blanket to wipe off any excess oil before dressing. Assist the client, if necessary.

30. Leave the room and provide privacy for the client.

31. **(CAUTION)** Wash your hands thoroughly with soap and water to remove oil.

32. Remove used linens from the table or bed and place them to be washed in the appropriate receptacle.

33. **(CAUTION)** Clean the table using a 1:5 solution of bleach and water.

PRACTICE LM21-1

Using Procedure Assessment Sheet LM21-1 in your Lab Activity Manual, practice performing a foot massage. Review the step-by-step procedure until you have mastered the skill. Follow your teacher's guidelines for completion of hands-on testing.

Procedure LM22-1 — One-Handed Instrument Transfer

When you practice one-handed instrument transfer, refer to the step-by-step guide in the following sections.

Equipment and Supplies

Dental tray • client • basic-setup • additional pen and palm grasp instruments

PREPROCEDURE

Before you begin, review these steps.

1. Gather needed equipment.
2. Prepare the treatment area.
3. Assemble the dental tray with the basic setup and additional pen and palm grasp instruments.
4. Seat the client and yourself.
5. (CAUTION) Wash your hands and put on protective glasses, mask and then gloves.

PROCEDURE

Keep the following points in mind when you use one-handed instrument transfer. Refer to Figure LM22-1.

6. Simultaneously pass the mirror and explorer, in their position of use, to the operator. Use two-handed transfer for this, with the mirror in your right hand and the explorer in your left.
7. From the dental tray, pick up the pen grasp instrument on the handle away from the working end.
8. Grasp between your thumb and index and middle fingers of the left hand.
9. Move the instrument to the transfer zone.
10. Receive the explorer with the little finger of your left hand.
11. Place the pen grasp instrument in the operator's hand in the position of use. Return the explorer to the tray or rotate it back into the passing position.
12. Repeat the process with the other pen grasp instruments.
13. From the dental tray, pick up the palm grasp instrument near the working end.
14. Grasp it between your thumb and index and middle fingers.
15. Receive the used instrument with the little finger of your left hand.
16. Place the palm instrument in the operator's hand in the position of use.
17. Return the used instrument to the tray.
18. During the procedure:
    - The operator is able to maintain a fulcrum.
    - The instrument is placed in the operator's hand firmly and distinctly.
    - The instrument is removed from the operator's hand distinctly and without hesitation.
    - The instruments are kept parallel to one another during transfer.
    - When receiving an instrument that will be needed immediately, rotate the instrument into passing position using the one-handed technique.

POSTPROCEDURE

When you have completed one-handed instrument transfer, do the following.

19. (CAUTION) Remove gloves, mask, and glasses. Wash your hands.
20. Dismiss the client.
21. (CAUTION) Return to the treatment room, put on utility gloves, and complete posttreatment aseptic procedures.

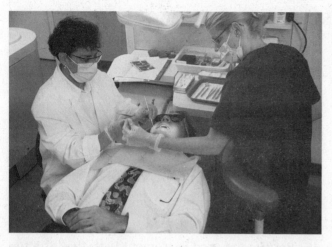

Figure LM22-1. Simultaneously transferring mirror and explorer.

PRACTICE LM22-1

Using Procedure Assessment Sheet LM22-1 in your Lab Activity Manual, practice one-handed instrument transfers. Review the step-by-step procedure until you have mastered the skill. Follow your teacher's guidelines for completion of hands-on testing.

Procedure LM22-2 | Using the Oral Evacuator

When you use an oral evacuator, refer to the step-by-step guide in the following sections.

Equipment and Supplies

Dental tray • client • basic tray setup

PREPROCEDURE

Before you begin, review these steps.

1. Gather needed equipment.

2. Prepare the treatment area.

3. Assemble the dental tray with a basic setup.

4. Seat the client.

5. (CAUTION) Wash your hands and put on protective glasses, mask, and then gloves.

PROCEDURE

Keep the following points in mind when you use an oral evacuator.

6. Place the oral evacuator in right hand using the thumb-to-nose grasp. See textbook Figure 22–68.

7. Position the oral evacuator appropriately.

   • For a procedure on maxillary right posterior, with the tip slightly distal and opening parallel to the lingual surface of the tooth being treated. See textbook Figure 22–70.

   • For a procedure on the maxillary left posterior, position the tip slightly distal, with the opening parallel to the buccal surface of the tooth being treated.

   • For a procedure on the facial surface of the maxillary or mandibular anterior area, position the tip parallel to the lingual surface

PROCEDURE LM22-2: Using the Oral Evacuator (continued)

of the tooth being treated, with the tip slightly beyond the incisal edge. See textbook Figure 22–69.

- For a procedure on the lingual surface of the maxillary or mandibular anterior area, position the tip parallel to the facial of the tooth being treated, with the tip slightly beyond the incisal edge.
- For a procedure on the mandibular right posterior, position the tip slightly distal, with the opening parallel to the lingual surface of the tooth being treated.
- For a procedure on the mandibular left posterior, position the tip slightly distal, with the opening parallel to the buccal surface of the tooth being treated.

8. Retract the cheek and tongue from the preparation area.
9. Remove all fluid and debris from the oral cavity.
10. When the dentist pauses to change burs or examine the tooth, rotate the evacuator opening toward the maxillary occlusal surface and clear away any excess fluid from the back of the mouth.

11. Maintain client comfort.
12. Use the air-water syringe to clear the mirror.

POSTPROCEDURE

When you have completed using an oral evacuator, do the following.

13. (CAUTION) Remove gloves, mask, and glasses. Wash your hands.
14. Dismiss the client.
15. (CAUTION) Return to the treatment room, put on utility gloves, and complete posttreatment aseptic procedures.

PRACTICE LM22-2

Using Procedure Assessment Sheet LM22-2 in your Lab Activity Manual, practice using an oral evacuator. Review the step-by-step procedure until you have mastered the skill. Follow your teacher's guidelines for completion of hands-on testing.

Procedure LM22-3 | Preparing the Anesthetic Syringe and Assisting with the Administration

When you prepare an anesthetic syringe and assist with the administration of topical and local anesthesia, refer to the step-by-step guide in the following sections.

PREPROCEDURE

Before you begin, review these steps.

1. Gather needed equipment.
2. Prepare the treatment area.
3. Assemble instruments and materials for specified procedure.
4. Seat the client.

5. (CAUTION) Wash your hands and put on protective glasses, mask and then gloves.

Equipment and Supplies

Basic setup • anesthetic syringe • anesthetic cartridges carpules • disposable anesthetic needle • topical anesthetic • cotton swab • needle recapping device (optional)

PROCEDURE

Keep the following points in mind when you prepare an anesthetic syringe and assist with the administration of topical and local anesthesia.

6. Prepare the anesthetic syringe. Do this out of the client's line of vision.

- Insert the cartridge into the syringe: Pull down on the thumb ring of the syringe, insert the rubber stopper end into the barrel of the syringe, and release the pressure on the thumb ring. See Figure LM22-2.
- Place the needle on the syringe: Remove the shorter, clear protective cap, push the exposed end of the needle through the opening in the hub of the anesthetic syringe. Be careful to keep the needle straight so that it will pierce the rubber diaphragm in the aluminum cap of the carpule. Screw the needle onto the hub.
- Gently tap the bottom of the thumb ring to engage the harpoon in the rubber stopper.
- Loosen and remove the colored needle cap.
- Express a few drops of solution to make sure that the syringe is functioning properly.
- Recap the needle, using the one-handed scoop technique, as shown in Figure LM22-3, or use a recapping device.

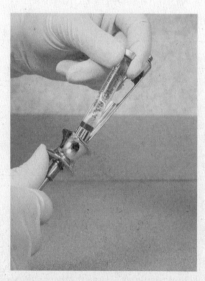

Figure LM22-2. Pull down on thumb ring to insert anesthetic carpule.

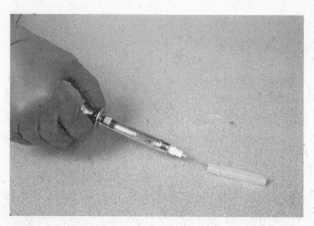

Figure LM22-3. Recapping a needle with the one-handed scoop technique.

7. Moisten a cotton swab with a small amount of topical anesthetic.

8. After the dentist is seated and has explained the procedure to the client, pass a 2 × 2 gauze pad to the dentist to use to dry the injection site.

9. Receive the gauze pad and pass the topical anesthetic on a moistened cotton swab.

10. After 1 to 2 minutes, the dentist will remove the cotton swab.

11. Pass the anesthetic syringe under the client's chin and place the thumb ring over the dentist's thumb.

12. Remove the needle guard while stabilizing the syringe in the dentist's hand.

13. Watch the client for any adverse reactions as the dentist slowly administers the anesthetic. Following the injection, the dentist usually recaps the needle with the scoop technique and places it on the dental tray.

14. Rinse and evacuate to remove any excess anesthetic solution.

POSTPROCEDURE

When the treatment or procedure is completed, do the following.

15. (CAUTION) Remove gloves, mask, and glasses. Wash your hands.

PROCEDURE LM22-3: Preparing the Anesthetic Syringe *(continued)*

16. Dismiss the client.

17. (CAUTION) Return to the treatment room and put on utility gloves.

18. (CAUTION) Disassemble the syringe:
- Unscrew the needle.
- Pull back on the thumb ring, pull down on the cartridge, and remove from syringe.
- Place the used needle and cartridge in the biohazardous sharps container.

19. (CAUTION) Complete all other posttreatment aseptic procedures.

PRACTICE LM22-3

Using Procedure Assessment Sheet LM22-3 in your Lab Activity Manual, practice preparing the anesthetic syringe and assisting with the administration of topical and local anesthesia. Review the step-by-step procedure until you have mastered the skill. Follow your teacher's guidelines for completion of hands-on testing.

Procedure LM22-4A — Preparing Alginate and Assisting with an Alginate Impression

When you prepare alginate and assist with an alginate impression, refer to the step-by-step guide in the following sections.

Equipment and Supplies

Basic setup • maxillary perforated impression tray, in several sizes • mandibular perforated impression tray, in several sizes • alginate canister • two alginate mixing bowls • alginate spatula • water measure cylinder • powder measure scoop • paper towels

PREPROCEDURE

Before you begin, review these steps.

1. Gather needed equipment.

2. Prepare the treatment area.

3. Assemble the instruments and materials for the procedure. See Figure LM22-4.

4. Seat the client in an upright position.

5. (CAUTION) Wash your hands and put on protective glasses and mask and then gloves.

6. Gently turn the canister over several times to fluff the alginate.

7. Measure the alginate powder for a mandibular impression and place it on a paper towel next to a bowl. Scoop powder from canister and gently tap and level the powder with the alginate spatula. Follow the manufacturer's directions and use their measuring scoop. Common measurements are 2 scoops for a mandibular impression and 3 scoops for a maxillary impression.

8. Repeat the procedure for a maxillary impression.

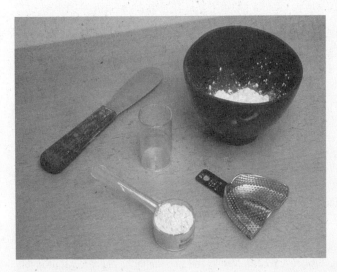

Figure LM22-4. Alginate set up.

9. Measure water for a mandibular impression and pour it into a bowl next to the 2 scoops.

10. Measure water for a maxillary impression and pour it into a bowl next to the 3 scoops.

11. Check the temperature of the water. Water temperature will affect the setting time of the alginate. It is best to use room-temperature water. Warmer water will speed up the setting time. Cooler water will slow it down.

PROCEDURE

Keep the following points in mind when you prepare alginate and assist with an alginate impression.

12. Explain the procedure to the client.

13. After the dentist has determined the correct size of tray, add the two scoops of powder to the water in the bowl.

14. Using a circular motion, with the tip of the spatula toward the bottom of the bowl, quickly incorporate all the powder into the water.

15. With the bowl in the palm of your hand, tilt the bowl toward you. Using a figure 8 motion, beat and press the alginate against the side of the bowl. See Figure LM22-5. Turn the bowl while

Figure LM22-5. Mixing and smoothing the alginate with the flat side of the spatula.

you mix. The mix should be creamy and smooth in 1 minute.

16. Gather the material into a single mass.

17. Place one-half of the material on each side of the impression tray. Press down and spread the material over the entire surface of the tray.

18. Wet your fingers and smooth the alginate.

19. Transfer the tray, with the tray handle directed toward the dentist.

20. While the impression is setting, clean the spatula. In 2 to 3 minutes, the material will be firm and not lose its form with finger pressure.

21. When the material is set, receive the impression from the dentist.

22. Repeat the process for the maxillary impression. Load the maxillary tray from the posterior, and load all the alginate at once.

POSTPROCEDURE

When you have completed preparing alginate and assisting with an alginate impression, do the following.

23. (CAUTION) Remove gloves, mask, and glasses. Wash your hands.

24. Dismiss the client.

25. (CAUTION) Return to the treatment room and put on utility gloves.

26. (CAUTION) Gently rinse the impressions under running water to remove any blood, saliva, or debris.

27. (CAUTION) Spray the impressions with an approved surface disinfectant.

28. (CAUTION) Unless the models will be poured immediately, wrap the impressions in a moistened paper towel and place them in a sealed plastic bag labeled with the client's name. When prepared this way, the impression can be safely transported to a dental laboratory or poured in the office later. Not all offices pour models.

PROCEDURE LM22-4A: Preparing Alginate and Assisting with an Alginate Impression *(continued)*

29. (CAUTION) Clean and disinfect the alginate bowls. Place any excess alginate in a trash container.

30. (CAUTION) Clean and sterilize the alginate spatula.

31. (CAUTION) Complete all other posttreatment aseptic procedures.

PRACTICE LM22-4A

Using Procedure Assessment Sheet LM22-4A in your Lab Activity Manual, practice preparing alginate and assisting with an alginate impression. Review the step-by-step procedure until you have mastered the skill. Follow your teacher's guidelines for completion of hands on testing.

Procedure LM22-4B Mixing and Assisting with an Elastomeric Impression

When you mix and assist with an elastomeric impression, refer to the step-by-step guide in the following sections. Note that this procedure is for taking an impression of a prepared tooth for a crown or bridge.

Equipment and Supplies

Basic setup • disposable quadrant tray • adhesive • impression material, base and accelerator • impression paste spatula • heavy paper mixing pad, about 6 × 9 inches • impression material syringe

PREPROCEDURE

Before you begin, review these steps.

1. Gather needed equipment.

2. Prepare the treatment area.

3. Assemble instruments and materials.

4. Seat the client.

5. (CAUTION) Wash your hands and put on protective glasses and mask and then gloves.

6. Coat the inside of the tray with adhesive.

7. Extrude equal lengths of the base and accelerator onto the paper mixing pad. The strips should be close together without touching. The accelerator strip is thinner than the base strip. Equal lengths of material, not equal amounts of material, are needed. Refer to Figure LM 22–6(a.)

8. Place the syringe tip on the impression paste syringe.

PROCEDURE

Keep the following points in mind when you mix and assist with an elastomeric impression.

9. When the dentist is ready to take the impression, mix the material: With the tip of the spatula, use a spiral motion, working from the top to the bottom of the strips to mix the accelerator into the base very quickly. Next, use the flat side of the spatula to thoroughly mix the material. This should take about 30 to 45 seconds. Refer to LM 22–6 (b.) and (c.)

10. Load the syringe: Using the back end of the syringe barrel, in short sweeping motions scoop the material up into the syringe. See Figure LM22-7.

11. Place the plunger in the syringe barrel and extrude the material into the tip.

12. Load the tray with the remainder of the material.

13. Pass the syringe to the dentist.

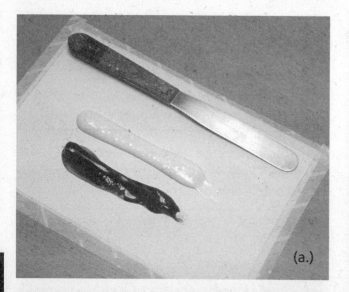

(a.)

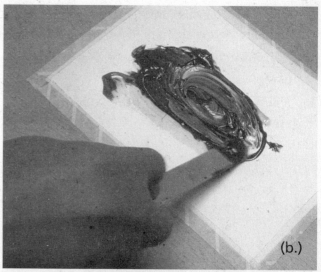

(b.)

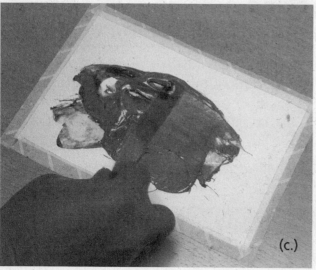

(c.)

Figure LM22-6. Mixing paste type impression materials.

14. Receive the syringe and pass the filled tray to the dentist.

15. The impression material will set in 6 to 10 minutes depending upon the type of material used.

POSTPROCEDURE

When you have completed mixing and assisting with an elastomeric impression, do the following.

16. Disassemble the syringe.

17. Remove excess material from the spatula and syringe. When the material is set, it will be rubbery and will peel off the spatula and syringe.

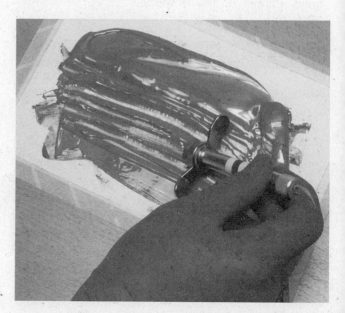

Figure LM22-7. Loading the impression material syringe.

PROCEDURE LM22-4B: Mixing and Assisting with an Elastomeric Impression *(continued)*

Brushes may be used to assist with cleaning the inside of the barrel of the syringe.

18. Tear off and dispose of the top sheet of the mixing pad.

19. (CAUTION) Clean and sterilize the syringe and spatula.

20. (CAUTION) Rinse, dry, and disinfect the impression.

21. (CAUTION) Place the impression in a labeled bag for transfer to the laboratory.

PRACTICE LM22-4B

Using Procedure Assessment Sheet LM22-4B in your Lab Activity Manual, practice mixing and assisting with an elastomeric impression. Review the step-by-step procedure until you have mastered the skill. Follow your teacher's guidelines for completion of hands-on testing.

Procedure LM22-4C Mixing Dental Plaster and Stone and Fabricating a Model

When you mix dental plaster and stone and fabricate a model, refer to the step-by-step guide in the following sections.

Equipment and Supplies

Rubber mixing bowl • plaster spatula • graduated cylinder to measure water • dental plaster or stone • scale • vibrator • plastic barrier • paper towels • impression • plastic or glass slab or tile

PREPROCEDURE

Before you begin, review these steps.

1. Gather needed equipment.

2. Place the plastic cover over the top of the vibrator.

PROCEDURE

Keep the following points in mind when you mix dental plaster and stone and fabricate a model.

3. (CAUTION) Wash your hands and put on mask and gloves.

4. Gently dry impression with air-water syringe.

5. Measure 30 mL of water for stone or 50 mL of water for plaster.

6. Pour the water into rubber mixing bowl.

7. Place the towel on the scale and weigh out 100 g of stone or plaster.

8. Pick up the towel and gradually slide the stone or plaster into the water.

9. Mix the water and powder together but DO NOT whip. Whipping will cause air bubbles to form.

10. Turn the vibrator to low or medium speed.

11. Place the mixing bowl on the vibrator; press down, and rotate the bowl to bring bubbles to the surface. Mixing and vibrating should be completed in less than 2 minutes.

12. Pick up the impression and place the tray edge near the handle on the vibrator.

13. With the spatula, place a small amount of plaster or stone in the posterior area on one side of the dental arch.

14. Tilt the tray to allow the plaster or stone to flow into the teeth around the arch.

15. Continue adding small increments until all tooth areas of the impression are covered.

16. Add larger increments until the entire impression is filled.

17. Place the remaining plaster or stone on a plastic or glass slab or tile. Shape into a base approxi-

PROCEDURE LM22-4C: Mixing Dental Plaster and Stone and Fabricating a Model (continued)

mately the same size as the impression tray and ½ to 1 inch thick.

18. Invert the filled impression onto the base without pushing into the base.

19. Hold the impression by the handle to keep it level while smoothing the base mix up into the inverted material. Do not cover the edges of the impression tray. If the edges of the impression tray are covered, the tray will be locked in place when the plaster hardens. Figure LM22-8 shows how to invert the impression onto the base.

20. Allow the model to set for 1 hour before separating.

POSTPROCEDURE

When you have finished mixing dental plaster and stone and fabricating a model, do the following.

21. Place any excess plaster in a trash container.

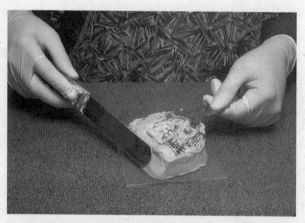

Figure LM22-8. Inverting the impression onto the base.

22. (CAUTION) Clean and disinfect the plaster bowl and spatula.

23. Rinse all plaster from the sink.

24. Remove and discard the vibrator cover.

25. (CAUTION) Remove your gloves and mask.

26. (CAUTION) Wash your hands.

27. Separating models:
   - (CAUTION) When models are set, put your gloves on again and use a lab knife to remove any excess plaster from around the margins of the impression tray.
   - Pull straight up on the tray handle to remove the impression from the model.

28. (CAUTION) If reusable trays were used, remove the impression material from the tray and clean and sterilize the tray.

29. (CAUTION) Remove gloves and wash your hands.

PRACTICE LM22-4C

Using Procedure Assessment Sheet LM22-4C in your lab activity manual, practice mixing dental plaster and stone and fabricating a model. Review the step-by-step procedure until you have mastered the skill. Follow your teacher's guidelines for completion of hands-on testing.

When you prepare amalgam and assist with an amalgam restoration, refer to the step-by-step guide in the following sections.

Equipment and Supplies

Amalgam tray setup • various instruments • anesthetic syringe

PREPROCEDURE

Before you begin, review these steps.

1. Gather needed equipment.
2. Prepare the treatment area.
3. Prepare amalgam tray setup. Refer to textbook Procedure 22D, Dental Tray Setups, for a complete listing of instruments and materials necessary for the tray.
4. Prepare the anesthetic syringe.
5. Read the amalgam manufacturer's directions for mixing time and speed and adjust the settings on the amalgamator.
6. Seat the client.
7. (CAUTION) Wash your hands and put on protective glasses, mask and then gloves.

PROCEDURE

Keep the following points in mind when you prepare amalgam and assist with an amalgam restoration.

8. Transfer the mouth mirror and explorer to dentist. The dentist always reexamines the area intended for treatment to verify that the treatment plan is correct.
9. Transfer a 2 × 2 gauze pad to the dentist for use in drying the injection site.
10. Receive the gauze pad and pass a cotton swab moistened with topical anesthetic.
11. Pass the anesthetic syringe.

12. Rinse and evacuate to remove any excess anesthetic solution.
13. A dental dam may be placed to isolate the treatment area.
14. The dentist uses the handpiece and burs to remove decay and prepare the cavity.
15. During cavity preparation, use the oral evacuator and air-water syringe, retract oral tissues, and adjust the light as needed to maintain a clear operating field.
16. Pass the explorer and hand cutting instruments as required.
17. When the cavity preparation is complete, the cavity is thoroughly rinsed and dried.
18. If required, mix bases or liners and transfer them to the dentist.
19. Assemble and transfer the matrix band if the cavity involves a proximal surface.
20. Activate the premeasured amalgam capsule by pressing the ends of the capsule together. This breaks a membrane in the capsule that separates the mercury and the silver alloy.
21. Place the amalgam capsule in the amalgamator and mix. Figure LM22-9 shows how to load the amalgam capsule in the amalgamator.
22. Open the capsule and drop the mix onto a squeeze cloth or an amalgam well.
23. Fill the amalgam carrier and transfer it to the dentist.
24. Transfer the amalgam condenser and refill the carrier. Repeat until the cavity is overfilled. It may be necessary to use more than one capsule depending on the size of the cavity.
25. Transfer the carving instrument (discoid-cleoid, Hollenback carver, burnisher) to shape the amalgam to the proper contour and contact with adjacent and opposing teeth.
26. Use the oral evacuator to remove excess amalgam as the dentist is carving.

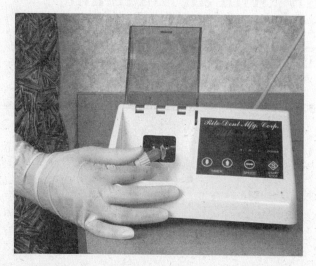

Figure LM22-9. Loading amalgam capsule in amalgamator.

27. Remove the rubber dam.

28. Transfer articulating paper to check the occlusion.

29. Rinse and evacuate.

30. Advise the client to avoid chewing on the area for several hours and to avoid hot drinks and food until numbness is gone.

POSTPROCEDURE

When you have completed preparing amalgam and assisting with an amalgam restoration, do the following.

31. (CAUTION) Remove gloves, mask, and glasses. Wash your hands.

32. Dismiss the client.

33. (CAUTION) Return to the treatment room and put on utility gloves.

34. (CAUTION) Disassemble the syringe and place the used needle and cartridge in the biohazardous sharps container.

35. (CAUTION) Put scrap amalgam in the container reserved for this purpose. Since mercury is a hazardous material, excess amalgam should not be thrown into the trash. It might end up in a landfill and possibly contaminate groundwater, or it might be incinerated and contaminate the air.

36. (CAUTION) Complete all other posttreatment aseptic procedures.

PRACTICE LM22-5A

Using Procedure Assessment Sheet LM22-5A in your Lab Activity Manual, practice preparing amalgam and assisting with an amalgam restoration. Review the step-by-step procedure until you have mastered the skill. Follow your teacher's guidelines for completion of hands-on testing.

Procedure LM22-5B | Preparing Composite and Assisting with a Composite Restoration

When you prepare composite and assist with a composite restoration, refer to the step-by-step guide in the following sections.

Equipment and Supplies

Composite resin tray setup

PREPROCEDURE

Before you begin, review these steps.

1. Gather needed equipment.

2. Prepare the treatment area.

PROCEDURE LM22-5B: Preparing Composite and Assisting with a Composite Restoration *(continued)*

3. Prepare the composite resin tray setup. Refer to textbook Procedure 22D for a complete listing of the instruments and materials to include.

4. Prepare the anesthetic syringe.

5. Read the composite manufacturer's directions.

6. Seat the client.

7. (CAUTION) Wash your hands and put on protective glasses, mask and then gloves.

PROCEDURE

Keep the following points in mind when you prepare composite and assist with a composite restoration.

8. Transfer the mouth mirror and explorer to the dentist.

9. Transfer a 2 × 2 gauze pad to the dentist for use in drying the injection site.

10. Receive the gauze pad and pass the topical anesthetic (moistened cotton swab).

11. Pass the anesthetic syringe.

12. Rinse and evacuate to remove any excess anesthetic solution.

13. A dental dam may be placed to isolate the treatment area.

14. The dentist uses the handpiece and burs to remove decay and prepare the cavity.

15. During cavity preparation, use the oral evacuator and air-water syringe, retract oral tissues, and adjust the light as needed to maintain a clear operating field.

16. Pass the explorer and hand cutting instruments as required.

17. When the cavity preparation is complete, the cavity is thoroughly rinsed and dried.

18. If required, mix bases or liners and transfer them to the dentist.

19. Transfer the acid etch syringe to the dentist.

20. Rinse and dry the tooth after approximately 15 to 30 seconds.

21. Plastic matrix strip is placed interproximally (between two teeth).

22. Place the bonding agent on the applicator tip and transfer it to the dentist.

23. Transfer the curing light to harden the bonding material. Figure LM22-10 illustrates a curing light. (CAUTION) The curing light is a very high-intensity light. Do not look directly at the light. Clients and dental staff can wear special glasses for protection.

24. Transfer the composite material. This is supplied in compules or unit doses, and can be expressed directly into the cavity, or a small amount from a larger syringe can be placed on small mixing pad and placed with a plastic instrument. Figure LM22-11 shows the ways in which composite may be supplied.

25. The dentist places the material, the matrix is pulled tightly around the tooth, and the material is light-cured.

26. Transfer sandpaper strips and discs, finishing burs, diamonds, and polishing points as needed for smoothing the restoration.

27. Remove the rubber dam.

28. Transfer articulating paper to check the occlusion.

29. Rinse and evacuate.

30. Advise the client to avoid chewing on the area for several hours and to avoid hot drinks and food until numbness is gone.

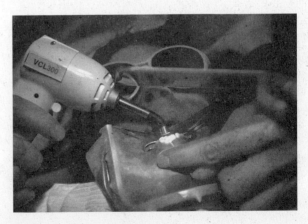

Figure LM22-10. Curing light.

PROCEDURE LM22-5B: Preparing Composite and Assisting with a Composite Restoration *(continued)*

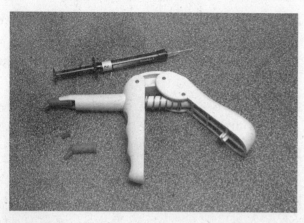

Figure LM22-11. Composite is supplied in syringe or in single dose compules.

POSTPROCEDURE

When you have completed preparing composite and assisting with a composite restoration, do the following.

31. (CAUTION) Remove gloves, mask, and glasses. Wash your hands.

32. Dismiss the client.

33. (CAUTION) Return to the treatment room and put on utility gloves.

34. (CAUTION) Disassemble the syringe. Place the used needle and cartridge in the sharps container.

35. (CAUTION) Complete all other posttreatment aseptic procedures.

PRACTICE LM22-5B

Using Procedure Assessment Sheet LM22-5B in your Lab Activity Manual, practice preparing composite and assisting with a composite restoration. Review the step-by-step procedure until you have mastered the skill. Follow your teacher's guidelines for completion of hands-on testing.

Procedure LM22-6A — Mixing Zinc Oxide Eugenol Cement

When you mix zinc oxide eugenol cement, refer to the step-by-step guide in the following sections.

Equipment and Supplies

Zinc oxide powder and eugenol liquid • powder scoop and liquid dropper (the appropriate ones for the specific material) • paper pad • cement spatula • plastic instrument • 2 × 2 gauze pad

PREPROCEDURE

Before you begin, review these steps.

1. Gather needed equipment.

2. Assemble the instruments and materials needed for the procedure.

3. Read the cement manufacturer's instructions. Some zinc oxide eugenol cements are two-paste systems. They are mixed in the same manner as calcium hydroxide. Refer to Procedure LM22-6B which discusses calcium hydroxide.

PROCEDURE LM22-6A: Mixing Zinc Oxide Eugenol Cement *(continued)*

PROCEDURE

Keep the following points in mind when you mix zinc oxide eugenol cement.

4. Fluff the powder in the closed bottle.

5. Measure the powder with the scoop and level it with the cement spatula. The amount of powder needed is determined by the amount of cement needed for the procedure.

6. Place the powder on the right side of the pad.

7. Replace the cap on the powder bottle.

8. Draw up the liquid into the dropper and replace the bottle cap.

9. Holding the dropper perpendicular to the pad, dispense drops close to the powder without touching the powder. Use one drop of liquid for each scoop of powder.

10. Divide the powder into two sections and then divide one section into two or three smaller sections.

11. Draw the larger section into the liquid and incorporate the powder using a figure 8 rotary motion.

12. Continue mixing in small increments of powder until the desired consistency is reached. For temporary luting, the mix should be creamy. As the spatula is lifted off the pad, the cement should follow the spatula for about 1 inch before breaking into a thin thread. For a base or temporary restoration, the cement should be puttylike and capable of being rolled into a ball. The dentist's preferences also dictate the consistency required. Mixing time is 1 to 1½ minutes.

13. Once mixing is completed, gather all material into one area.

14. Remove excess cement from the spatula with a 2 × 2 gauze pad.

15. Hold the pad and a clean 2 × 2 gauze pad at the client's chin and pass the plastic instrument to the dentist.

POSTPROCEDURE

When you have completed mixing and placing zinc oxide eugenol cement, do the following.

16. Remove excess cement from the plastic instrument.

17. Tear off the top sheet from the paper pad and throw it away.

18. Disinfect all surfaces touched during the procedure. This includes the exterior of bottles and the dropper.

19. Sterilize the instruments.

PRACTICE LM22-6A

Using Procedure Assessment Sheet LM22-6A in your Lab Activity Manual, practice mixing zinc oxide eugenol cement. Review the step-by-step procedure until you have mastered the skill. Follow your instructor's guidelines for completion of hands-on testing.

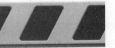

PROCEDURE TROUBLESHOOTING

Mixing Cements

It is very difficult to remove hardened cement from instruments. The best practice is to remove any excess cement from instruments immediately after use with moistened 2 × 2 gauze pad. Alcohol or orange solvent may help to remove any hardened cement.

Procedure LM22-6B — Mixing Calcium Hydroxide Cement

When you mix calcium hydroxide cement, refer to the step-by-step guide in the following sections.

Equipment and Supplies

Calcium hydroxide base and catalyst paste tubes • small paper mixing pad • small spatula, ball-ended instrument, or explorer • 2 × 2 gauze pad

PREPROCEDURE

Before you begin, review these steps.

1. Gather needed equipment.

2. Read the cement manufacturer's instructions.

PROCEDURE

Keep the following points in mind when you mix calcium hydroxide cement.

3. Express very small, equal amounts of both the catalyst and the base in close proximity to one another on the mixing pad. Finished mix will be about the size of the surface of a pencil eraser. Refer to Figure LM22-12.

4. Replace the caps on both tubes.

5. Using a circular motion, quickly (10 to 15 seconds) mix the two pastes together until the color is uniform.

6. Remove excess cement from the mixing instrument with a 2 × 2 gauze pad.

7. Hold the mixing pad and a clean 2 × 2 gauze pad at the client's chin and pass the ball-ended instrument or an explorer to the dentist.

POSTPROCEDURE

When you have completed mixing and placing calcium hydroxide cement, do the following.

8. Remove excess cement from the placement instrument.

9. Tear off the top sheet from the paper pad and throw it away.

10. Disinfect all surfaces touched during the procedure. Include the exteriors of paste tubes.

11. Sterilize the instruments.

PRACTICE LM22-6B

Using Procedure Assessment Sheet LM22-6B in your Lab Activity Manual, practice mixing calcium hydroxide cement. Review the step-by-step procedure until you have mastered the skill. Follow your teacher's guidelines for completion of hands-on testing.

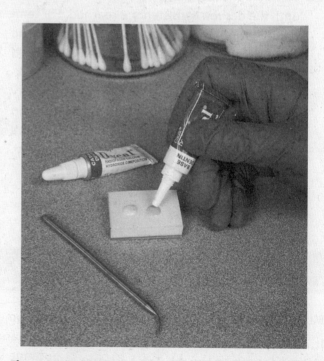

Figure LM22-12. Calcium hydroxide. Express small, equal amounts of catalyst and base.

Procedure LM22-6C Mixing Polycarboxylate Cement

When you mix polycarboxylate cement, refer to the step-by-step guide in the following sections.

Equipment and Supplies

Polycarboxylate powder and dispenser • polycarboxylate liquid, either a squeeze bottle or a calibrated syringe. See Figure LM22-13 • treated paper pad • cement spatula • plastic instrument • 2 × 2 gauze pad

PREPROCEDURE

Before you begin, review these steps.

1. Gather needed equipment.
2. Read the cement manufacturer's instructions.

PROCEDURE

Keep the following points in mind when you mix polycarboxylate cement.

3. Fluff the powder in the closed bottle.
4. Measure the powder using the dispenser supplied by manufacturer.
5. Place the powder on the right side of the pad.
6. Replace the cap on the powder bottle.
7. Hold the bottle or syringe perpendicular to the pad. Dispense drops close to the powder without touching the powder. Follow the manufacturer's directions for the appropriate number of drops or calibrations per scoop of powder.
8. Incorporate all the powder into the liquid at once.
9. Mix quickly using a folding motion and some pressure. Finish mixing within 45 seconds.
10. For luting, the mix should be creamy. As the spatula is lifted off the pad, the cement should follow the spatula for about 1 inch before breaking into a thin thread. For a base, the liquid is decreased and the mix will be glossy but the consistency will be tacky and stiff.
11. Once mixing is completed, gather all material into one area. Use the material immediately before the mix becomes dull and stringy.
12. Remove excess cement from the spatula with a moist 2 × 2 gauze pad.
13. For luting, use a plastic instrument to coat the internal surfaces of the crown or bridge. Transfer the crown or bridge to the dentist occlusal side up.
14. If you are using polycarboxylate as a base, hold the slab and a clean 2 × 2 gauze pad at the client's chin and pass the plastic instrument to the dentist.

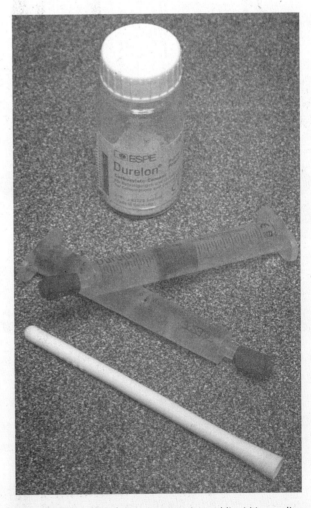

Figure LM22-13. Polycarboxylate powder and liquid in a calibrated syringe.

PROCEDURE LM22-6C: Mixing Polycarboxylate Cement (continued)

POSTPROCEDURE

When you have completed mixing and placing polycarboxylate cement, do the following.

15. Remove excess cement from the plastic instrument.

16. Tear off the top sheet from the paper pad and throw it away.

17. Disinfect all surfaces touched during procedure (including the exteriors of bottles and the dropper).

18. Sterilize the instruments.

PRACTICE LM22-6C

Using Procedure Assessment Sheet LM22-6C in your Lab Activity Manual, practice mixing calcium hydroxide cement. Review the step-by-step procedure until you have mastered the skill. Follow your teacher's guidelines for completion of hands-on testing.

Procedure LM22-6D Mixing Glass Ionomer Cement

When you mix glass ionomer cement, refer to the step-by-step guide in the following sections.

Equipment and Supplies

Glass ionomer powder and liquid • powder scoop • paper pad or glass slab • cement spatula • plastic instrument • 2 × 2 gauze pad

PREPROCEDURE

Before you begin, review these steps.

1. Gather needed equipment.

2. Read the cement manufacturer's instructions.

PROCEDURE

Keep the following points in mind when you mix glass ionomer cement.

3. Fluff the powder in the closed bottle.

4. Measure the powder with the scoop and level it with the cement spatula. The amount of powder needed is determined by the amount of cement needed for the procedure and by the manufacturer's recommendations.

5. Place the powder on the right side of the pad.

6. Replace the cap on the powder bottle.

7. Holding the dropper or liquid bottle perpendicular to the pad, dispense the recommended amount of liquid close to the powder without touching the powder.

8. Replace the cap on the liquid immediately, to prevent evaporation.

9. With the spatula, add the powder to the liquid in small, even increments.

10. Incorporate the powder using a figure 8 rotary motion. Complete mixing in 60 seconds.

11. Once mixing is complete, gather all material into one area. Manipulation time is an additional 2 minutes while the surface of the cement remains glossy.

12. Remove excess cement from the spatula with a 2 × 2 gauze pad.

13. For luting, use a plastic instrument to thinly coat the internal surfaces of the crown or bridge. Transfer the crown or bridge to the dentist occlusal side up.

14. If you are using glass ionomer as a base or restorative material, hold the slab and a clean 2 × 2 gauze pad at the client's chin. Pass the plastic instrument to the dentist.

PROCEDURE LM22-6D: Mixing Glass Ionomer Cement (continued)

POSTPROCEDURE

When you have completed mixing and placing glass ionomer cement, do the following.

15. Remove excess cement from the plastic instrument.

16. Tear off the top sheet from the paper pad and throw it away.

17. Disinfect all surfaces touched during the procedure, including the exterior of bottles.

18. Sterilize the instruments.

PRACTICE LM22-6D

Using Procedure Assessment Sheet LM22-6D in your Lab Activity Manual, practice mixing glass ionomer cement. Review the step-by-step procedure until you have mastered the skill. Follow your teacher's guidelines for completion of hands-on testing.

Procedure LM22-7A | Manual Processing of Dental Radiographs

When you process dental radiographs manually, refer to the step-by-step guide in the following sections.

Equipment and Supplies

Safety glasses and gloves • paper towel • stirring rod • film rack and marking pen • timer

PREPROCEDURE

Before you begin, review these steps.

1. Gather needed equipment.

2. (CAUTION) Put on safety glasses and gloves.

3. Fill the water tank.

4. Stir the developer, rinse the stirring rod thoroughly, and stir the fixer.

5. Check the temperature of the developer. Adjust the water temperature until the developer is 68°F.

6. Cover the work surface with a paper towel.

7. Label the film rack with client's name and date.

8. Turn on safelights and turn off overhead lights.

PROCEDURE

Keep the following points in mind when you process dental radiographs manually.

9. Open the outer film packet. Remove the inner paper packet. Without touching the film inside, pull back the paper wrapping and drop the film onto the towel. Continue with all film packets.

10. (CAUTION) Dispose of all contaminated film packets.

11. (CAUTION) Remove gloves and wash and dry your hands.

12. Attach each film to the film rack. Keep the films parallel to one another to avoid having them touch.

13. Smoothly immerse the film rack into the developer tank (left side of the tank).

14. Slowly agitate, or raise the rack up and down, several times.

15. Hook the rack on the edge of the developer tank. Place the cover on the processing tank.

16. Set the timer for 4½ minutes.

PROCEDURE LM22-7A: Manual Processing of Dental Radiographs (continued)

17. When the timer rings, remove the rack from the developer. Place the film in the rinsing section, the middle portion of the processing tank. Agitate slowly for 30 seconds.

18. Smoothly immerse the film rack in the fixer tank, or right side of the tank. Agitate it carefully, hook the rack over the edge of the tank, and replace the cover.

19. Set the timer for 10 minutes.

20. When the timer rings, remove the rack from the fixer. Place the rack in the rinsing section, hook the rack over the edge of the tank, and replace the cover.

21. Set the timer for 20 minutes.

22. When the timer rings, remove the rack, and hang it to dry. (CAUTION) Do not handle the films until thoroughly dry.

23. When the films are dry, place them in a labeled mount.

POSTPROCEDURE

When you have completed processing dental radiographs manually, do the following.

24. Dry off all work surfaces.

25. When you have finished processing for the day, turn off the water and drain the rinsing tank.

26. Replace the tank cover.

27. Turn off the safelights.

PRACTICE LM22-7A

Using Procedure Assessment Sheet LM22-7A in your Lab Activity Manual, practice manual processing of dental radiographs. Review the step-by-step procedure until you have mastered the skill. Follow your teacher's guidelines for completion of hands-on testing.

Procedure LM22-7B Mounting Dental Radiographs

When you mount dental radiographs, refer to the step-by-step guide in the following sections.

Equipment and Supplies

Film mount • processed radiographs • view box

PREPROCEDURE

Before you begin, review these steps.

1. (CAUTION) Wash your hands.
2. Gather needed equipment.
3. Turn on the view box.

PROCEDURE

Keep the following points in mind when you mount dental radiographs. Also see Figure LM22-14.

4. Label the film mount with client's name, the dentist's name, and date.
5. Place all films on the work surface, with the dot rounding up.
6. Locate the four bitewings. Both maxillary and mandibular crowns will be on the film.
7. Mount the bitewings:
   - The bitewing closest to the center of the mount has both premolars.
   - The bitewing toward the outside of the mouth has the second and third molars.
   - The occlusal plane is curved as if "smiling."
8. Locate the six anterior films. The length of the teeth is in the same direction as the length of the film.
9. Mount the anterior films:
   - The maxillary teeth are larger.
   - The maxillary cuspid is the longest tooth in the mouth.
   - Place the incisal edge of the films toward the middle of the mount.

- Place the roots of the maxillary teeth toward the top and the roots of the mandibular teeth toward the bottom edges of the mount.

10. Locate the eight posterior films and mount them. The following points will help you determine where the posterior films should be placed on the mouth.
    - The maxillary molars have three roots that are not clearly distinct.
    - The mandibular molars have two roots, a distinct mesial and a distinct distal root.
    - The roots generally curve toward the distal.
    - The occlusal plane is curved as if "smiling."
    - The film closest to the center of the mount shows both premolars.
    - The film toward the outside of the mount shows the second and third molars.
    - The teeth on the film are oriented as in the mouth, with the roots of the maxillary teeth at the top and the roots of mandibular teeth at the bottom.

11. Review the entire mount for accuracy.

POSTPROCEDURE

When you have completed mounting dental radiographs, do the following.

12. Place the radiographs in the client's chart.
13. Turn off the view box.

PRACTICE LM22-7B

Using Procedure Assessment Sheet LM22-7B in your Lab Activity Manual, practice mounting dental radiographs. Review the step-by-step procedure until you have mastered the skill. Follow your teacher's guidelines for completion of hands-on testing.

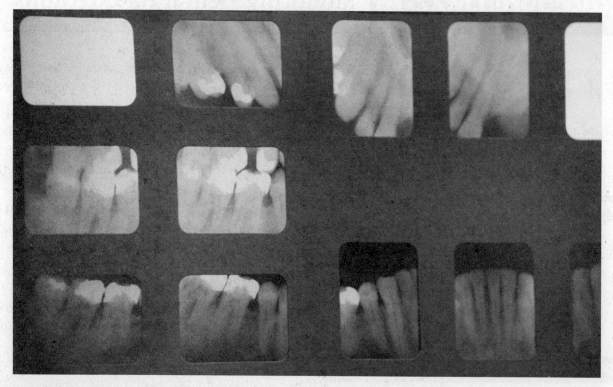

Figure LM22-14. Dental X-ray series.

Procedure LM23-1 — Performing a Fecal Examination

A **fecal examination** is commonly performed in veterinary hospitals as a diagnostic test for parasites. Parasites found in the stool or fecal material of an animal indicate that an organism is living in the animal's intestines. This can be very harmful to the animal's health.

Various types of parasite ova (eggs) and larvae (the early forms of a parasite) can infect an animal. A veterinary technician should be knowledgeable about the appearance of these parasites. He or she should know how to operate a microscope and a **centrifuge**. The centrifuge is used to spin and separate the specimen. This prepares it for viewing under a microscope.

Before you begin this procedure, review Procedure 3C, "Operating a Microscope," found in Chapter 3 and Procedure 24E4, "Microscopic Urine Analysis," in Chapter 24. The Preprocedure and Procedure parts of this last Procedure discuss the operation of a centrifuge. It takes time to learn to recognize the types and appearances of parasites. Ask for help from a trained veterinary professional. You can use a photographic chart to help you begin to recognize ova and parasites found in an animal's fecal sample.

When you perform a fecal examination, follow the step-by-step guide given in the following sections.

Equipment and Supplies

Clean, dry centrifuge tubes • flotation solution • cover slips • microscope slides

PREPROCEDURE

Before you begin performing a fecal examination, review these steps.

1. Be sure that you have correctly identified which animal needs to be checked for internal parasites.

2. Gather needed equipment.

3. (CAUTION) Put on gloves.

4. Collect a fresh fecal sample from the animal. If the sample is already in the refrigerator, make sure that it is properly identified.

(CAUTION) Evaluate only samples that are properly labeled. Using the wrong sample will cause reporting errors.

PROCEDURE

As you begin the procedure, keep this list on hand for reference.

5. Examine the feces as to color, texture, form, and the presence of mucus, blood, or tapeworm segments. Normal dog stool is cylindrical and solid. It is usually brown in color with no blood, mucus, or parasites. Occasionally, undigested food items such as grass, corn, and other foreign objects may be present. It is not unusual for articles of clothing to pass through the digestive tract of a dog.

6. Note any abnormalities on the report form or in the animal's record.

7. Use an applicator stick or tongue depressor to place a small amount of fecal material on a slide and add a drop of saline.

8. Mix the feces with the saline using the application stick or tongue depressor.

9. Examine the slide under low power on a microscope. Observe for the characteristic movement associated with protozoan organisms.

10. Look for the presence of any parasite larvae or eggs.

11. Place a gumball-sized fecal mass in a cup and add 20 mL of flotation solution. Mix them together until the liquid turns brown.

12. Pour the liquefied feces through a strainer or cheesecloth into a 15 mL-test tube. Fill the test tube.

13. (CAUTION) Place the tube in a centrifuge. Balance the centrifuge with another tube filled with water directly across from it.

14. Operate the centrifuge for 3 to 5 minutes at 1500 rpm.

15. Remove the tube from the centrifuge and place it in a test tube rack.

16. Add flotation solution to fill the tube, if necessary, so that the fluid is just over the top. This will float the parasite eggs to the top of the solution.

17. Place a 22 mm-square cover slip over the top of the tube. Leave it in place for 5 minutes.

18. Place the cover slip in the center of a clean, dry microscope slide.

19. Place the slide on the microscope stage. Examine it under low power for the presence of larva or eggs.

20. Reexamine the entire slide under high power.

21. Note any positive findings on a report sheet or in the animal's medical record.

22. Place the microscope slide in the glass waste receptacle.

23. (CAUTION) Thoroughly wash out the test tube and place it in the drying rack.

24. (CAUTION) Thoroughly rinse the strainer.

25. Turn off the microscope light and replace the microscope dust cover.

26. (CAUTION) Remove your gloves and wash your hands.

POSTPROCEDURE

Once you have completed the examination, do the following.

PRACTICE LM23-1

Using Procedure Assessment Sheet LM23-1 in your Lab Activity Manual, practice performing a fecal examination. Review the step-by-step procedure until you have mastered the skill. Follow your teacher's guidelines for completion of hands-on testing.

Procedure LM23-2 | Performing a Urinalysis on a Dog

A **urinalysis** is a series of tests performed on urine. Results help the veterinarian determine whether the animal has a urinary tract infection or another disease that causes changes in the urine. It is a quick and easy procedure that requires attention to detail. The microscopic examination requires specialized training to identify the cells and other structures. To perform a urinalysis you will need to be familiar with the **refractometer (TS meter)**. This is a small telescope-like device that allows you to determine the **specific gravity** of a solution. The specific gravity is the density of the urine. If the specific gravity is out of the normal range, this can indicate kidney or other diseases.

When you perform a urinalysis on a dog, follow the step-by-step guide given in the following sections.

Equipment and Supplies

Gloves • urine container • leash • dropper or pipette • refractometer • reagent strips • pen and medical record • centrifuge • centrifuge tube(s) • microscope • microscope slide • coverslip or stain

PREPROCEDURE

Before you begin performing a urinalysis on a dog, review these steps.

PROCEDURE LM23-2: Performing a Urinalysis on a Dog *(continued)*

1. Gather needed equipment.

2. Take the dog for a walk on a leash.

3. Take a clean, dry container for urine collection. You may attach the container to a stick that is 2 to 3 feet long.

4. Allow the dog to urinate for a few seconds and then place the container under the urine stream. You need only ¼ to ½ ounce of urine. This is 7 to 15 cc or mL.

5. Return the dog to its enclosure.

6. (CAUTION) Wash your hands.

7. (CAUTION) Label the urine container with the name of the animal and the date.

8. Take the sample to the lab for analysis. If the analysis will not be done for several hours, place the container in the lab refrigerator.

PROCEDURE

As you begin the procedure, keep this list on hand for reference.

9. Examine the urine sample for color, transparency, and odor. Normal dog urine is clear yellow to almost colorless. The darkest urine is seen in the morning. As the dog continues to drink during the day, the urine becomes diluted and has little color. Medications can cause urine to appear green or blue. A red color usually indicates bleeding, which is common in urinary tract diseases.

10. Note any abnormalities on the proper report sheet or in the animal's medical record.

11. If you are using a sample that has been in the refrigerator, allow it to come to room temperature before testing.

12. Using a dropper or pipette, place a drop of urine on the prism cover glass of a refractometer (TS meter).

13. Close the cover plate over the urine and hold the refractometer up to the light. Look in the eyepiece as you would with a telescope.

14. You will see a light-dark interface. Read the value for the **specific gravity** that is intersected by the light-dark interface. The value will be between

1.000 and 1.055. Figure LM23-1 shows the light-dark interface on a refractometer.

15. Record the value on your report sheet or in the animal's record.

16. (CAUTION) Clean the refractometer according to the manufacturer's recommendations.

17. (CAUTION) Open a bottle of urine reagent strips, remove one strip, and close the jar immediately. Review the directions on the bottle. Figure LM23-2 shows part of the scale on a reagent strip jar.

18. Insert the strip into the urine so that all the colored squares are covered.

19. Remove the strip and hold it in a horizontal position, tapping it slightly on the edge of the jar.

20. Compare the colors of the squares with the colors on the chart on the reagent strip bottle. Each color corresponds to a certain value indicated on the bottle.

21. Record the values on the report sheet or in the animal's record.

22. Dispose of the reagent strip.

23. (CAUTION) Remove gloves if worn and wash your hands thoroughly.

24. (CAUTION) Put 5 to 7 mL of urine in a centrifuge tube and place it in a centrifuge.

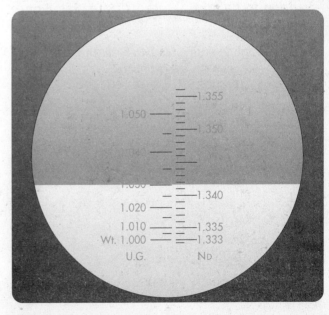

Figure LM23-1. The light dark interface on a refractometer. What is the value of this solution?

PROCEDURE LM23-2: Performing a Urinalysis on a Dog *(continued)*

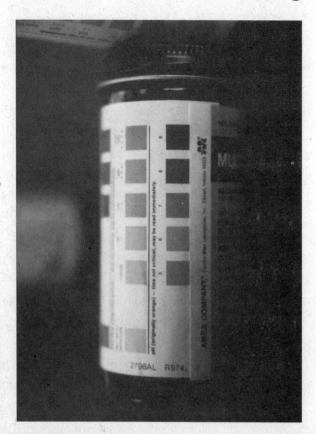

Figure LM23-2. The reagent strip jar has a scale on the side indicating what each color change means.

See Figure LM23-3. Fill a similar sized tube filled to the same level with water. Place the tube directly across from the urine tube. This is done to balance the centrifuge. See Figure LM23-4.

25. Centrifuge the urine for 2 to 5 minutes at 1000 to 2000 rpm. See Figure LM23-5.

26. Once the centrifuge stops, remove the urine-filled tube. Pour off the **supernatant**, leaving only a drop or two in the tube. The supernatant is the liquid lying above the layer of precipitated insoluble material after a specimen has been centrifuged. See Figure LM23-6.

27. Gently flick the bottom of the tube with your finger, to suspend the urine sediment in the remaining few drops.

28. Using a pipette or dropper, place a drop of the sediment suspension on a clean, dry microscope slide.

29. You may choose to add a stain or place a cover slip on top of the slide that contains the sediment suspension.

30. Examine the slide under low power on a microscope. Note the cells and other structures. You may want to use high power for smaller objects. If a photographic chart is available, compare the objects to the chart or ask a veterinary professional or instructor for assistance. Record the results on the proper form or in the animal's medical record.

POSTPROCEDURE

Once you have completed the procedure, do the following.

31. (CAUTION) Clean the lab area.

32. (CAUTION) Make sure that the top is securely on the reagent strip bottle.

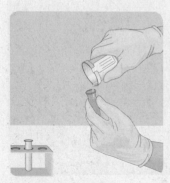

Figure LM23-3. Put urine in centrifuge tube.

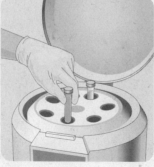

Figure LM23-4. Put tube of water across from tube of urine.

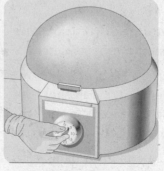

Figure LM23-5. Set timer on centrifuge.

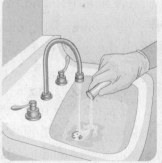

Figure LM23-6. Pour off supernatant.

33. Make sure that you have turned off the microscope light.

34. Place the dust cover over the microscope.

35. (CAUTION) Remove your gloves and wash your hands.

Procedure LM23-3 — Administering a Medication by Subcutaneous Injection

Vaccinations and other medications are administered to animals by the subcutaneous route. Remember that **subcutaneous** means "under the skin." Only sterile medications and equipment should be used for this procedure. Figure LM23-7 shows a technician administering a subcutaneous injection.

When you administer a medication by subcutaneous injection, follow the step-by-step guide in the following sections.

Equipment and Supplies

Pen • treatment sheet • medication • syringe and needle • alcohol moistened cotton

PREPROCEDURE

Before you begin the procedure, review the following steps.

1. Gather needed equipment.

2. Check with your supervisor or the treatment chart to determine which animal needs medication. Verify the medication and the amount to be given.

3. (CAUTION) Locate the drug. Determine how many cubic centimeters (cc) or milliliters (mL) are required. Double-check the name of the dog and amount of medication to be administered.

4. Obtain the appropriate size syringe and determine the size of hypodermic needle to use. You will usually use a 3-cc syringe and 22-gauge 1-inch needle. Figure LM23-8 shows a typical syringe used to administer a subcutaneous injection to an animal.

5. Wipe the rubber area on top of the vial with cotton moistened with alcohol.

6. Remove the needle guard and attach it firmly to the hub of the syringe. Draw the plunger back.

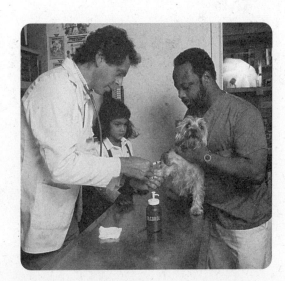

Figure LM23-7. The technician is administering a subcutaneous injection while the veterinary assistant restrains the dog.

PROCEDURE LM23-3: Administering a Medication by Subcutaneous Injection (continued)

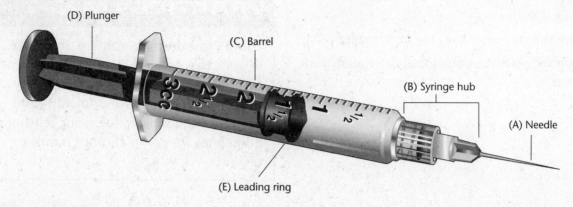

Figure LM23-8. This is the syringe most commonly used for a subcutaneous injection of an animal. Can you name the size, gauge, and needle size?

Fill the syringe with the volume of air equal to the volume of drug to be administered.

7. Insert the needle through the rubber area and inject the air. Figure LM23-9(a.) shows how to do this.

8. Turn the needle and bottle upside down, keeping the tip of the needle below the level of the medication. Pull the plunger back until the correct volume of medication enters the syringe. Refer to Figure LM23-9(b.).

9. **(CAUTION)** Remove the needle from the vial. Hold the syringe with the needle upright. Flick it with your finger to move any air to the top. Keeping the syringe upright, push the plunger to expel any excess air from the syringe.

10. **(CAUTION)** Check the medication amount again before administering the injection.

PROCEDURE

As you begin administering a subcutaneous injection, keep this list on hand.

11. **(CAUTION)** Have someone restrain the animal.

12. **(CAUTION)** Wipe an area of the skin between the animal's shoulder blades with cotton moistened with alcohol.

13. Gently tent the skin by pulling it away from the animal.

14. Insert the needle through the skin at a 45° angle. Do this quickly.

15. **(CAUTION)** Pull slightly back on the plunger, making sure that no blood appears in the needle hub. If you see blood, the needle tip is in a blood vessel and not just under the skin. Never inject medication if you see blood in the needle hub. Medication injected directly into the bloodstream can cause serious or even fatal consequences.

16. If you do not see any blood, completely depress the plunger to administer the medication. If you see blood, remove the needle and use another location.

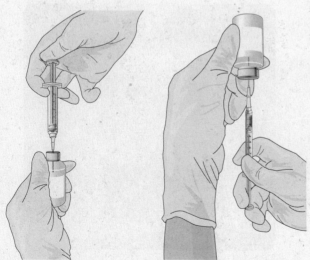

Figure LM23-9A and B. (a.) Insert needle and inject air. (b.) Pull back plunger for correct amount of medication.

PROCEDURE LM23-3: Administering a Medication by Subcutaneous Injection (continued)

17. Remove the needle from the animal.

18. (CAUTION) Place the needle in the proper biohazardous waste container. Figure LM23-10 shows a biohazardous waste container.

19. Place the syringe in a trashcan, or follow the procedures of your facility.

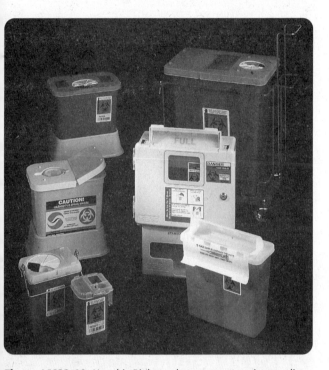

Figure LM23-10. Use this Biohazardous waste container to dispose of contaminated waste.

POSTPROCEDURE

Once you have administered the injection, do the following.

20. Return the animal to its cage.

21. Return the drug to its proper storage place.

22. (CAUTION) Clean up the area where you have been working.

23. (CAUTION) Wash your hands.

24. Record the medication and the dose administered.

25. Mark the procedure as completed on the treatment sheet.

PRACTICE LM23-3

Using Procedure Assessment Sheet LM23-3 in your Lab Activity Manual, practice administering a medication by subcutaneous injection. Review the step-by-step procedure until you have mastered the skill. Follow your teacher's guidelines for completion of hands-on testing.

Procedure LM24-1 — Performing the Test for Infectious Mononucleosis

A rapid test exists for infectious mononucleosis and can be performed by the Medical Laboratory Assistant (MLA). Infectious mononucleosis is an acute disease caused by the Epstein-Barr virus (EBV) or cytomegalovirus (CMV). The disease is characterized by fever, weakness, lymphadenopathy, hepatosplenomegaly, and atypical lymplocytes that resemble monocytes. The client may have the usual dominant symptoms of unexplained fever, fatigue, and sore throat. A rapid test, which can be completed in about 15 minutes, will help the physician diagnose the disease.

When you perform the test for infectious mononucleosis, refer to the step-by-step guide in the following sections.

Equipment and Supplies

The mononucleosis test kit • timer • biohazardous materials container • disposable capillary tubes • blood or plasma • gloves • face shield

PREPROCEDURE

Before you begin, review these steps.

1. Gather needed equipment.
2. (CAUTION) Wash your hands and put on gloves and a face shield.
3. Review the client's request form.
4. Label the tubes with client's name.
5. Verify that the controls have been run for the day and are within the correct range. Controls must be run daily.
6. If the controls have not been run, review the manufacturer's directions and run the controls. In some cases, your supervisor must check final results of the controls.
7. Confirm that the test kit has been brought to room temperature.
8. Check the expiration date of the kit.

PROCEDURE

Keep the following points in mind when you perform the test for infectious mononucleosis.

9. Fill a disposable capillary tube to the calibration mark with serum or plasma.
10. Drop the specimen (serum or plasma) onto the test slide.
11. (CAUTION) Immediately dispose of the capillary tube in a biohazardous materials container.
12. Mix reagents carefully by rolling the bottle gently between the palms of your hands.
13. Hold the dropper in a vertical position. Be careful not to touch the dropper to the slide.
14. Follow the manufacturer's directions for adding reagents.
15. Use a clean stirrer for each area to avoid cross-contamination.
16. Follow the manufacturer's directions for timing and observation of **agglutination**.

POSTPROCEDURE

Once you have completed the test, do the following.

17. (CAUTION) Disinfect the work area.
18. (CAUTION) Remove the gloves and face shield and wash your hands.
19. Record the test results in the client's record or on a lab form.

PRACTICE LM24-1

Using Procedure Assessment Sheet LM24-1 in your Lab Activity Manual, practice performing the test for infectious mononucleosis. Review the step-by-step procedure until you have mastered the skill. Follow your teacher's guidelines for completion of hands-on testing.

Many results obtained from chemical reagent strips must be confirmed or must have a follow-up test for specific substances. Therefore, the reagent test strips can be thought of as screening tests.

When the glucose test on the reagent strip is positive, most laboratories automatically do another test to confirm the presence of sugar. This test is called the copper reduction test. It confirms the presence and measures the quantity of certain sugars in the client's urine. These sugars include lactose, galactose, and glucose. The amount and type of sugars indicate the presence and severity of a disease affecting the metabolism of sugar, such as diabetes mellitus or diabetes insipidus. The test is also used to screen for galactosuria in children 2 years or younger. Increased levels of galactose are present in the urine of clients who lack an enzyme that metabolizes galactose.

Each laboratory has a procedure for performing these confirmatory tests. To confirm the quantity of sugar in urine, a confirmation tablet containing copper sulfate, citric acid, sodium hydroxide, and sodium carbonate is used. The sugars—lactose, glucose, and galactose—give up electrons easily in a chemical reaction and are called reducing sugars. The color of the reaction helps determine the quantity of sugar in the urine.

> When you test urine for glucose using copper reduction, refer to the step-by-step guide in the following sections.

Equipment and Supplies

Confirmation tablets • dropper • test tubes • distilled water • test tube rack • color chart • fresh urine sample • timer • gloves • face shield

PREPROCEDURE

Before you begin, review these steps.

1. Gather needed equipment.
2. Check the expiration date of the tablets.

3. (CAUTION) Wash your hands and put on gloves.
4. (CAUTION) Put on a face shield.

PROCEDURE

Keep the following points in mind when you test urine for glucose using copper reduction.

5. Gently swirl the container to mix the specimen. Aspirate the urine into the disposable dropper. Squeeze the dropper bulb before placing it in the urine. When you release the bulb, the urine will be drawn into the dropper tip.

6. Put the tube in the rack. Hold the dropper vertically and add the amount of urine and water specified by the manufacturer's directions.

7. Remove a tablet from the bottle by pouring the tablet into the bottle cap.

8. (CAUTION) Tap the tablet into the test tube and recap the container tightly. Do not touch the tablet.

9. Observe the entire reaction to avoid missing a rapid pass-through phase. A rapid pass-through happens when the glucose level is so high that it goes beyond the orange color that indicates the highest level of glucose. If you miss this phase, you may obtain a result that indicates a trace of glucose instead of a high level.

10. When the bubbling stops, follow the timing precisely, using the manufacturer's directions. Then gently shake the tube to mix the entire contents.

11. Immediately compare the color of the specimen with the five-drop color chart. Results are recorded as trace, 1+, 2+, 3+, or 4+.

12. If an orange color appears briefly during the reaction, rapid pass-through has occurred, and the test must be repeated using the alternate color procedure and chart.

PROCEDURE LM24-2A: Testing Urine for Glucose Using Copper Reduction *(continued)*

POSTPROCEDURE

When you have completed testing urine for glucose using copper reduction, do the following.

13. (CAUTION) Disinfect the work area.

14. Return items to their proper storage location.

15. Remove the face shield and gloves.

16. (CAUTION) Wash your hands.

17. Record the results in the client's chart or on a lab form.

PRACTICE LM24-2A

Using Procedure Assessment Sheet LM24-2A in your Lab Activity Manual, practice testing urine for glucose using copper reduction. Review the step-by-step procedure until you have mastered the skill. Follow your teacher's guidelines for completion of hands-on testing.

Procedure LM24-2B | Testing Urine for Protein Using the Sulfosalicylic Acid Precipitation Test

When protein is found in the urine using a reagent strip, a follow-up test is performed. The sulfosalicylic acid precipitation test confirms the presence of protein in the urine. Proteinuria (excess protein in the urine) is one of the first signs of renal disease. A slight amount of protein is normally present in the urine, but large amounts may be pathological or indicate disease.

When you test urine for protein using the sulfosalicylic acid precipitation test, refer to the step-by-step guide in the following sections.

Equipment and Supplies

3 percent sulfosalicylic acid • clear test tubes • rack • dropper • centrifuge tube • gloves • face shield • cleaning solution

PREPROCEDURE

Before you begin, review these steps.

1. Gather needed equipment.

2. (CAUTION) Wash your hands and put on gloves.

3. (CAUTION) Put on a face shield.

4. If the urine is cloudy, filter the specimen or use a centrifuged specimen.

PROCEDURE

Keep the following points in mind when you test urine for protein using the sulfosalicylic acid precipitation test.

5. Using a clear test tube in a rack and the dropper, mix equal amounts of urine and 3 percent sulfosalicylic acid.

6. (CAUTION) Observe for cloudiness. Cloudiness indicates the presence of protein.

7. Record the results. The test is reported according to the degree of cloudiness as negative, trace, 1+, 2+, 3+, or 4+.

POSTPROCEDURE

When you have completed the test, do the following.

8. (CAUTION) Disinfect the work area.

9. Return items to their proper storage location.

10. Remove gloves and face shield.

11. (CAUTION) Wash your hands.

12. Record the results in the client's chart or on a lab form.

PROCEDURE LM24-2B: Testing Urine for Protein *(continued)*

PRACTICE LM24-2B

Using Procedure Assessment Sheet LM24-2B in your Lab Activity Manual, practice testing urine for protein using the sulfosalicyclic acid precipitation test. Review the step-by-step procedure until you have mastered the skill. Follow your teacher's guidelines for completion of hands-on testing.

Procedure LM24-2C Performing a Pregnancy Test

This test detects the presence or absence of human chorionic gonadotropin (HCG) in the urine. HCG is found in the urine during pregnancy. A first-morning urine specimen is the best for pregnancy testing. This is when the concentration of HCG is the highest. These tests are often used in physician office laboratories (POLs), but they have a high rate of false positives and false negatives because of problems with technique. Be sure to follow the manufacturer's directions exactly.

When you perform a pregnancy test, refer to the step-by-step guide in the following sections.

Equipment and Supplies

The urine specimen • pregnancy test kit • clean slides • disposable mixing sticks • timer • disposable droppers • gloves • face shield • cleaning solution

PREPROCEDURE

Before you begin, review these steps.

1. Gather needed equipment.

2. Check the expiration date of the kit.

3. Allow the test kit to come to room temperature, if the manufacturer specifies it.

4. (CAUTION) Wash your hands and put on gloves and face shield.

PROCEDURE

Keep the following points in mind when you perform a pregnancy test.

5. Label the test tube with the client's name and label the control tubes.

6. Follow manufacturer's guidelines exactly regarding timing and methods.

7. Read the results using the color comparison charts or examples in the directions.

POSTPROCEDURE

When you have performed the pregnancy test, do the following.

8. (CAUTION) Disinfect the work area.

9. Return items to their proper storage location.

10. Remove the face shield and gloves.

11. (CAUTION) Wash your hands.

12. Record the results in the client's chart or on a lab form.

PRACTICE LM24-2C

Using Procedure Assessment Sheet LM24-2C in your Lab Activity Manual, practice performing a pregnancy test. Review the step-by-step procedure until you have mastered the skill. Follow your teacher's guidelines for completion of hands-on testing.

Procedure LM24-3 — Collecting a Capillary Blood Sample

Capillaries are tiny blood vessels that connect small arteries and veins. Capillary collection is an easy way to obtain a small amount of blood. This method is used most commonly for clients, such as young children, whose veins are too small for a phlebotomy.

MLAs and phlebotomists are responsible for the proper collection of capillary specimens. With adults and children, the usual site is the middle or ring finger. With infants, the lab assistant may use the great toe or heel.

This blood collection technique requires a puncture of the skin with sharp devices known as lancets. Automatic puncturing devices are more commonly used.

Frequently, this sample is collected at the client's side and is another example of point-of-care testing. Capillary samples are requested and obtained most often for glucose, hematocrit, and hemoglobin tests. For further testing, the capillary blood may be collected in small containers. It is important to identify a small sample properly because there is little of the specimen remaining for repeat procedures.

When you collect a capillary blood sample, refer to the step-by-step guide in the following sections.

Equipment and Supplies

Sterile disposable lancets or automated equipment with disposable platforms • alcohol swabs • sterile gauze pads • nonallergenic adhesive strip • tubes for requested test • sealing clay or caps for capillary tubes • pen • gloves • face shield • cleaning solution

PREPROCEDURE

Before you begin, review these steps.

1. Gather needed equipment.

2. Review the requisition and calculate the amount of sample needed.

3. If more than one tube of blood is required, arrange microtubes in the order of the draw. Refer to Tables LM24-1 and LM24-2 on page B-73.

4. Introduce yourself and identify client.

5. Verify the client information, and explain the procedure.

6. Have the client sit in a comfortable position in a collection chair or lie comfortably in bed with their hand and arm resting on the bed.

7. (CAUTION) Wash your hands and put on gloves and a face shield.

PROCEDURE

Keep the following points in mind when you collect a capillary blood sample.

8. Load the lancet device with a sterile lancet.

9. Select a puncture site on the side of the middle finger of the nondominant hand or on the heel for an infant. See Figure LM24-1(a.)

10. Rub the area to promote circulation. If the client's fingers are very cold, warm them first. Apply a warm, moist washcloth or paper towel to the area.

PROCEDURE LM24-3: Collecting a Capillary Blood Sample *(continued)*

Table LM24-1 Order of Draw for Multiple Tubes Using a Vacuum Tube System

1. Sterile specimens (blood culture tubes)
2. Plain tubes (red-topped)
3. Coagulation tubes (light blue-topped)
4. Other anticoagulants (in order of top color):

   - Green
   - Lavender
   - Yellow
   - Gray

Table LM24-2 Order of Draw for Filling Tubes Using a Syringe System

1. Sterile specimens (blood culture tubes)
2. Coagulation tubes (light blue-topped)
3. Other anticoagulants (in order of top color):

   - Lavender
   - Green
   - Gray
   - Yellow

4. Plain tubes (red-topped)

Note: Anticoagulated tubes should be filled before other tubes, before the specimen in the syringe has a chance to clot.

11. Clean the site with alcohol and let it air-dry, or dry it with sterile gauze. Do not blow on the skin to accelerate drying. You may contaminate the skin with microorganisms.

12. With your nondominant forefinger and thumb, grasp the client's finger on the sides near the puncture site.

13. Remove the sterile lancet from the package or remove the plastic tip. Do not touch the point of the lancet and do not lay it on the work surface. This will cause contamination. If the lancet or plastic tip becomes contaminated, discard it and obtain a new one.

14. Hold the lancet at a right angle to the client's finger and make a rapid, deep puncture across the fingerprint on the fingertip. The puncture should not be parallel to the fingerprint. This is shown in Figure LM24-1(b.).

15. **(CAUTION)** Dispose of the lancet and tip cover immediately in a sharps container.

16. Wipe away the first drop of blood using sterile gauze or cotton ball.

17. Use gentle pressure to start the blood flow. Do not apply too much pressure. This may cause tissue fluid to mix with blood and dilute the sample. If this happened, the test results would be incorrect. Figure LM24-2 shows the correct finger puncture position.

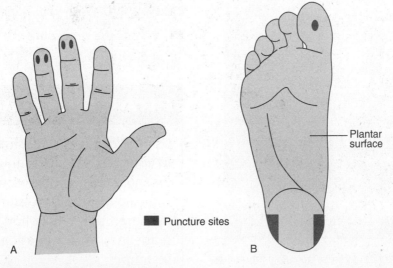

■ Puncture sites

Plantar surface

A   B

Figure LM24-1(a.) Puncture sites for capillary blood sample.

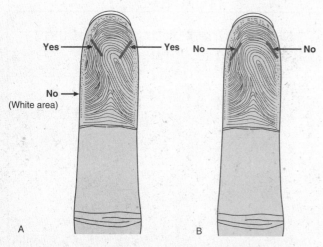

Figure LM24-1(b.) A dermal puncture should be done across the fingerprint. Which of these is correct?

18. Collect the samples in the capillary tubes or micro blood collection tubes. Hold the tube horizontally by the colored end to the drop of blood. Allow the tube to fill. Do not allow air bubbles to enter the tube or touch the tube to the skin. If this occurs, discard the tube and start with a new tube.

19. Seal the tubes with clay and place them in a test tube. Figure LM24-3 shows how to seal the tubes.

20. Mix by gently rotating any microtubes that contain an anticoagulant.

21. Apply pressure to the puncture site and apply a nonallergenic adhesive strip if needed.

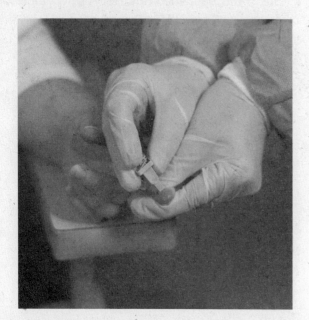

Figure LM24-2. Gloves are worn for most laboratory procedures including this capillary puncture.

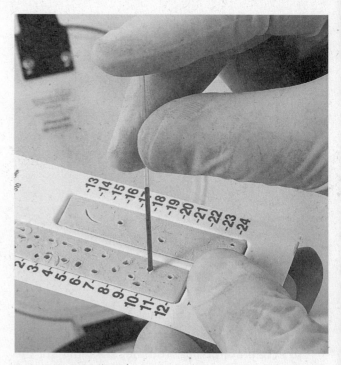

Figure LM24-3. Press the end of the tube into the clay sealant.

22. Label all tubes with the client's name, date, and other information required.

23. Thank and dismiss the client.

POSTPROCEDURE

When you have collected a capillary blood sample, do the following.

24. (CAUTION) Disinfect the work area.

25. Return items to their proper storage location.

26. (CAUTION) Remove the face shield and gloves.

27. (CAUTION) Wash your hands.

28. Record the procedure in the client's chart or on a lab form.

PRACTICE LM24-3

Using Procedure Assessment Sheet LM24-3 in your Lab Activity Manual, practice collecting a capillary blood sample. Review the step-by-step procedure until you have mastered the skill. Follow your teacher's guidelines for completion of hands-on testing.

Procedure LM24-4 Performing a Hematocrit

A **hematocrit** is a screening test that determines the presence of anemia. The word hematocrit also applies to the percentage of red blood cells per total volume of blood.

A small tube of blood is placed in a microhematocrit centrifuge and spun for several minutes. Centrifugal force separates the blood into three layers: plasma, buffy coat, and packed red blood cells. (See Figure LM24-4.) The buffy coat is a thin, white layer consisting of white blood cells and platelets. The amount of packed red blood cells is measured to determine the percentage of red blood cells in the blood.

The microhematocrit centrifuge is the most common device used to test for red blood cells in the blood. It requires less blood and can be done in a shorter period of time than other available tests.

When you perform a hematocrit, refer to the step-by-step guide in the following sections.

Equipment and Supplies

EDTA anticoagulated blood specimen tube or plain capillary tubes • microhematocrit centrifuge • gloves • face shield • cleaning solution

PREPROCEDURE

Before you begin, review these steps.

1. Gather needed equipment. Be certain that the microhematocrit centrifuge has been tested for accurate speed.

2. Obtain an EDTA anticoagulated blood specimen tube. EDTA is a special additive in a blood specimen tube that prevents the blood from coagulating.

3. (CAUTION) Wash your hands and put on a face shield and gloves.

PROCEDURE

Keep the following points in mind when you perform a hematocrit.

4. Gently mix the EDTA anticoagulated blood. For a capillary specimen, proceed to step 5.

5. Fill two plain capillary tubes three-quarters full with anticoagulated blood or blood from a capillary puncture site.

6. Seal the dry end of each tube with sealing clay. Refer to Figure LM24-4.

7. Place the tubes opposite each other to balance the microcentrifuge. Make sure that the sealed ends are secure against the rubber tubing.

8. (CAUTION) Note the numbers on the centrifuge slots and record them, along with the client's name.

9. Secure the locking top, fasten the lid down, and lock.

10. Set the timer and adjust the speed as needed. Follow the manufacturer's guidelines for time and speed.

11. (CAUTION) Allow the centrifuge to come to a complete stop. Unlock the lids.

12. Remove the tubes immediately.

13. Read the microhematocrit values. Depending on the equipment used in your facility, the cen-

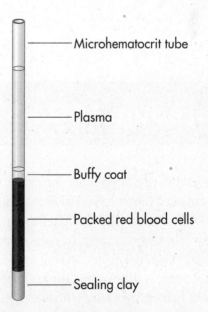

Figure LM24-4. Why should the sealed ends of the capillary tubes be pointing outward when centrifuging?

PROCEDURE LM24-4: Performing a Hematocrit (continued)

trifuge may have a built-in reader. A separate reader may be used. Figure LM24-5 shows a built-in reader. You will locate the bottom line of packed red blood cells.

14. Average the results of the two capillary tube readings. Expected are:
female 38 to 47%
male 40 to 54%

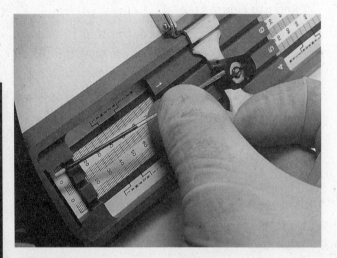

Figure LM24-5. This built-in microhematocrit reader is used to determine the microhematocrit value after centrifuging.

15. Dispose of the capillary tubes in a biohazardous sharps container.

POSTPROCEDURE

When you have performed a hemocrit, do the following.

16. **(CAUTION)** If any tubes have broken during the procedure, be certain to carefully clean and decontaminate the centrifuge.

17. Return items to their proper storage location.

18. **(CAUTION)** Disinfect the work area.

19. **(CAUTION)** Remove the face shield and gloves and wash your hands.

20. Record the results in the client's record or on a lab record.

PRACTICE LM24-4

Using Procedure Assessment Sheet LM24-4 in your Lab Activity Manual, practice measuring hematocrit. Review the step-by-step procedure until you have mastered the skill. Follow your teacher's guidelines for completion of hands-on testing.

Procedure LM24-5   Performing a Hemoglobin Test

A hemoglobin test determines the oxygen-carrying ability of the red blood cells. The word **hemoglobin** means blood protein. This protein has the ability to combine with and transport oxygen to body cells. Hemoglobin also assists in carrying carbon dioxide from the body cells to the lungs. The normal amounts of hemoglobin vary with age, sex, diet, altitude, and disease. Expected amounts are usually between 12 to 18 g/dl.

A hemoglobinometer is used to measure the amount of hemoglobin in the blood. Before the blood can be tested in the hemoglobinometer, it must be hemolyzed. This process destroys the red blood cells and releases the hemoglobin into the specimen to be tested.

When you perform a hemoglobin test, refer to the step-by-step guide in the following sections.

PROCEDURE LM24-5: Performing a Hemoglobin Test (continued)

Equipment and Supplies

The hemoglobinometer • hemolysis applicator • chamber • cover glass • needed reagents • alcohol preps • gauze squares • automatic or manual lancet device • biohazardous materials container • sharps container • face shield • gloves • cleaning solution

PREPROCEDURE

Before you begin, do the following.

1. Gather needed equipment.

2. Introduce yourself to the client.

3. (CAUTION) Identify the client, verify information, and explain the procedure.

4. Seat the client in a comfortable position in collection chair.

5. (CAUTION) Wash your hands and put on a face shield and gloves.

PROCEDURE

Keep the following points in mind when you perform a hemoglobin test.

6. Prepare the hemoglobinometer following the manufacturer's instructions.

7. Clean the site with alcohol.

8. Follow the procedure for a capillary puncture.

9. Wipe away the first drop of blood.

10. Place a drop of blood on the chamber slide or hemoglobin instrument.

11. Follow the guidelines for proper calculation of the client's hemoglobin. This will usually include the following steps:

    • Rotate the hemolysis applicator on the slide until the specimen turns from red and cloudy to clear. This usually takes 30 seconds.

    • Cover the chamber with the cover glass.

    • Insert the chamber into the hemoglobinometer, turn on the light, view the specimen, and note the heading.

12. (CAUTION) Dispose of the waste in the biohazardous waste container, and dispose of the sharps in appropriate container.

13. Thank and dismiss the client.

POSTPROCEDURE

When you have completed the hemoglobin test, do the following.

14. (CAUTION) Disinfect the work area.

15. Return items to their proper storage location.

16. (CAUTION) Remove gloves and face shield and wash your hands.

17. Record the test results in the client's medical record or on a lab form.

PRACTICE LM24-5

Using Procedure Assessment Sheet LM24-5 in your Lab Activity Manual, practice measuring hemoglobin. Review the step-by-step procedure until you have mastered the skill. Follow your teacher's guidelines for completion of hands-on testing.

A complete blood count (CBC) is a diagnostic test that requires a blood smear. A complete blood count measures the red and white blood cells in the blood. Once the blood smear is made, it is usually sent to a hospital or reference laboratory. In the laboratory, a medical laboratory technician or medical technologist completes the test.

The smear may be stained and used for a differential count. In a differential count, the number and percentage of each of five different types of white blood cells are determined. Each type of white blood cell has a specific function. The presence or absence of each type helps to determine a diagnosis.

When you make a blood smear, refer to the step-by-step guide in the following sections. Also refer to Figure LM24-6, illustrations A through D.

Equipment and Supplies

Equipment needed for a capillary or venous blood draw • clean glass slides with frosted ends • pencil • laboratory request form • biohazardous sharps container • biohazardous materials container • gloves • face shield • cleaning solution

PREPROCEDURE

Before you begin, review these steps.

1. Gather needed equipment.

2. Label the slides with the client's name and date on the frosted end of two slides.

3. Review the request form to verify the test ordered.

4. Introduce yourself to the client.

5. (CAUTION) Identify the client, verify information, and explain the procedure.

6. Have the client sit in a comfortable position in a collection chair or lie comfortably in bed with their hand and arm rested on the bed.

7. (CAUTION) Wash your hands and put on gloves and face shield.

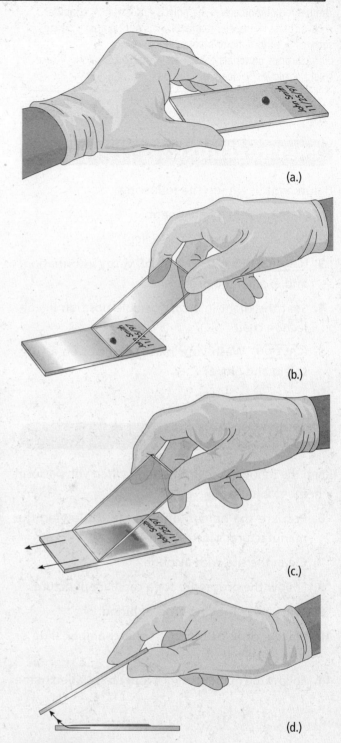

(a.)

(b.)

(c.)

(d.)

Figure LM24-6.
(a.) Place a small drop of blood ¼ inch from frosted end of slide.
(b.) Hold the second glass slide at a 45° angle from the first slide.
(c.) Place the upright (spreader) slide against the first slide and draw the spreader slide against the drop of blood.
(d.) Move the angled slide toward the frosted end and gently spread out the blood.

PROCEDURE LM24-6: Making a Blood Smear *(continued)*

PROCEDURE

Keep the following points in mind when you make a blood smear.

8. Obtain the blood specimen using the method preferred in your facility—venipuncture, butterfly puncture, or capillary puncture.

9. Place a small drop of blood approximately ¼ inch from the frosted end of each glass slide. Be sure to place the labeled side of the slide up. If you are performing a capillary puncture, do not allow the client's finger to touch the slide. (Figure LM24-6(a.))

10. Hold the corners of the frosted end of one slide on a flat surface. With your other hand, hold the second glass slide at a 45° angle. (Figure LM24-6(b.))

11. Place the upright (spreader) slide against the first one and draw the spreader slide against the drop of blood. The blood should spread across the edge of the spreader slide in a straight line. (Figure LM24-6(c.))

12. Move the angled slide toward the frosted end and gently spread out the blood. This will distribute the blood evenly across the slide. (Figure LM24-6(d.))

13. Allow the blood smear to air-dry.

14. Place the blood smear in appropriate container, along with a completed lab form.

15. If a CBC has been ordered, the EDTA tube should accompany the blood slide.

16. Recheck the puncture site for bleeding, bruising, or swelling.

17. Thank and dismiss the client.

POSTPROCEDURE

When you have made the blood smear, do the following.

18. (CAUTION) Immediately dispose of all biohazardous materials in the biohazardous waste container. All lancets go into the sharps container.

19. (CAUTION) Disinfect the work area.

20. (CAUTION) Remove the gloves and face shield and wash your hands.

21. Record the test results in the client's record or on a lab form.

PRACTICE LM24-6

Using Procedure Assessment Sheet LM24-6 in your Lab Activity Manual, practice making a blood smear. Review the step-by-step procedure until you have mastered the skill. Follow your teacher's guidelines for completion of hands-on testing.

Procedure LM24-7   Manual Method for Counting Cells

Occasionally the physician needs to know a client's red or white blood cell count immediately. If this is the case, you may count the blood cells manually. Performing the test in the office laboratory is convenient to both the physician and the client.

It is important that all health care personnel in the laboratory use the same counting and reporting system to ensure accuracy.

The same basic procedure can be used to count white blood cells, red blood cells, platelets, and sperm cells. Depending on the purpose of the test,

PROCEDURE LM24-7: Manual Method for Counting Cells *(continued)*

different diluting fluids and areas on the hemocytometer are used. The hemocytometer is a machine that counts blood cells. Hemo—blood cyto—cell, and meter—to measure.

When you use the manual method for counting blood cells, refer to the step-by-step guide in the following sections. Also see Figure LM24-7(a).

Equipment and Supplies

Hand tally counter • microscope hemocytometer and glass coverslip • disposable self-filling diluting pipette with a plastic reservoir prefilled with exact amount of diluting solution • pad • pen • gloves • face shield • cleaning solution

PREPROCEDURE

Before you begin, review the following steps.

1. Gather needed equipment.
2. **(CAUTION)** Wash and dry your hands.
3. **(CAUTION)** Put on gloves and a face shield.

PROCEDURE

Keep the following points in mind when you use the manual method for counting blood cells.

4. Place the hemocytometer on the lowered microscope stage under low-power magnification.
5. Center the ruled area over the opening in the stage.
6. Adjust the light so that you can see the cells to be counted.
7. Follow the correct path sequence for counting cells to avoid counting cells twice or missing them altogether. See Figure 24-7(b.)
8. When you have finished one area, record the number.
9. Return the tally to zero, move to the next square, and count the cells using the same sequence.
10. For white blood cells, the numbers counted each square should not vary by more than 10 cells. For red blood cells, the numbers should not vary by

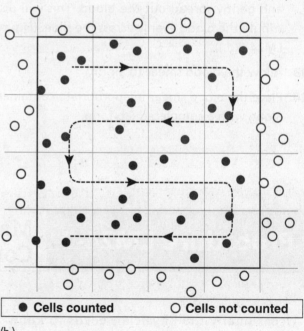

(a.)

(b.)

Figure LM24-7.
(a.) Use the grid to count the cells.
(b.) How many cells are counted on this grid? Why were certain cells excluded?

more than 20 cells. If this happens, wash the chamber, refill it, and count again.

11. Total the cells counted and average the numbers from both sides of the chamber.

12. Calculate the results following the instructions for your counting instrument.

POSTPROCEDURE

When you have completed counting blood cells using the manual method, do the following.

13. Record the results in the client's record or on a lab form.

14. (CAUTION) Disinfect the work area.

15. (CAUTION) Remove your gloves and wash your hands.

PRACTICE LM24-7

Using Procedure Assessment Sheet LM24-7 in your Lab Activity Manual, practice the manual method for counting blood cells. Review the step-by-step procedure until you have mastered the skill. Follow your teacher's guidelines for completion of hands-on testing.

Procedure LM24-8 — Collecting a Venous Blood Sample

When you collect a venous blood sample, refer to the step-by-step guide in the following sections.

Equipment and Supplies

Tubes • syringe and needle or evacuated system • needle and adapter • alcohol wipes • tourniquet • nonallergenic tape • marker • biohazardous materials container • biohazardous sharps container • sterile gauze pads • gloves • face shield • cleaning solution

PREPROCEDURE

Before you begin, review these steps.

1. Check the requisition form to determine the tests ordered. Calculate the amount of specimen needed and select the correct tubes for the tests ordered.

2. Gather needed equipment.

3. Check all tubes for expiration dates. Arrange the tubes in the order of draw according to the method to be used. (See Tables LM24-1, LM24-2)

4. (CAUTION) Wash and dry your hands and put on gloves and a face shield.

5. Introduce yourself to the client.

6. (CAUTION) Identify the client, verify information, and explain the procedure to the client.

7. Seat the client in a comfortable position in the collection chair or have the client lie comfortably in bed.

8. Make sure that both arms will be well supported in a slightly downward position.

9. Select the venipuncture site by palpating the antecubital space. (See Figure LM24-8(a).)

10. Ask the client to open and close his or her hand several times to make the veins more prominent. You may tie a tourniquet at this time to help locate the vein. (See Figure LM24-8(b).)

11. Use your index finger to locate the median vein and trace the path of the vein. Judge the depth of the vein. Do not use your thumb to palpate. If you do this, you will be feeling your own

PROCEDURE LM24-8: Collecting a Venous Blood Sample *(continued)*

pulse. Remove the tourniquet. (See Figure LM24-8(c.))

12. Determine the method that you will use for the venipuncture—evacuated tubes or syringe. Based upon method used, make sure that all necessary equipment is available.

13. **CAUTION** Do not remove shield from the needle at this time.

PROCEDURE

Keep the following points in mind when you collect a venous blood sample.

14. **CAUTION** Clean the venipuncture site by starting in the center and working in a circular pattern using alcohol prep pads. Do not recontaminate the area.

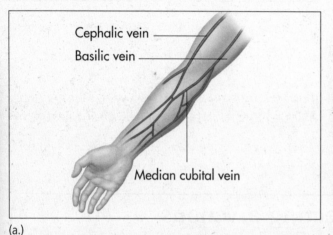

(a.)

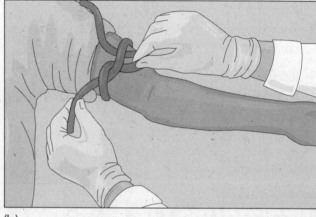

(b.)

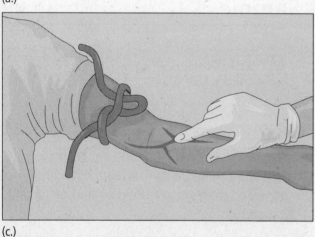

(c.)

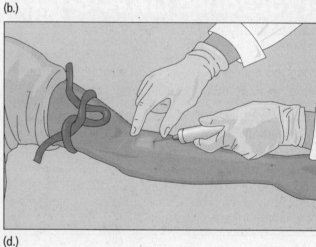

(d.)

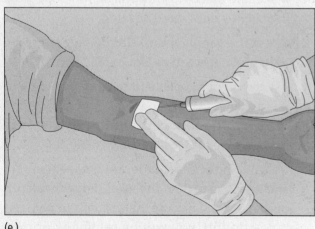

(e.)

Figure LM24-8.
(a.) Palpate antecubital space to locate vein.
(b.) Apply a tourniquet.
(c.) Locate the median vein and trace its path with your index finger.
(d.) Draw the skin tightly over the site and insert the needle quickly and smoothly at a 15° angle.
(e.) Remove tourniquet and place sterile gauze over the site to withdraw the needle.

15. Tie the tourniquet 3 to 4 inches above the client's elbow. Do not recontaminate the area with the tourniquet.

16. Remove the needle sheath.

17. Hold the evacuated system adapter, or syringe, in your dominant hand. Keep your thumb on the top and your fingers underneath.

18. Grasp the client's arm with your nondominant hand while using your thumb and forefinger to draw the skin tightly over the site. This will help to anchor the vein.

19. Insert the needle quickly and smoothly through the skin and into the vein, with the bevel of the needle up at a 15° angle, aligned parallel to the vein (Figure LM24-8(d.)). If you are using an evacuated system, push the tube onto the needle inside the adapter holder. Be sure not to move the needle after entering the vein. Allow the tube to fill completely. If you are using a syringe, slowly pull back the plunger of the syringe with your nondominant hand. Be sure not to move the needle after entering the vein. Allow the syringe to fill completely, or to the amount needed.

20. Remove the evacuated tube from the adapter smoothly and insert the next tube, or remove the needle from the vein.

21. (CAUTION) Release the tourniquet when the venipuncture is complete, BEFORE you remove the needle from the arm.

22. (CAUTION) Place sterile gauze over the site at the time you withdraw the needle. (Figure LM24-8(e.))

23. Instruct the client to apply direct pressure on the puncture site with a sterile gauze pad. The client may elevate the arm.

24. (CAUTION) Dispose of the evacuated needle immediately in a biohazardous sharps container. Do not recap used needles.

25. If you are using an evacuated system, gently invert the tubes with anticoagulants to mix thoroughly with the blood. If you are using a syringe, transfer the blood to tubes that have been placed in a rack. Figure LM24-9 shows how to transfer blood from a syringe. Gently invert any tubes containing anticoagulants.

26. (CAUTION) Dispose of the syringe and needle in a sharps container. Do not recap used needle.

27. Label the tubes with the client's name, date, time, and any other information needed. This may include your initials, the tests requested, and whether the client was fasting. A sample is shown in Figure LM24-10.

28. (CAUTION) Check the puncture site for bleeding.

29. Apply a hypoallergenic bandage.

30. Thank and dismiss the client.

POSTPROCEDURE

When you have collected a venous blood sample, do the following.

31. (CAUTION) Disinfect the area.

32. Return items to their proper storage location.

33. (CAUTION) Remove gloves and face shield and wash your hands.

34. Complete the laboratory requisition and label the specimen. Figure LM24-10 shows how to label the specimen.

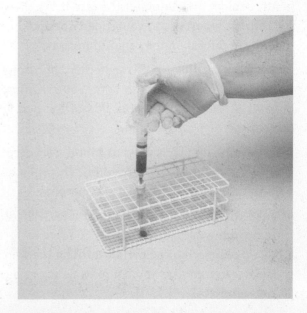

Figure LM24-9. Why is it important to use proper technique when transferring blood from a syringe to a vacuum tube?

PROCEDURE LM24-8: Collecting a Venous Blood Sample *(continued)*

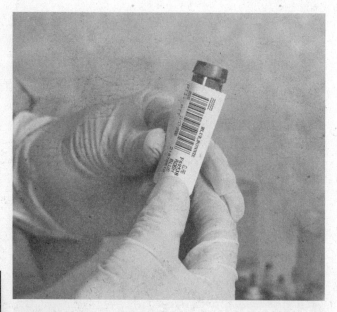

Figure LM24-10. Proper identification of clients and accurate labeling of specimens are essential. Computer labels may be available.

PROCEDURE TROUBLESHOOTING

Performing Phlebotomy

When you perform phlebotomy, you should consider these points in order to obtain a proper specimen with the least amount of difficulty.

1. If the client refuses to have his or her blood drawn, gently explain the reason for the test. If the client still refuses, report this to your supervisor and document the refusal on the requisition form.

2. Make sure that the client is seated or lying comfortably. If a client begins to faint, you can stand in front of the chair or at the side of the bed to protect the client from falling.

3. A hematoma, which is mass of blood, can occur during the phlebotomy procedure. This may be painful to the client. To avoid a hematoma:

   a. Take the tourniquet off the arm BEFORE you remove the needle.

   b. Avoid puncturing completely through the vein.

   c. Never attempt a venipuncture twice at or near the same site.

If a hematoma occurs, release the tourniquet, pull the needle out, and apply firm pressure. If the client complains of pain, apply an ice pack.

4. Select a venipuncture site that is free of lesions, abrasions, edema, and scar tissue. Do not perform venipuncture on the arm affected by a mastectomy or intravenous (IV) infusion.

5. If you do not immediately obtain blood after inserting the needle into the vein, and if the needle position appears correct, try the following:

   a. If you are using an evacuated tube, change it. The vacuum may have failed.

   b. Reposition the needle slightly by either turning the bevel or gently advancing the needle. Do not advance the needle more than halfway into the client's vein and do not probe.

   c. If these methods do not work, try another site.

A butterfly collection set, also known as a winged infusion set, is used for older clients and children who have small and/or fragile veins. The butterfly set is attached to an evacuated tube or, less commonly, to a syringe. Figure LM24-11 illustrates a butterfly assembly.

Butterfly collection allows you to lower the needle insertion angle. The system is sterile. The procedure is done using surgical or sterile technique. Follow all rules and regulations established by your facility. Maintain standard precautions.

> When you perform a butterfly blood collection, refer to the step-by-step guide in the following sections.

Equipment and Supplies

Tourniquet • antiseptic preps • sterile gauze pads • syringe • evacuated tube holder • butterfly needle set • blood collection tubes • biohazardous sharps container • nonallergenic bandage • pen • gloves • face shield • cleaning solution

PREPROCEDURE

Before you begin, review these steps.

1. Gather needed equipment.
2. Check the requisition and calculate the amount of sample needed.
3. Arrange the tubes in the order of the draw.
4. Introduce yourself to the client.
5. Identify the client, verify information, and explain the procedure.
6. (CAUTION) Wash your hands and put on gloves and a face shield.
7. Seat the client in a comfortable position in a collection chair or in bed with arm resting on the bed.
8. Make sure that both arms will be well supported in a slightly downward position.
9. Select a vein at the bifurcation usually at the back of the hand. The bifurcation is the site where a vein divides.

10. (CAUTION) Use gauze and clean the venipuncture site by starting in the center. Work in a circular pattern. Do not recontaminate the site.

PROCEDURE

Keep the following points in mind when you perform a butterfly blood collection. Also refer to Figure LM24-12.

11. Remove the butterfly device from the package.
12. Attach the butterfly device to the syringe or evacuated tube holder.
13. Insert the first tube into the evacuated tube holder.

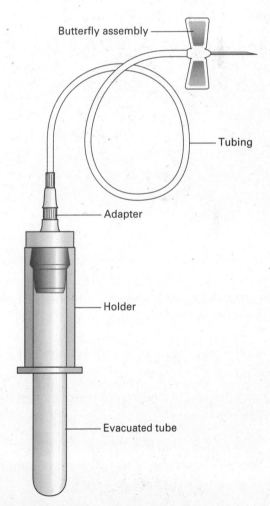

Butterfly assembly

Tubing

Adapter

Holder

Evacuated tube

Figure LM24-11. What is the advantage of using this butterfly assembly when performing venipuncture?

PROCEDURE LM24-9: Performing a Butterfly Blood Collection
(continued)

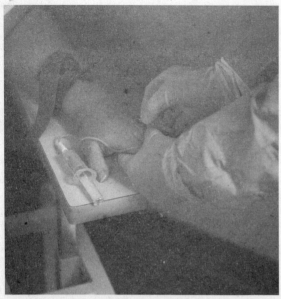

(a.)

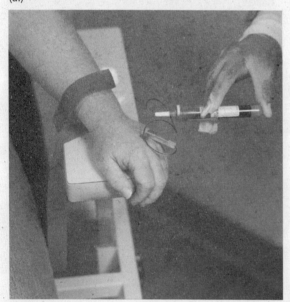

(b.)

Figure LM24-12. Hold the wings back on the butterfly assembly when performing venipuncture.

14. Apply a tourniquet to the client's wrist, just proximal to the wrist bone.

15. Hold the client's hand in your nondominant hand with the fingers lower than the wrist.

16. Using your thumb, pull the client's skin tightly.

17. With the needle at a 10 to 15° angle and the bevel up, align the needle with the vein.

18. Gently thread the needle up the lumen, or center of the vein.

19. Push the blood collection tube onto the end of the adapter or draw blood into the syringe.

20. Release the tourniquet when blood appears in the tube or syringe. Be careful to keep the needle in place.

21. Keep the tube and holder in a downward position so that the tube will fill from the bottom up.

22. Place a gauze pad over the puncture site and gently remove the needle.

23. (CAUTION) Immediately dispose of the needle and tubing in a sharps container. See Figure LM24-13.

24. Label the tubes with the client's name, date, time, and any other information needed. This may include your initials, the tests requested, and whether the client was fasting.

25. Check the puncture site for bleeding.

26. Apply a hypoallergenic bandage.

27. Thank and dismiss the client.

POSTPROCEDURE

When you have completed the butterfly blood collection, do the following.

28. (CAUTION) Disinfect the area.

29. Return items to their proper storage location.

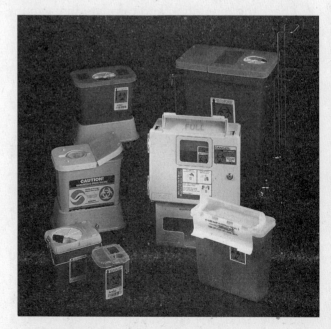

Figure LM24-13. Why is this container used?

PROCEDURE LM24-9: Performing a Butterfly Blood Collection

(continued)

30. **(CAUTION)** Remove gloves and face shield and wash your hands.

31. Complete the laboratory requisition.

32. Record the procedure in the client's chart or on a lab form.

PRACTICE LM24-9

Using Procedure Assessment Sheet LM24-9 in your Lab Activity Manual, practice performing a butterfly blood collection. Review the step-by-step procedure until you have mastered the skill. Follow your teacher's guidelines for completion of hands-on testing.

Procedure LM24-10 | Performing an Erythrocyte Sedimentation Rate Test

An erythrocyte sedimentation rate (ESR) test measures the rate at which erythrocytes or red blood cells will separate from plasma and settle to the bottom of a calibrated tube. This test is a good indicator of inflammation. It helps to diagnose conditions like infections, arthritis, tuberculosis, hepatitis, cancer, multiple myeloma, and lupus erythematosus.

When you perform an erythrocyte sedimentation rate test, refer to the step-by-step guide in the following sections.

Equipment and Supplies

The blood sample with EDTA anticoagulant • ESR tube and rack • timer • pipette to fill the ESR tube • gloves • face shield • cleaning solution

PREPROCEDURE

Before you begin, review these steps.

1. Gather needed equipment. The erythrocyte sedimentation rack is shown in Figure LM24-14.

2. Check the expiration date of the reagents.

3. **(CAUTION)** Wash your hands and put on gloves and a face shield.

4. Ensure the sedimentation rack is on a level surface.

PROCEDURE

Keep the following points in mind when you perform an erythrocyte sedimentation rate test.

5. Mix the blood sample.

6. Fill the pipette with blood and insert the tip of the pipette in the bottom of the tube.

7. Slowly fill the tube while moving the pipette to the top of the tube. Avoid air bubbles.

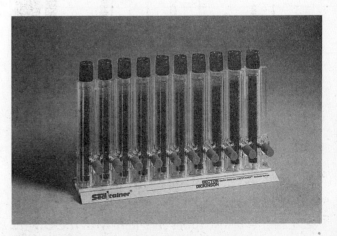

Figure LM24-14. What does the ESR test indicate?

8. Place the tube in the rack without jarring the rack.

9. Set the timer as instructed by the manufacturer.

10. Record the number of the client's tube for identification.

11. Measure the distance the erythrocytes have fallen after the specified time. The ESR scale measures from 0 at the top to 100 at the bottom. Each line is 1 mm.

POSTPROCEDURE

When you have completed the erythrocyte sedimentation rate test, do the following.

12. (CAUTION) Disinfect the work area.

13. Remove the face shield and gloves.

14. (CAUTION) Wash your hands.

15. Record the ESR result in the client's record or on a lab form.

PRACTICE LM24-10

Using Procedure Assessment Sheet LM24-10 in your Lab Activity Manual, practice the procedure for the erythrocyte sedimentation rate test. Review the step-by-step procedure until you have mastered the skill. Follow your teacher's guidelines for completion of hands-on testing.

Procedure LM24-11 Performing a Cholesterol Test

Cholesterol is one of the lipids (fats) normally found in the blood. A physician may order a screening test to determine whether the total cholesterol is increased or decreased. An elevated reading may be a symptom of liver malfunction, hypothyroidism, or atherosclerosis.

When you perform a cholesterol test, refer to the step-by-step guide in the following sections.

Equipment and Supplies

All equipment needed for a capillary or venous blood draw • laboratory request form • biohazardous sharps container • biohazardous materials container • gloves • face shield • cholesterol screening test

PREPROCEDURE

Before you begin, review these steps.

1. Gather needed equipment.

2. Label the test tubes or slides with the client's name and the controls.

3. Review the request form to verify the test ordered.

4. Introduce yourself to the client.

5. Identify the client, verify information, and explain the procedure.

6. Seat the client in a comfortable position in a collection chair or have the client lie comfortably in the bed with the arm supported.

7. (CAUTION) Wash your hands and put on gloves and a face shield.

PROCEDURE

Keep the following points in mind when you perform a cholesterol test.

8. Obtain the blood specimen required for the test procedure.

9. Follow the manufacturer's directions for the proper method for testing.

PROCEDURE LM24-11: Performing a Cholesterol Test *(continued)*

10. Do not touch a reagent pad with your fingers or the client's finger.

11. Give the client a clean gauze square to hold over the puncture site.

12. Read the result.

13. Recheck the puncture site.

14. Thank and dismiss the client.

POSTPROCEDURE

When you have completed the cholesterol test, do the following.

15. (CAUTION) Immediately dispose of all biohazardous materials in the biohazardous container. Put all lancets in the biohazardous sharps container.

16. Return items to their proper storage location.

17. Disinfect the work area.

18. (CAUTION) Remove gloves and face shield and wash hands.

19. Record the test results in the client's record or on a lab form.

PRACTICE LM24-11

Using Procedure Assessment Sheet LM24-11 in your Lab Activity Manual, practice performing a cholesterol test. Review the step-by-step procedure until you have mastered the skill. Follow your teacher's guidelines for completion of hands-on testing.

Procedure LM24-12 | Determining ABO Group

The determination of a client's ABO, or blood type, is rarely done outside a blood bank. This test determines the presence of A or B antigens on red blood cells. Blood type determines what can be donated by client or received by client. Testing with a known antiserum and observing for the presence or absence of agglutination confirms the client's blood type. Agglutination occurs when the antigen on the client's red blood cells corresponds to the antibody. When the antigen is not present on the red blood cells, no agglutination will occur. The different blood groups are listed below.

- Type A blood agglutinates with anti-A antiserum but does not agglutinate with anti-B antiserum.
- Type B blood agglutinate with anti-B antiserum but does not agglutinate with anti-A antiserum.
- Type O blood does not agglutinate with either anti-A or anti-B antiserum.
- Type AB blood agglutinates with both anti-A and anti-B antiserum.

Be sure to establish that it is lawful and within the laboratory regulations before you perform any diagnostic laboratory test. These regulations have been made for quality assurance purposes.

When you determine ABO group, refer to the step-by-step guide in the following sections.

Equipment and Supplies

Three glass slides with frosted ends • anti-A and anti-B serum • applicator sticks • manual or automatic lancets and device • alcohol preps • sterile gauze squares • marker • gloves • face shield • cleaning solution

PREPROCEDURE

Before you begin, review these steps.

1. Gather needed equipment.

2. Review the request form to verify the test ordered.

PROCEDURE LM24-12: Determining ABO Group (continued)

3. Check the expiration date of the reagents.

4. Introduce yourself to the client.

5. (CAUTION) Identify the client, verify information, and explain the procedure.

6. Have the client sit in a comfortable position in a collection chair or lie comfortably in bed with their hand and arm supported on the bed.

7. (CAUTION) Wash your hands and put on gloves and a face shield.

8. Label the slides in the frosted area with client's name.

9. Verify that the controls have been run for the day and that they are within the correct range.

PROCEDURE

Keep the following points in mind when you determine ABO group.

10. Place one drop of anti-A serum on slide 1. Place one drop of anti-B serum on slide 2. Place one drop of anti-A serum and anti-B serum on slide 3.

11. Follow the procedure for a capillary puncture. Be sure to allow the site to air-dry.

12. Wipe away the first drop of blood with a sterile gauze square.

13. Place one large drop of blood on each of the three prepared slides.

14. Cover the puncture site with a sterile gauze square and instruct the client to apply gentle pressure to the site.

15. Mix the antiserum and blood thoroughly, using a clean applicator stick for each slide.

16. Read and interpret the results of the reaction of each slide. Agglutination or clumping indicates a positive reaction.

17. Recheck the puncture site.

18. Thank and dismiss the client.

POSTPROCEDURE

When you have completed determining the ABO group, do the following.

19. (CAUTION) Immediately dispose of all biohazardous materials in the biohazardous waste container. Put all lancets in the sharps container.

20. (CAUTION) Disinfect the work area.

21. Remove the gloves and face shield and wash your hands.

22. Record the test results in the client's record or on a lab form.

PRACTICE LM24-12

Using Procedure Assessment Sheet LM24-12 in your Lab Activity Manual, practice determining the ABO group. Review the step-by-step procedure until you have mastered the skill. Follow your teacher's guidelines for completion of hands-on testing.

Procedure LM24-13 Determining Rh Blood Factor

A client's Rh factor is rarely determined outside a blood bank. This test determines the presence of D antigens on the surface of red blood cells. This is based on the presence or absence of agglutination with anti-D antiserum. D antigens represent the Rh factor in the blood (the letter D is used for simplicity). Anti-D antiserum contains antibodies that react with these antigens when mixed together on a slide.

- Rh-positive blood agglutinates with anti-D antiserum.

PROCEDURE LM24-13: Determining Rh Blood Factor *(continued)*

- Rh-negative blood does not agglutinate with anti-D antiserum.

   When you determine the Rh blood factor, refer to the step-by-step procedure in the following sections.

Equipment and Supplies

Glass slides with frosted ends • anti-D serum • applicator sticks • manual or automatic lancets and device • alcohol preps • sterile gauze squares • marker

PREPROCEDURE

Before you begin, review these steps.

1. Gather needed equipment.
2. Review the requisition to verify the test ordered.
3. Check the expiration date of the reagents.
4. Introduce yourself to the client.
5. Identify the client, verify information, and explain the procedure.
6. Have the client sit in a collection chair or lie in bed with the hand and arm supported on the bed.
7. (CAUTION) Wash your hands and put on gloves and a face shield.
8. Label the slides in the frosted area with client's name.
9. Verify that the controls have been run for the day and that they are within the correct range
10. Label one slide D and one slide C.
11. Place one drop of anti-D serum on the D slide.
12. Place one drop of control reagent on the C slide.

PROCEDURE

Keep the following points in mind when you determine the Rh blood factor. Follow the procedure for a capillary puncture. Be sure to allow the site to air-dry.

13. Wipe away the first drop of blood with a sterile gauze square.
14. Add two drops of the client's blood to each slide.
15. Thoroughly mix the blood with the anti-D serum. Use a clean applicator stick for each slide.
16. Read the results immediately. Agglutination on the slide indicates a positive reaction.
17. Recheck the puncture site.
18. Thank and dismiss the client.

POSTPROCEDURE

When you have determined the Rh blood factor, do the following.

19. (CAUTION) Immediately dispose of all biohazardous materials in the biohazardous materials container. Put all lancets in the sharps container.
20. (CAUTION) Disinfect the work area.
21. (CAUTION) Remove gloves and face shield and wash your hands.
22. Record the test results in the client's record or on a lab form.

PRACTICE LM24-13

Using Procedure Assessment Sheet LM24-13 in your Lab Activity Manual, practice determining the Rh factor. Review the step-by-step procedure until you have mastered the skill. Follow your teacher's guidelines for completion of hands-on testing.

Procedure LM26-1 — Adult PA Chest Radiographic Film Evaluation Procedure

Equipment and Supplies

Developed PA chest radiograph • view box

PREPROCEDURE

1. Gather needed equipment and obtain the completed film to be evaluated.

PROCEDURE

2. Place developed PA chest radiograph on view box. Make sure that the radiograph is placed correctly for viewing with the normal heart shadow falling on the right side of the lung field as you look directly at the PA chest radiograph. See Figure LM26-1. The radiographer is responsible for correct placement of radiographs on view boxes. Generally, images on the view box are placed as if the client were standing in the upright anatomical position facing forward with palms out toward the radiologist. The position is the same as when two people are facing each other in an upright position. The right hand of one person faces directly opposite the other person's left hand and vice versa.

3. Make sure there are no visible radiopaque items, or artifacts, within the chest area of consideration. Review the Troubleshooting box on page B-93.

4. Evaluate the contrast of the film. Contrast should be adequate to demonstrate anatomy. High contrast films have great differences between adjacent densities. They tend to be more black and white in appearance. This makes it difficult to see through the thicker anatomical parts. For example, the heart is superimposed over the thoracic spine. Low contrast films have fewer differences between adjacent densities. They appear gray or washed out. It is difficult to see details inside thinner anatomical parts such as soft tissues.

5. Make sure that the density is adequate to demonstrate anatomy. A radiograph that has too much density is darker than desired and represents overexposure. One that is too light represents underexposure. In both instances, important chest anatomy may be difficult to see.

6. Make sure that the film size and placement is correct. It is supposed to be 14×17 inches placed lengthwise.

7. Make sure that the essential anatomical structures are on the film. The entire lung field should be present. Check to make sure that the top areas of both lungs (apices) and the bottom areas of the lungs (bases) are displayed on the film without their edges cut off. Also, check to make sure that both right and left lateral sides of the lungs are displayed without their edges cut off.

8. Make sure that the correct letter marker is displayed in the correct location. The placement of the right "R" letter marker in the upper right-hand corner of the cassette corresponds with the client's right side. If the radiograph were placed correctly on the view box, then the "R" would be facing opposite your left side.

9. Make sure that there is appropriate collimation. A thin white border of about ¼ inch or more around the edge of the chest radiograph is an indication that collimation was applied adequately. In larger patients, this may be difficult to achieve without intentionally cutting off the edge of the lung fields. A major responsibility of the radiographer is to collimate to the part being radiographed to ensure that adequate radiation protection is provided.

10. Make sure that motion is not visible on the radiograph. Motion on a radiograph is easy to spot because anatomy appears blurred.

11. Make sure that the chest is not rotated.

12. Make sure that the chest is centered onto the film.

PROCEDURE LM26-1: Adult PA Chest Radiographic Film Evaluation Procedure *(continued)*

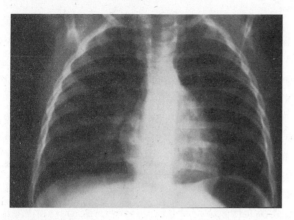

Figure LM26-1. When a PA chest radiograph is placed correctly on the view box which way is the heart shadow supposed to fall?

13. Make sure that the client's correct identification data has been stamped on the film identification corner. At this point in the radiographic procedure, if the radiographic film evaluation of the PA chest is satisfactory, then the radiographer takes the PA chest radiograph to the radiologist

for a diagnostic reading. If the film evaluation is not satisfactory, a repeat film is taken.

POSTPROCEDURE

14. Once a correct film has been completed, place in the appropriate area for the radiologist to review and create a diagnostic report.

PRACTICE LM26-1

Using Procedure Assessment Sheet LM26-1 in your Lab Activity Manual, practice adult PA chest radiographic film evaluation procedure. Review the step-by-step procedure until you have mastered the skill. Follow your teacher's guidelines for completion of hands-on testing.

PROCEDURE TROUBLESHOOTING

A radiographer must troubleshoot many problems. A frequent problem is ruling out artifacts. Anything on the final image other than the anatomy of the patient may be misinterpreted by the radiologist as disease or trauma. Physical artifacts are radiopaque items that block X-rays from reaching the film. (See Figure LM26-2.) Most artifacts are obvious, like the impression of a metal zipper that is superimposed onto a client's skull radiograph because the patient did not remove a garment before being radiographed. Or, the impression of metal sutures on a client's chest radiograph because of prior open heart surgery.

Some screen and film artifacts may not be so obvious. These may cause an inaccurate diagnosis because they can mimic disease or trauma. Screen artifacts can occur when dust, hair, and other debris

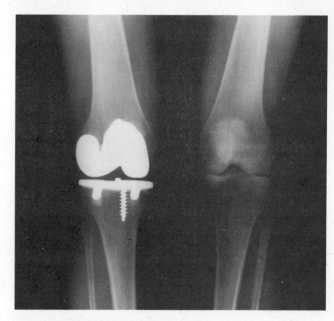

Figure LM26-2. Can you identify the artifact in this radiograph?

PROCEDURE LM26-1: Adult PA Chest Radiographic Film Evaluation
Procedure (continued)

get inside and rest between the screens and the X-ray film. The shadows that result may cause a false positive diagnosis by the radiologist or the client's physician.

Improper handling of the film or the film processor may also cause film artifacts. Film artifacts can create films that are fogged or contain pressure artifacts like fingerprints or static electricity marks.

When examining a radiograph for artifacts, the radiographer must isolate any potential artifacts, note them for the radiologist, identify their cause, and take the necessary precautions to eliminate them.

Transposition is another problem. It is an abnormality that results in anatomy that is normally found on the left side of the body being found on the right side and vice versa. Transposition occurs during a person's embryonic development. For example, the "normal" PA chest radiograph when displayed properly on a view box shows the heart on the left side. But, when transposition is identified in the client, the heart may be seen on the right side. This is a good example of why it is essential to properly mark the right or left side of the body when radiographic exposures are made. Otherwise, abnormalities like transposition may go undetected.

Before the optometrist or ophthalmologist performs an examination, eye drops are often used. Some eye drops dilate the pupil and cause the client to have difficulty seeing. Eye drops are also used to treat certain conditions such as infections and **glaucoma**. Glaucoma is a disease in which the pressure inside the eye increases to a dangerous level. This can lead to blindness. Eye drops may also be used to lubricate the eyes or as protection from diseases.

Great care should be taken when instilling eye drops. You should be aware of what the drops are for and instill them correctly. For example, some medications should only be put in one eye; others may have a different amount put in each eye. Eye drops are usually prescription medication. Depending upon your position, you may be trained to instill certain types of prescription and nonprescription medications.

Equipment and Supplies

Medication • client record • gloves • facial tissue • over-the-counter saline eye drops (for laboratory practice)

PREPROCEDURE

1. Gather needed equipment.

2. Check the expiration date on the medication bottle. Date the medication bottle the first time it is used. After eye medication is opened, it is usually only used for two weeks to prevent contamination. Check the appearance of the medication. Do not use any medication that looks abnormal.

3. Verify the medication order from the bottle and the client's chart. Make sure you know how many drops to place in each eye. When checking the medication order or bottle, remember the abbreviations: OD = right eye, OS = left eye, OU = both eyes, gt = drop, and gtt = drops.

4. **(CAUTION)** Wash your hands and put on gloves.

PROCEDURE

5. **(CAUTION)** Identify the client and explain the procedure.

6. Have the client sit or lie on his or her back with the head tilted back and towards the affected eye or the eye in which you will be placing the drops. This is done so that the excess medication flows away from the tear duct and from the other eye.

7. **(CAUTION)** Remove the dropper from the medication container. If necessary, draw the medication into it. Be careful not to touch the tip of the dropper or bottle onto any surface or the skin. This would cause the medication to be contaminated and it could not be used.

8. Hold the dropper or bottle in your dominant hand, the one you use for writing.

9. With a tissue in the other hand, pull the lower lid down till you see the conjunctival sac. This will be a pocket of tissue between the eye and eyelid. See Figure LM27-1.

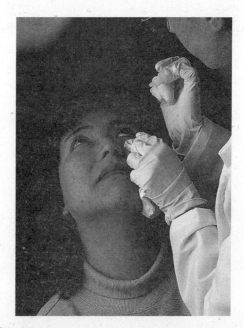

Figure LM27-1. Have the client tilt head back and toward the eye being treated. Why is this position used?

10. **CAUTION** Have the client look up and away. This helps to prevent the client from seeing the medication as it is instilled and may prevent blinking.

11. Rest the palm of your dominant hand on the client's forehead and instill the drops into the conjunctival sac. Resting your hand on the client's forehead will help steady it so the drops are placed in the correct location of the eye. Hold the tip of the dropper about ½ inch from the eye. Be careful not touch the eye or place eye drops directly on the colored portion of the eye. Never touch the eye, eyelid, or eye lashes with the tip of the bottle. See Figure LM27-2.

12. Release the lower eyelid and have the client blink to distribute the medication.

13. If medication went outside the eye, gently pat the skin from the inside to the outside of the eye with a tissue or allow the client to do so. Do not rub the eye.

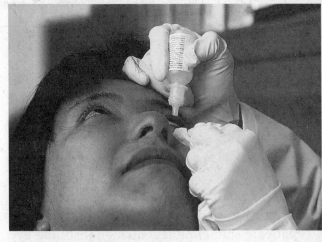

Figure LM27-2. Hold the bottle ½ inch from the eye when instilling eye drops. What standard precautions should be taken when instilling eye drops?

17. **CAUTION** Remove your gloves and wash your hands.

18. Clean the area and put your equipment away.

POSTPROCEDURE

14. **CAUTION** Discard any medication in the dropper before inserting it back into the bottle. If the dropper has become contaminated, obtain a new one.

15. Recap the bottle.

16. Record the procedure.

PRACTICE LM27-1

Using Procedure Assessment Sheet LM27-1 in your Lab Activity Manual practice instilling eye drops. Review the step-by-step procedure until you have mastered the skill. Follow your teacher's guidelines for completion of hands-on testing.

Procedure LM28-1 | Evaluating Client Charts

When you evaluate client charts, refer to the step-by-step guide in the following sections.

Equipment and Supplies

New labels and chart forms • pens • markers or rubber stamps • paper clips • stapler

PREPROCEDURE

1. Gather needed supplies.

PROCEDURE

Keep the following points in mind when you evaluate client charts.

2. After obtaining the medical record to be evaluated, determine whether it is active, inactive, or closed according to the policy of your office.

3. Check all pages in the record to confirm that the client's name is on each page and that the record is in reverse chronological order.

4. Securely add any loose pages that may have been hurriedly placed in the medical record. Again, make sure that the client's name is clearly written on each page.

5. If the record is considered active, add new or blank pages if necessary.

6. If the record is inactive, mark the front of the record according to the policy of your office. According to office policy, alphabetically or numerically file it in the appropriate inactive file cabinet.

7. If the record is closed, mark or stamp the front of the record as closed and file it in the area where closed files are kept. Usually, closed files are kept in storage facilities that may be off the premises. Patient charts are required to be kept for 7 years.

POSTPROCEDURE

When you have completed evaluating client charts, do the following.

8. Record inactive and closed files in a medical record logbook or cross-reference file. If a client whose record has been appropriately filed as inactive or closed becomes an active client, the cross-reference or logbook will make finding old records easier.

9. After evaluating the medical record, return the chart to the filing cabinet appropriately.

PRACTICE LM28-1

Using Procedure Assessment Sheet LM28-1 in your Lab Activity Manual, practice evaluating client charts. Review the step-by-step procedure until you have mastered the skill. Follow your teacher's guidelines for completion of hands-on testing.

Procedure LM28-2 — Completing Insurance Forms

When you complete insurance forms, refer to the step-by-step guide in the following sections.

Equipment and Supplies

The client's medical record • the superbill or encounter form filled out by the physician • the medical office fee schedule reference material from the provider • pen • typewriter • software program designed to electronically complete the CMS-1500 • ICD and CPT coding books • a blank CMS-1500 form for each claim being filed

PREPROCEDURE

1. Gather needed supplies.

2. Check the encounter form or superbill, textbook Figure 28-5, for accuracy and completeness. Refer to the medical record if necessary to determine an accurate physician diagnosis and treatments given if the information is not clearly indicated on the encounter form.

3. Refer to the ICD and CPT coding books to determine the accuracy of the assigned codes according to the superbill. If no codes were assigned, use the coding books to determine the most appropriate codes. Coding is discussed in Chapter 29, "Health Information."

4. Check the client medical record for:
   - Insurance information including a copy of the client's insurance card, front and back.
   - A form signed by the client giving permission to release confidential information to the insurance provider. This is needed in order to submit the claim for reimbursement.
   - A form signed by the client giving permission to have the payment from the insurance provider sent to the medical office and not to the client. Remember: The client may not be the policyholder. He or she may be the dependent of the policyholder. In addition, for minor children under the age of 18, the parent must sign all forms giving permission to release information about the care and treatment of the child.

PROCEDURE

Keep the following points in mind when you complete insurance forms.

5. Use a black or blue pen, a typewriter, or a computer with insurance software. Fill in the name of the insurance company and the address to which the form will be sent in the top righthand corner.

6. Continue filling out the CMS-1500, textbook Figure 28-6, as follows:
   - **Box 1:** Place a check mark in the appropriate box.
   - **Box 2:** Insert the client's last name, first name, and middle initial.
   - **Box 5:** Insert the client's address, street address, city, state, and ZIP code.
   - **Box 3:** Fill in the client's sex and date of birth.
   - **Box 6:** Indicate the relationship of the client to the insured or policyholder.
   - **Box 8:** Indicate the status of the client as appropriate.
   - **Box 10:** Always check No for each of the three questions related to the reason for the visit to the medical office unless the questions are applicable. Do not leave this box blank.
   - **Box 1a:** Fill in the insured or policyholder identification number. The insurance provider assigns this number. The number may be similar to the client's social security number. Fill it in as indicated on the insurance card and include any extra letters or numbers.
   - **Box 4:** Fill in the policyholder's last name, first name, and middle initial.
   - **Box 7:** Complete the policyholder's address including the street address, city, state, and ZIP code. If the policyholder and client live at the same location, the word "Same" may be inserted in box 7.
   - **Box 11:** If the group number is noted on the insurance card, use it in this box. However, if no group number is given, leave this box blank.

PROCEDURE LM28-2: Completing Insurance Forms (continued)

- **Box 11a:** If the insured or policyholder is not the client, or patient, fill in the policyholder's sex and date of birth in this box.
- **Box 11b:** Give the name of the employer or the school, if the policyholder is a full-time student, on this line.
- **Box 11c:** Leave this box blank. The name of the insurance company will be printed in the top righthand corner of the form.
- **Box 11d:** If the client, or patient, is covered by another insurance plan, check the Yes box and go to the 9 form locators. If another insurance company does not cover the patient, check the No box and leave the 9 form locators blank.
- **Box 12:** If the medical record contains a form signed by the client giving permission to release medical information to the insurance company, write the words "Signature on file" in this box. If no signed form is in the client's medical record, the client must sign on this blank line before the insurance claim form can be processed.
- **Box 13:** This box is commonly referred to as the "Assignment of benefits" line. Again, if the client has signed a form indicating permission to do so, write in the words "Signature on file," indicating that any reimbursement from the insurance company should be sent to the medical office instead of the client.
- **Boxes 14 through 20:** Leave these boxes blank unless you have been specifically instructed by the insurance company to complete them.
- **Box 21:** Indicate the numerical diagnosis code on the lines provided in this box. The CMS form allows for a total of 4 diagnosis codes to be entered.
- **Boxes 22 and 23:** Leave these boxes blank unless you are specifically instructed by the insurance company to complete them.
- **Box 24:**
  a. **Column A:** For each line used for procedural codes, write in the date when service was provided on the lines in the column, even if all procedures were administered on the same day. Leave the "To" columns blank.
  b. **Column B:** Using place of service codes, fill in the code determined by the location where service was provided. For services provided in the medical office, the office has a POS, or place of service, code of 11, as shown in your textbook.
  c. **Column C:** The TOS, or type of service, code is another numerical code assigned to describe the type of service provided. Unless otherwise instructed by the specific insurance provider, leave this column blank.
  d. **Column D:** Using the CPT book if needed, fill in the correct procedural codes and modifiers, if appropriate, in the blanks provided.
  e. **Column E:** For each procedural code listed, indicate the most appropriately linked diagnostic code in this column by writing in the number 1, 2, 3, or 4 located beside the diagnostic codes in Box 21. Do not repeat the diagnostic codes in these boxes.
  f. **Column F:** Using the office fee schedule, fill in the appropriate charges for the corresponding procedural codes in column D. Figure LM28-1 shows a fee schedule.
  g. **Column G:** Indicate the number of days or units in this column by writing in the correct number. Usually, you will use the number 1. Do not leave column blank.
  h. **Column, H, I, J, and K:** Leave these columns blank unless you have been specifically instructed to fill them in by insurance providers.
  i. **Box 25:** Write in the physician or practice employee identification number (EIN) or federal tax ID number or the physician's social security number. Depending on the number used, place a check mark in the appropriate box indicating SSN or EIN.
- **Box 26:** Leave this box blank.
- **Box 27:** If the form is being completed for a government-sponsored insurance plan, indicate

Fee Schedule

Service Rendered	CPT	Fee
New Patient		
Minimal OV	99201	$50
Low OV	99202	$65
Detailed OV	99203	$90
Moderate OV	99204	$130
High OV	99205	$170
Established Patient		
Minimal OV	99211	$26
Low OV	99212	$39
Detailed OV	99213	$53
Moderate OV	99214	$78
High OV	99215	$120
Procedures		
Urinalysis, non-automated, w/scope	81000	$14
Culture	87086	$35
Routine venipuncture	36415	$14
Destruction of lesion	54050	$88
Cystourethroscopy	52000	$352
Visceral vascular study, Duplex scan	93975	$370
Vasectomy	55250	$615
Prostate biopsy	55700	$380
Uroflowmeter	51741	$96
Acidic Acid	99070	$25

Figure LM28-1. Sample fee schedule needed to complete claim form.

Yes or No according to whether the physician has agreed to accept the assignment, or payment, in full. Other insurance plans permit this box to be left blank.

- **Box 28:** Total the charges in column F and put the total amount due in this box.
- **Box 29:** If the client made a payment such as a co-payment, co-insurance, or deductible, indicate the amount paid on this line. If no payment was received from the client, write in zeros.
- **Box 30:** Subtract box 29 from box 28 and place the balance on this line.
- **Box 31:** The physician must sign the CMS before it leaves the office.
- **Box 32:** Leave this line blank.
- **Box 33:** Indicate the physician's name and full address in this box. In the bottom of the box, write in the physician's identification number and group number if appropriate.

7. Check the completed form for accuracy. To demonstrate the willingness of the medical office to be compliant, some offices have a system in which another employee checks the forms. This provides for as much accuracy as possible and demonstrates to any outside auditing agency that the office is trying as much as possible to avoid committing unintentional fraud.

POSTPROCEDURE

When you have completed an insurance form, do the following.

8. After verifying that the CMS-1500 form is accurately and completely filled out, make a copy. Place the original into an envelope and mail it. If the form has been completed electronically, save the document in a separate file and either print it out to mail or submit it electronically.

9. Note the claim information in the claims register, shown in Figure LM28-2. Place the copy of the CMS in a separate file or binder usually called the claims pending file.

10. Make a note on the client's ledger card or electronic financial record indicating that an insurance form was sent, the date, and the amount billed.

11. Within 6 to 8 weeks, depending on the insurance provider, an EOB should arrive along with a reimbursement check. If the claim has been denied or if there is a problem with the completion of the form, this will be indicated on the EOB. Correct the problem or begin the appeals process as soon as possible and resubmit the claim form.

12. If an EOB has not been received in a timely manner, follow up with the insurance provider to determine the cause for the delay.

13. When payment has been made and received by the medical office, remove the copy of the claim form from the claims pending file, attach the EOB, and place them in a separate file for inactive insurance claims. Do not discard these forms.

PROCEDURE LM28-2: Completing Insurance Forms (continued)

They might be needed for reference if a question arises at a later date.

14. Indicate the payment on the office day sheet and individual client account ledger.

15. Process the check received from the insurance provider for deposit into the medical practice bank account.

16. Bill the client for any balance due or notify the billing and collections specialist of a balance due.

PRACTICE LM28-2

Using Procedure Assessment Sheet LM28-2 in your Lab Activity Manual, practice completing insurance forms. Review the step-by-step procedure until you have mastered the skill. Follow your teacher's guidelines for completion of hands-on testing.

Patient's Name	Insurance Company	Claim Filed		Payment Received		Difference (owed by patient)
		Date	Amount	Date	Amount	

Figure LM28-2. One way to keep track of submitted insurance claim forms is by maintaining a claims register. How can an organized system of tracking claims forms already submitted prevent fraud?

Procedure LM29-1 | Documenting Health Care

This procedure gives you the opportunity to practice documenting health care.

PREPROCEDURE

1. Before you begin, obtain a sample client chart from your supervisor for evaluation.

PROCEDURE

Inspect the documentation to verify that it meets these standards:

2. Records must be complete and dated.
3. Records must be legible.
4. Entries must be signed.
5. Changes must be clearly made.

POSTPROCEDURE

6. List each of the four standards cited in the Procedure. Next to each standard, write a statement of how you evaluated the standard when you examined the discharge summary.

PRACTICE LM29-1

Using Procedure Assessment Sheet LM29-1 in your Lab Activity Manual, practice diagnostic coding. Review the step-by-step procedure until you have mastered the skill. Follow your teacher's guidelines for completion of hands-on testing.

Procedure LM29-2 | Billing Review

This procedure gives you the opportunity to practice verifying billing information.

PREPROCEDURE

1. Before you begin, study the encounter form in Figure LM29-1 and the UB-92 form shown in Figure LM29-2.

PROCEDURE

Follow the instructions in the list below.

2. Compare the data in the Patient Identification Information section of the encounter form with the corresponding data on the UB-92. Verify that all data is correctly reported on the claim form. Write down any incorrect items.

3. Compare the data in the Insurance Information section of the encounter form with the corresponding data on the UB-92. Verify that all data is correctly reported on the claim form. Write down any incorrect items.

4. Compare the data in the Procedures and Services section of the encounter form with the corresponding data on the UB-92. Verify that all data is correctly reported on the claim form. Write down any missing or incorrect items.

5. Based on your review, calculate the total charge amount.

POSTPROCEDURE

6. Compare your findings with the answers your instructor will give you.

PROCEDURE LM29-2: Billing Review *(continued)*

Figure LM29-1. Encounter Form—Inpatient Hospitalization.

ENCOUNTER FORM - INPATIENT HOSPITALIZATION

PATIENT IDENTIFICATION INFORMATION

Name	Address	City/State/Zip	Admission Date	Time
Bernard Schwartz	33 Mountain Ave	Belmont NY 12813	9-21-2002	5:45 p.m.

Telephone	Sex	Marital Status	Birthdate	Discharge Date	Time
716-555-2689	M	Married	8-1-1933	9-23-2002	2:45 p.m.

Medical Record No.	Patient Control No.	Internal Control No.	SS No.
99-13-33	48026028001	23516	020-25-9463

Occupation	Employer Name/Address/Telephone Number
Retired	N/A

INSURANCE INFORMATION

Name of Insurance	Insurance ID No.	Group Name	Group No.	Payer Code
Medicare Part A	020529463A	N/A	A	MC

Address of Insurance Company	Accept Assignment (Y or N)	Provider No.
PO Box 90302, Albany NY 22021	Y	56298

PROCEDURES/SERVICES, ICD-9-CM OR HCPCS CODES AND CHARGES

Injection	15.85	ECG	260.00
Chest X-ray	77.35	Cardiology services	700.00
Inhalation service	20.20	ER fee	416.00*
Inpatient semi-private bed (2 days)	890.00		
		*Includes 78.00 professional component charge	
		Note: 760.00 deductible applies to Medicare A	

PRINCIPAL DIAGNOSIS/ICD-9-CM CODE	ADMITTING DIAGNOSIS/ICD-9-CM CODE	
Shortness of Breath	786.09	Shortness of Breath	786.09

SECONDARY DIAGNOSES/ICD-9-CM CODES

INPATIENT PROCEDURES/ICD-9-CM CODES/DATES

PROVIDER OF CARE	PROVIDER ID NUMBER
Robert A. Handlerman, MD	2365218

PRACTICE LM29-2

Using Procedure Assessment Sheet LM29-2 in your Lab Activity Manual, practice verifying billing information. Review the step-by-step procedure until you have mastered the skill. Follow your teacher's guidelines for completion of hands-on testing.

Figure LM29-2. A complete UB-92 Form.

Procedure LM31-1 | Donning Sterile Gloves

Sterile gloves are used for invasive procedures that are done on parts of the body that are considered sterile. Sterile parts of the body are those not exposed to the outside of the body. They include the abdominal cavity, urinary bladder, uterus, and blood vessels. Sterile gloves should be worn during dressing changes or any procedure in which you are going to touch non-intact skin or a sterile part of the body.

If a procedure requires a sterile field, you should prepare the field prior to donning sterile gloves. See Procedure LM31-2. Once you put on sterile gloves you cannot touch anything that is not sterile.

Equipment and Supplies

Sterile gloves • clean surface above waist level

PREPROCEDURE

1. Gather needed equipment. Gloves come in four sizes, S, M, L and XL. Check the package for tears and make sure the expiration date has not passed.
2. (CAUTION) Wash your hands. Perform a surgical scrub if required.

PROCEDURE

3. Peel the outer wrap off the gloves and place the inner wrapper on a clean surface above waist level.
4. Position the gloves so the cuff end is closest to your body.
5. Carefully open the package touching only the flaps. Use instructions if available provided on inner package. Avoid reaching over the sterile inside of the inner package. Follow these steps if instructions are not provided:
   - Open the package so the first flap is opened away from you.
   - Pinch the corner and pull to one side.

   - Place your fingertips under the side flaps and gently pull until the package is completely open.
6. Use the non-dominant hand and grasp the inside cuff of the opposite glove. This is the folded edge. Do not touch on the outside of the glove. If you are right-handed you should use your left hand to put on the right glove first, and vice versa.
7. Holding the glove at arm's length and waist level, insert your dominant hand into the glove, with your palm facing up. Be careful not to let the outside of the glove touch any other surface.
8. With the sterile gloved hand, slip your gloved fingers into the cuff of the other glove. Pick up the other glove touching only the outside. Do not touch any other surfaces.
9. Pull the glove up and onto your hand. Make sure the sterile gloved hand does not touch the ungloved hand. Adjust the fingers as necessary, touching only glove to glove. Do not adjust the cuffs. There is a risk of contamination from your bare forearms.

POSTPROCEDURE

10. Keep your hands in front of you between your shoulders and your waist. If you move your hands out of this area they are considered contaminated.
11. If contamination or the possibility of contamination occurs, change gloves. Never take a chance. If there is any possibility of contamination, remove and change your gloves.
12. Remove gloves the same way you remove clean gloves by carefully touching only the inside. See Chapter 3, "Safety and Infection Control Practice."
13. (CAUTION) Clean the area and put equipment away.
14. (CAUTION) Wash hands.

PROCEDURE LM31-1: Donning Sterile Gloves *(continued)*

PRACTICE LM31-1

Using Procedure Assessment Sheet LM31-1 in your Lab Activity Manual, practice donning sterile gloves. Review the step-by-step procedure until you have mastered the skill. Follow your teacher's guidelines for completion of hands-on testing.

PROCEDURE TROUBLESHOOTING

Sterile Technique

1. Contact of a sterile area or article with an unsterile article renders it unsterile.

2. If there is a doubt about the sterility of an article or area, it is considered unsterile.

3. Unused opened sterile supplies must be discarded or re-sterilized.

4. Packages are wrapped or sealed in such a way that they can be opened without contamination.

5. The edges of wrappers (1 inch margin) covering sterile supplies, outer lips of bottles, or flasks containing sterile solutions are not considered sterile.

6. When a sterile surface or package becomes wet it is considered contaminated.

7. Reaching over a sterile field when you are not wearing sterile clothing contaminates the area.

8. When wearing sterile gloves keep your hands between your shoulders and your waist to maintain sterility.

9. Even in a sterile gown, your back is considered contaminated; do not turn your back on a sterile field.

Procedure LM31-2 — Preparing a Sterile Field and Opening Sterile Packages

A sterile field is an area used during surgical asepsis or sterile technique that is free of microorganisms. Sterile fields are prepared for surgical or other invasive procedures. To maintain sterility throughout this procedure, follow the surgical technique troubleshooting steps. See the Troubleshooting Box in Procedure LM31-1.

Equipment and Supplies

Sterile packages (commercially prepared) or sterile packages wrapped in linens (with four corners for opening) • cleaning solution • sterile drape

PROCEDURE LM31-2: Preparing a Sterile Field and Opening Sterile Packages (continued)

PREPROCEDURE

1. Gather needed equipment.

2. Check the expiration date and the sterilization indicator on the packages.

3. (CAUTION) Clean and disinfect the tray or counter to be used.

4. (CAUTION) Wash your hands.

PROCEDURE

5. Create a sterile field using a commercially prepared sterile field or a sterile instrument pack. Follow these steps:
   - Place the sterile package on the tray or counter, with the first flap pointing away from you.
   - Unfold the outmost fold away from yourself.
   - Unfold the sides of the package one at a time. Touch only the outside of the sterile package.
   - Open the last flap towards yourself.

6. Open packaged sterile packages to place on the sterile field.
   - Check to ensure you have the correct item or instrument.

- Stand away from the sterile field.
- Grasp the package flaps and pull apart about halfway.
- Hold the package over the sterile field with the opening down and with a quick movement pull the flap completely open, dropping the sterile item on the field.

POSTPROCEDURE

7. Apply sterile gloves after sterile field is completed.

8. Assist or perform sterile procedure as required.

9. (CAUTION) Clean the area and wash your hands.

PRACTICE LM31-2

Using Procedure Assessment Sheet LM31-2 in your Lab Activity Manual, practice preparing a sterile field and opening sterile packages. Review the step-by-step procedure until you have mastered the skill. Follow your teacher's guidelines for completion of hands-on testing.

Procedure LM32-1 | Taking a Diet History

PREPROCEDURE

Before you begin taking a diet history, review these steps.

1. Gather needed equipment.

2. Review the client's medical history so that you understand why the client is hospitalized or has been referred for nutrition counseling. You can obtain this information from the client's medical chart, from a nurse, or from the client.

3. Introduce yourself to the client. Explain why you will be asking questions about his or her usual diet and how you will use this information.

PROCEDURE

Ask the following questions when you take the diet history.

4. How many meals and snacks does the client eat in an average day?

5. How many servings does the client eat from each of the following food groups on most days?
   • Grains—breads, cereals, rice, pasta, and other grains
   • Fruits—fresh, canned, dried, juices
   • Vegetables—fresh, canned, frozen, or juice
   • Dairy products—milk, yogurt, and cheese
   • Protein foods—meat, poultry, fish, eggs, dried beans and peas, nuts, and seeds

6. Does the client have any **food intolerances** or allergies? Food intolerance means that the body has trouble digesting or handling some compo-

nent of food. For instance, some people have discomfort (stomach pain, gas, diarrhea) when they eat foods that have lactose in them. Lactose is the natural sugar found in milk and milk products. A **food allergy** is sensitivity to food that involves the body's immune system. Foods that cause an allergic reaction should be avoided completely.

7. Does the client avoid any specific foods or food groups? For example, a client following a vegetarian diet may avoid all meats, dairy products, and eggs. Other clients may avoid certain foods for cultural reasons.

8. Does the client have any problems with eating? These may include chewing problems related to condition of teeth or dentures. There may be swallowing problems, or problems with a dry mouth or taste changes.

9. Does the client follow a special diet prescribed by a doctor or dietitian, such as a low-fat or low-sodium diet?

10. Does the client take any medications? These may include vitamin, mineral, or herbal supplements. Medications can cause side effects that may affect the ability and desire to eat. When taken in large doses, vitamin and mineral supplements can cause harm. Herbal supplements can interfere with the body's ability to use medications and nutrients properly.

11. Where does the client obtain food? The answer to this question can reveal information about where the client usually eats, such as in restaurants, in cafeterias, at home, or at a food shelter.

12. Does the client ever skip meals? If the answer to this question is yes, ask whether the client skips meals for any of the following reasons:
    • Not enough food or money to buy food
    • No transportation to grocery stores
    • No working appliances (stove or kitchen utensils) available to prepare foods

PROCEDURE LM32-1: Taking a Diet History *(continued)*

- No place to store perishable foods (refrigerator or freezer)
- No access to food shelters or congregate meal programs

13. What is the client's level of physical activity? This may be activity involved with an occupation, household activities such as shopping, cleaning, and walking up and down stairs. The activity may be regularly scheduled exercise.

14. What foods and beverages does the client consume, and in what amounts, in a 24-hour period?

16. Review the 24-hour dietary recall form if appropriate. Count the number of servings from each food group and compare the results with the recommended number of servings from each food group for the client's age, gender, and activity level. Refer to Chapter 8, "Nutrition," for a description of the food groups, serving sizes, and recommended daily servings.

17. Give the information you obtained from the diet history and the food group evaluation to the client's registered dietitian for further evaluation.

POSTPROCEDURE

Once you have taken the diet history, check the following list to be sure that you have covered everything.

15. Review the client's answers to the diet history questions. Clarify any answers that are not clear.

PRACTICE LM32-1

Using Procedure Assessment Sheet LM32-1 in your Lab Activity Manual, practice taking a diet history. Review the step-by-step procedure until you have mastered the skill. Follow your instructor's guidelines for completion of hands-on testing.

PART C

Procedure Assessment for Additional Career Skills

First Aid and CPR

PROCEDURE LM4-1:
Amputation

PROCEDURE ASSESSMENT

Procedure Steps	Suggested Points	Self Practice	Peer Practice	Peer Testing	Final Testing	Total Earned
PREPROCEDURE						
1. Gather needed equipment.	6					
2. Ensure scene is safe and wear latex or vinyl gloves.	7					
3. Call EMS.	7					
4. Check client's level of responsiveness and ABCs .	8					
PROCEDURE						
5. Control all major external bleeding.	7					
6. Treat the client for shock. See Procedure 4H in your textbook, "First Aid for Shock."	8					
7. If possible, retrieve amputated part with your gloved hand.	7					
8. Provide first aid to the part that remains. Apply a tourniquet to control life-threatening bleeding only.	7					
9. Wrap the amputated part with a sterile gauze dressing or other clean cloth.	7					
10. Place the amputated part in a waterproof plastic bag or other waterproof container.	7					
11. Place the bag or container containing the part on ice.	8					
12. Keep the part cool but do not freeze it.	7					
13. Comfort and reassure client while waiting the arrival of EMS.	6					
POSTPROCEDURE						
14. Send amputated part with client to hospital.	8					
TOTAL POSSIBLE POINTS	100					

Comments: _____

_____

_____

_____

_____

Signatures: _____   Date: _____

SCORING   *See Preface for scoring instructions.*

Name _____ Date _____

Emergency Medical Services

PROCEDURE LM13-1A:
Preparing an Oxygen Cylinder

PROCEDURE ASSESSMENT

Procedure Steps	Suggested Points	Self Practice	Peer Practice	Peer Testing	Final Testing	Total Earned
PREPROCEDURE						
1. Gather needed equipment.	5					
2. Place cylinder in upright position and stand it to one side.	4					
PROCEDURE						
3. Remove protective seal from valve of cylinder.	4					
4. Keep the plastic valve.	3					
5. Open cylinder's valve for less than a second.	5					
6. Select the appropriate flow meter.	6					
7. Place cylinder's nylon O-ring on the regulator's oxygen port.	5					
8. Align regulator's pins with cylinder's valve inlets.	6					
9. Tighten the "T-screw."	5					
10. Open cylinder's main valve all the way, then close it a half turn.	6					
11. Check for leaks.	6					
• If there's a leak, turn off valve and bleed oxygen from regulator.	1					
• Once it's bled, remove regulator and repeat steps starting at step 7.	1					
12. If there's no leak, attach oxygen tubing and delivery device, turn on flow meter, and adjust flow to prescribed rate.	7					
13. Apply delivery device to client.	8					
14. Secure cylinder or lay it down.	6					
POSTPROCEDURE						
15. Remove delivery device from client.	7					
16. Turn off oxygen's main valve.	5					
17. Disconnect flow device from regulator.	5					
18. Turn on flow meter and bleed, or discharge, residual oxygen from regulator.	5					
TOTAL POSSIBLE POINTS	**100**					

PROCEDURE LM13-1A: Preparing an Oxygen Cylinder *(continued)*

Comments: _____

_____

_____

_____

_____

_____

_____

_____

Signatures: _____ Date: _____

SCORING *See Preface for scoring instructions.*

Emergency Medical Services

PROCEDURE 13-1B:
Providing Oxygen

--- **PROCEDURE ASSESSMENT** ---

Procedure Steps	Suggested Points	Self Practice	Peer Practice	Peer Testing	Final Testing	Total Earned
PREPROCEDURE						
1. Gather needed equipment.	4					
2. Determine need for oxygen use.	4					
• Client must have spontaneous adequate air exchange to safely use this device.						
3. Follow appropriate infection control practices.	4					
PROCEDURE						
(for Nonrebreather Mask)						
4. Remove nonrebreather mask and tubing from packaging.	2					
5. Uncoil tubing and the reservoir bag and tubing.	2					
6. Connect female connector of tubing to nipple of oxygen source flow meter.	3					
7. Turn on oxygen cylinder valve; adjust flow meter between 12 and 15 liters per minute.	3					
8. Place thumb over one-way inlet valve between mask and reservoir bag, until bag becomes fully inflated.	2					
9. Remove thumb from valve.	2					
10. Explain to client that you're going to place him on oxygen.	3					
11. Place mask over client's nose and mouth.	3					
• Slip elastic strap over client's head so strap is between each ear and back of client's head.						
12. Tighten elastic strap as needed.	2					
13. Squeeze metal strip across nose to achieve a better seal.	3					
• If better seal is achieved, reservoir bag will remain partly inflated when client breathes in.						
14. If bag completely flattens, increase flow of oxygen.	3					
15. Monitor client's status.	3					

PROCEDURE LM13-1B: Providing Oxygen *(continued)*

Procedure Steps	Suggested Points	Self Practice	Peer Practice	Peer Testing	Final Testing	Total Earned
PROCEDURE						
(for Nasal Cannula)						
16. Remove nasal cannula from packaging.	2					
17. Uncoil tubing.	2					
18. Connect female connector of tubing to nipple of oxygen source flow meter.	3					
19. Turn on oxygen cylinder valve; adjust flow meter to between 2 and 6 liters per minute.	5					
• Never exceed the 6 liters per minute flow rate with a cannula.						
20. Check that oxygen properly flows from cannula's prongs.	4					
21. Tell client you're going to place him on oxygen.	3					
22. Hold loop part of cannula in front of client's face so prongs are oriented on upper side of loop.	3					
23. Orient curvature of prongs so that tips face upward.	3					
24. Point tips of prongs toward each nostril and insert them.	4					
25. Hold loop at nose to keep prongs inserted.	2					
• With other hand, carefully pass one side of loop over and behind ear on one side of client's head.	2					
26. Continue to hold inserted prongs in nostrils.	2					
• Pass other loop over and behind ear on other side of client's head.	2					
27. Once loop is over each ear, grasp loop at neck.	2					
• Advance plastic fastener up under client's chin until bottom of loop is held firmly in place.	3					
28. Recheck loop. Ensure it's firmly in place but not uncomfortable.	3					
POSTPROCEDURE						
29. Carefully remove oxygen delivery device from client.	4					
30. Turn off oxygen at flow meter and cylinder valve.	3					
31. Bleed flow meter dry.	3					
32. Replace cylinder if pressure is 500 psi or below.	2					
TOTAL POSSIBLE POINTS	**100**					

PROCEDURE LM13-1B: Providing Oxygen *(continued)*

Comments: _____
_____
_____
_____
_____
_____
_____
_____

Signatures: _____ Date: _____

SCORING *See Preface for scoring instructions.*

Name _____ Date _____

Emergency Medical Services

PROCEDURE LM13-2A:
Manual Stabilization of the Head and Neck

PROCEDURE ASSESSMENT

Procedure Steps	Suggested Points	Self Practice	Peer Practice	Peer Testing	Final Testing	Total Earned
PREPROCEDURE						
1. Determine if client requires head/neck stabilization.	12					
• Once applied, manual stabilization cannot be released until client is completely immobilized on long spine board.						
PROCEDURE						
• Client is sitting up:						
a. Position yourself behind client's head.	11					
b. Grasp both sides of client's head with both hands and spread your fingers over sides of head.	12					
c. Hold head motionless. Don't allow client to move head.	12					
• Client is lying on back, face up:						
a. Kneel behind client's head.	11					
b. Grasp both sides of client's head with both hands and spread your fingers over sides of head.	12					
c. Hold head motionless. Don't allow client to move head.	12					
• If client is in another position, adapt the procedure so that head can remain motionless.	9					
POSTPROCEDURE						
2. Maintain stabilization until client is completely immobilized on long spine board.	9					
TOTAL POSSIBLE POINTS	**100**					

Comments: _____
_____
_____
_____
_____

Signatures: _____ Date: _____

SCORING   *See Preface for scoring instructions.*

Emergency Medical Services

PROCEDURE LM13-2B:
Applying Cervical Collars

PROCEDURE ASSESSMENT

Procedure Steps	Suggested Points	Self Practice	Peer Practice	Peer Testing	Final Testing	Total Earned
PREPROCEDURE						
1. Gather needed equipment.	6					
2. Ensure scene is safe. Tell client not to move head or neck.	5					
3. Have a partner place himself behind client's head.	3					
• Ask partner to apply manual stabilization to client's head/neck.	4					
• Continue manual stabilization without interruption.	4					
4. Perform initial assessment.						
• Without moving client's neck or with assistance from another, obtain general impression of client's condition and injuries.	5					
• Evaluate airway, breathing, signs of circulation, and level of responsiveness.	5					
• Assess motor and sensory abilities in all four extremities.	5					
5. Examine head and neck for signs of injury.	3					
6. Measure correct size of cervical collar.						
• Determine collar size by measuring height between top of shoulder and tip of chin when head is in neutral, inline position.	4					
• Use your fingers to measure shoulder to chin distance.	4					
• Ensure chin piece won't lift client's chin and hyperextend neck.	3					
• Ensure collar isn't too small or too tight.	3					
PROCEDURE						
• If client is sitting:						
a. Your partner maintains inline stabilization of head/neck.	3					
b. You properly angle collar for placement.	4					
c. Then position collar bottom under chin and lower jaw.	4					
d. Set collar in place around neck.	4					
e. Secure Velcro straps on collar.	3					
f. Ask partner to spread fingers and maintain manual support for head/neck until client is completely immobilized on spinal immobilization device.	3					

PROCEDURE LM13-2B: Applying Cervical Collars *(continued)*

Procedure Steps	Suggested Points	Self Practice	Peer Practice	Peer Testing	Final Testing	Total Earned
• If client is lying:						
a. Your partner kneels at client's head/neck, applies manual stabilization to head/neck, and continues stabilization without interruption.	3					
b. You position collar in place.	4					
c. Then position collar bottom under chin and lower jaw.	4					
d. Set collar around neck.	4					
e. Secure Velcro straps on collar.	3					
f. Ask partner to spread fingers and maintain manual support for head/neck until client is completely immobilized on spinal immobilization device.	3					
POSTPROCEDURE						
7. Monitor client until transported to medical facility.	4					
TOTAL POSSIBLE POINTS	**100**					

Comments: _____

_____

_____

_____

_____

_____

_____

_____

_____

Signatures: _____   Date: _____

SCORING   *See Preface for scoring instructions.*

Emergency Medical Services

PROCEDURE LM13-3:
Emergency Childbirth During a Normal Delivery

PROCEDURE ASSESSMENT

Procedure Steps	Suggested Points	Self Practice	Peer Practice	Peer Testing	Final Testing	Total Earned
PREPROCEDURE						
1. Gather needed equipment.	3					
2. Evaluate expectant mother:						
• Ask mother her name, age, and expected due date.	1					
• Labor for a first birth is typically much longer than for a second birth.						
• Ask mother how long she's been in labor and how often contractions occur.	2					
a. When contractions last 30 seconds to 1 minute and are 2 to 3 minutes apart, delivery is imminent.						
• Ask mother if she has bled or discharged mucus.	1					
• Ask mother if her amniotic sac has ruptured.	1					
• Ask, "Do you feel the need to move your bowels?"	2					
a. If "Yes," this usually means baby has moved into birth canal.						
b. Don't allow mother to use bathroom.						
• Check mother to see if she is crowning; if so, birth is imminent.	2					
• During contraction, feel mother's abdomen.	2					
a. If it's very hard, delivery is underway.						
• Take vital signs.	2					
3. Observe for signs of imminent delivery.	3					
• Crowning is present.						
• Contractions are closer than 2 minutes apart and last from 30 to 90 seconds.						
• Client feels baby's head moving down birth canal.						
• Client's abdomen is very hard.						
4. Prepare the mother.						
• You put on gloves, gown, and face shield.	3					
a. First Responders and EMTs should follow strict standard precaution guidelines to protect themselves from exposure.						

PROCEDURE LM13-3: Emergency Childbirth During a Normal Delivery (continued)

Procedure Steps	Suggested Points	Self Practice	Peer Practice	Peer Testing	Final Testing	Total Earned
• Place mother on bed or floor.						
a. Elevate buttocks with blankets or pillows.	2					
b. Have mother lie with knees drawn up and legs spread apart.	2					
c. If possible, raise up her back.	1					
• Remove mother's clothing below waist and her underpants.	1					
• Drape both legs, knees, and abdomen with clean sheets or towels.	2					
• Position someone at mother's head.	1					
• Position all OB supplies near you and within easy reach.	2					

PROCEDURE

Procedure Steps	Suggested Points	Self Practice	Peer Practice	Peer Testing	Final Testing	Total Earned
5. Deliver baby.						
• Position yourself so you have a clear view of vaginal opening.	2					
• Calmly speak to mother throughout delivery.	2					
• Have person at head take vital signs and monitor mother for vomiting.	2					
• Position gloved hand at opening of vagina when baby's head begins to appear.	3					
• As head delivers, spread your fingers evenly over bony part of skull.	3					
a. Avoid soft areas of skull.						
• Continue to support head, but don't allow it to pop out.	2					
a. As head delivers, have suction available.	2					
• With towel in other hand, support tissue between mother's vagina and anus to help prevent tearing as baby's head delivers.	3					
• If amniotic sac hasn't ruptured by the time the head delivers, tear it with your fingers and pull membrane away from baby's mouth and nose.	3					
• Once head has delivered, check if umbilical cord is wrapped around baby's neck.	1					
a. If cord is around neck, use your fingers to slip it over head.	2					
b. If that isn't possible, carefully clamp cord in two places and cut between clamps.	2					

PROCEDURE LM13-3: Emergency Childbirth During a Normal Delivery *(continued)*

Procedure Steps	Suggested Points	Self Practice	Peer Practice	Peer Testing	Final Testing	Total Earned
• Suction baby's airway with bulb syringe as soon as head delivers.	3					
a. Compress bulb before placing it in baby's mouth	2					
b. Always suction mouth first, then nostrils.	2					
c. Continue to support head with one hand as you suction airway.	1					
• Help deliver first shoulder by exerting gentle downward pressure on head.	3					
• Help deliver second shoulder by gently guiding head upwards.	3					
• As torso and full body are born, support newborn with both hands.	2					
a. Be sure to grasp feet as they are born.	2					
b. Remember that newborns are very slippery.						
• After delivery, immediately clean and dry newborn's head, face, and torso.	3					
• Wrap baby in warm, dry, clean blanket or sheet.	2					
a. Position baby on side with head slightly lower than body.	2					
b. You may have to periodically suction infant's airway.						
• Record date and time of baby's birth.	1					
POSTPROCEDURE						
6. Ask your partner to monitor and complete assessment of newborn.	2					
7. Observe mother for delivery of placenta.	3					
8. After placenta delivers, wrap it in towel and put in plastic bag.	2					
9. Place two sanitary napkins over vaginal opening.	2					
10. Have client lower her legs and massage the uterus.	3					
11. Transport mother and baby to hospital for evaluation.	2					
TOTAL POSSIBLE POINTS	**100**					

PROCEDURE LM13-3: Emergency Childbirth During a Normal Delivery *(continued)*

Comments: _____

_____

_____

_____

_____

_____

_____

_____

Signatures: _____   **Date:** _____

SCORING   *See Preface for scoring instructions.*

Name _____ Date _____

The Physician's Office

PROCEDURE LM15-1:
Measuring Blood Glucose Using a Glucometer

········ **PROCEDURE ASSESSMENT** ········

Procedure Steps	Suggested Points	Self Practice	Peer Practice	Peer Testing	Final Testing	Total Earned
PREPROCEDURE						
1. Gather needed equipment.	4					
2. Wash your hands.	6					
3. Review glucometer operator's manual if necessary.	2					
4. Perform quality control check on glucometer.	3					
• Use a test strip and/or control solution.	2					
5. Note expiration date on testing strips.	6					
• Don't use strips if expiration date has passed.						
6. Review request form to verify test ordered.	3					
PROCEDURE						
7. Identify client by asking his/her full name.	6					
8. Explain procedure to client.	5					
9. Put on gloves and choose one of client's fingers for capillary stick.	6					
• Finger should be free of bruises, scars, calluses, cuts, or sores.						
10. Clean finger with antiseptic wipe.	4					
• Quickly puncture chosen site with capillary stick.	4					
11. Dispose of stick in biohazard sharps container.	6					
12. Remove first drop of blood with clean gauze or tissue.	4					
13. Squeeze second drop of blood onto testing strip.	4					
• Place strip into glucometer at appropriate time.	4					
• Check instructions; you may have to remove first drop of blood before you insert testing strip into glucometer.	4					
• You can use small pipette to transfer blood from finger to strip.	3					
14. Glucometer will beep when it's done processing specimen.	2					
15. Blood glucose amount will appear in digital display window.	2					
• If number is less than 20 or greater than 300, or if something other than a number appears, repeat test.						

PROCEDURE LM15-1: Measuring Blood Glucose Using a Glucometer *(continued)*

Procedure Steps POSTPROCEDURE	Suggested Points	Self Practice	Peer Practice	Peer Testing	Final Testing	Total Earned
16. Put used gauze or tissue and testing strip in biohazard container.	6					
17. Turn off glucometer and put in storage cabinet.	4					
18. Remove gloves and wash hands.	6					
19. Record procedure and blood glucose amount in client's record.	4					
TOTAL POSSIBLE POINTS	100					

Comments: _____
_____
_____
_____
_____
_____
_____
_____
_____

Signatures: _____ Date: _____

SCORING *See Preface for scoring instructions.*

The Physician's Office

PROCEDURE LM15-2:
Assisting with Minor Office Surgery

············· P R O C E D U R E A S S E S S M E N T ·············

Procedure Steps	Suggested Points	Self Practice	Peer Practice	Peer Testing	Final Testing	Total Earned
PREPROCEDURE						
1. Wash hands and gather needed equipment.	5					
2. Check client's medical record for signed consent form.	3					
3. Identify client by asking his/her full name.	3					
4. Instruct client on clothing removal, gown, and draping.	2					
5. If so instructed by physician, shave or clean surgical area.	2					
PROCEDURE						
6. Take all equipment to exam room.	4					
7. Put sterile drape on mayo stand from back to front of tray.	3					
8. Don't let top of sterile drape touch anything.	3					
• Don't let your arms pass over sterile field.	2					
9. A 1-inch border around drape is considered nonsterile. Don't touch any other area of drape without gloves on.	3					
10. Don't talk or cough over sterile drape.	3					
11. Add articles to sterile field by gently flipping items in peel-apart packages onto drape.	2					
12. Leave nonsterile items on side table for easy access.	2					
13. Put on sterile gloves and straighten items on sterile field.	4					
• Or, use sterile transfer forceps.						
14. Remove gloves and discard them.	2					
15. Place second sterile drape over sterile field (tray), from front to back.	2					
• Don't touch any nonsterile surfaces with drape.	3					
16. A 1-inch border and top of drape are considered nonsterile.						
17. Push tray to side by grasping mayo stand on bottom.	2					
• Don't touch sterile drapes.	2					
18. Tell physician that client and supplies are ready.	3					

PROCEDURE LM15-2: Assisting with Minor Surgery *(continued)*

Procedure Steps	Suggested Points	Self Practice	Peer Practice	Peer Testing	Final Testing	Total Earned
19. Help physician by:						
• Holding basin for used instruments.	2					
• Opening sterile items for physician.	2					
• Putting other items in sterile field as needed.	2					
20. Reassure client as needed.	3					
POSTPROCEDURE						
21. Apply antibiotic ointment, sterile dressing, and tape to surgical area if so ordered.	3					
22. Help client get dressed, if necessary.	2					
23. Tell client how to care for surgical area.	4					
• Tell client when to return for suture removal, etc.	2					
24. Put on clean gloves and clean exam room.	5					
• Discard disposable items in proper containers.	3					
• Sanitize and disinfect work surfaces and tables.	4					
• Put away unused items.	2					
25. Take nondisposable instruments to utility room.	2					
• Sanitize, disinfect, and prepare them for sterilization process.	4					
26. Remove gloves and wash hands.	5					
TOTAL POSSIBLE POINTS	**100**					

Comments: _____

_____

_____

_____

_____

_____

_____

_____

Signatures: _____   Date: _____

SCORING   *See Preface for scoring instructions.*

The Physician's Office

PROCEDURE LM15-3:
Removing Sutures

PROCEDURE ASSESSMENT

Procedure Steps	Suggested Points	Self Practice	Peer Practice	Peer Testing	Final Testing	Total Earned
PREPROCEDURE						
1. Wash hands and gather needed equipment.	7					
PROCEDURE						
2. Identify client by asking his/her full name.	7					
3. Explain procedure to client.	6					
4. Put on clean gloves, remove dressings, and discard them in biohazard waste container.	7					
5. Inspect wound for redness, swelling, drainage, and approximation.	5					
• If you see problems, tell physician before removing sutures.	4					
6. If wound is well-healed, determine number of sutures to be removed.	4					
7. Clean wound with antiseptic solution and sterile gauze.	5					
8. Pick up thumb forceps in nondominant hand.	3					
• Pick up suture scissors in dominant hand.	3					
9. Using forceps, lift one suture by knot.	5					
• Slip curved end of scissors under suture closest to skin and cut suture.	4					
10. Pull suture with forceps until it's completely removed from skin.	5					
11. Put suture onto 2- by 2-inch gauze pad.	5					
12. Continue procedure until all sutures are removed.	4					
13. Count sutures on gauze pad and discard pad in biohazard waste container	7					
POSTPROCEDURE						
14. Discard disposable items or sanitize and disinfect nondisposable items.	7					
15. Remove gloves and wash hands.	7					
16. Record procedure and note condition of wound in client's record.	5					
TOTAL POSSIBLE POINTS	**100**					

Comments: _____

_____

_____

_____

_____

_____

_____

Signatures: _____   **Date:** _____

SCORING   *See Preface for scoring instructions.*

The Physician's Office

PROCEDURE LM15-4:
Opening Medication Vials and Ampules

P R O C E D U R E   A S S E S S M E N T

Procedure Steps	Suggested Points	Self Practice	Peer Practice	Peer Testing	Final Testing	Total Earned
PREPROCEDURE						
1. Wash hands and gather needed equipment.	8					
2. Look up drug in reference book.	4					
• Note normal dosages and route of administration.	3					
• Note any contraindications.	3					
• Alert physician about any questions or concerns before you prepare or administer medication.	3					
3. Get correct medication from storage area.	6					
4. Check medication label carefully against physician's order.	8					
PROCEDURE						
5. To open a medication vial:						
• Take medication vial to well-lit, clean area.	7					
• Remove plastic cap on bottle by snapping it off with your fingers.	6					
• If vial is multiple-dose vial, under plastic cap it will have rubber diaphragm that can be punctured more than once.	6					
• If vial is single-dose vial, it won't have rubber diaphragm.	6					
6. To open a medication ampule:						
• Take ampule and 2 × 2 inch gauze pad to clean, well-lit area.	7					
• Put on clean gloves.	8					
• Hold ampule by bottom and gently tap top to remove medication that may be trapped inside ampule.	3					
• Hold bottom of ampule with your nondominant hand and put gauze around neck of ampule.	3					
• Gently but firmly break ampule at scored area on neck of ampule where top and bottom meet.	4					

PROCEDURE LM15-4: Opening Medication Vials and Ampules *(continued)*

Procedure Steps POSTPROCEDURE	Suggested Points	Self Practice	Peer Practice	Peer Testing	Final Testing	Total Earned
7. Discard glass stem of ampule in biohazard sharps container.	8					
8. Prepare medication for administration.	7					
TOTAL POSSIBLE POINTS	100					

Comments: _____

_____

_____

_____

_____

_____

_____

_____

Signatures: _____ Date: _____

SCORING   *See Preface for scoring instructions.*

Name _____   Date _____

The Physician's Office

PROCEDURE LM15-5:
Aspirating Medication from Vials and Ampules

············ **PROCEDURE ASSESSMENT** ············

Procedure Steps	Suggested Points	Self Practice	Peer Practice	Peer Testing	Final Testing	Total Earned
PREPROCEDURE						
1. Gather needed equipment and wash hands.	5					
2. Calculate dosage ordered.	5					
• Check your calculation at least 2 times.	3					
• If you're uncertain, ask someone else to check your calculation.	3					
3. Assemble needle and syringe without contaminating them.	3					
4. Refer to Procedure LM15-4 for opening the vial or ampule.	2					
PROCEDURE						
5. To aspirate medication from a vial:						
• Clean top of vial with antiseptic wipe.	3					
• Remove needle cap and put it on clean counter.	3					
• Pull back on plunger of syringe until an amount of air equal to amount of medication to be withdrawn is obtained.	3					
• Inject this air into vial through rubber stopper.	2					
• Lift vial so it's upside down with needle inside vial.	3					
• Use your dominant hand to pull back on plunger of syringe. Keep bevel of needle under fluid of medication at all times.	2					
• Pull back on plunger until more than correct amount of medication has been drawn into syringe.	3					
• If any bubbles appear in syringe, firmly tap outside of syringe to move them to top, near hub of needle.	4					
• Gently push any extra medication and air bubbles out of syringe and into vial until correct dosage is obtained in syringe.	3					
• Remove needle from vial and recap vial by scooping the needle cap onto needle. Don't use 2 hands to recap needle.	5					
6. To aspirate medication from an ampule:						
• Open ampule according to Procedure LM15-4.	2					
• Remove needle from needle cap and put it on clean counter.	3					

PROCEDURE LM15-5: Aspirating Medication from Vials and Ampules) *(continued)*

Procedure Steps	Suggested Points	Self Practice	Peer Practice	Peer Testing	Final Testing	Total Earned
• Pick up ampule with one hand and quickly invert it.	2					
• Insert needle into ampule. Don't inject air into ampule.	3					
• Keeping bevel of needle under fluid, slowly pull back on plunger and withdraw medication.	3					
• Remove needle from ampule and check for air bubbles.	4					
• Holding needle and syringe in dominant hand, gently tap syringe to move bubbles to top of syringe and push excess medication and air out of syringe.	3					
• Use needle guard or recap needle by using scooping technique. Don't use 2 hands to recap needle.	5					
POSTPROCEDURE						
7. Check label on vial or ampule for accuracy at least 3 times:	5					
• First, when you get medication from storage area.	3					
• Second, before you withdraw medication from ampule or vial.	3					
• Third, after you aspirate medication.	3					
8. Discard single-dose vials in proper waste container or replace multiple-dose vials in proper storage area.	4					
9. Discard stem and base of ampules in biohazard sharps container.	5					
TOTAL POSSIBLE POINTS	**100**					

Comments:

_____

_____

_____

_____

_____

_____

_____

_____

_____

Signatures: **Date:**

SCORING   *See Preface for scoring instructions.*

The Physician's Office

PROCEDURE LM15-6:
Reconstituting Powder Medication for Injection

············· P R O C E D U R E   A S S E S S M E N T ·············

Procedure Steps	Suggested Points	Self Practice	Peer Practice	Peer Testing	Final Testing	Total Earned
PREPROCEDURE						
1. Get correct medication from storage area.	4					
2. Verify medication against physician's order.	7					
• Refer to reference book as needed.						
3. Determine amount of diluent to be used.	5					
• Check against medication information insert or reference book.	4					
4. Gather needed supplies.	4					
5. Wash your hands.	7					
PROCEDURE						
6. Open vials containing medication and diluent. See Procedure LM15-4.	3					
7. Wipe tops of vials with alcohol wipe.	4					
8. Assemble needle and syringe without contaminating them.	4					
9. Remove needle cap and put it on clean counter.	3					
10. Pull back on plunger of syringe until amount of air is equal to amount of diluent to be used.	5					
11. Insert needle into vial of diluent and invert vial using nondominant hand.	4					
12. Push plunger so that air in syringe is inserted into vial.	4					
13. Remove proper amount of diluent by pulling back on plunger.	5					
• Remove any air bubbles and withdraw needle from diluent vial.						
14. Insert needle and syringe containing diluent into medication vial.	4					
15. Inject diluent into vial containing powder.	4					
16. Without aspirating any medication, remove syringe and needle and discard them in biohazard sharps container.	7					
17. Roll vial between hands to mix powder completely with diluent.	3					

PROCEDURE LM15-6: Reconstituting Powder Medication for Injection (continued)

Procedure Steps POSTPROCEDURE	Suggested Points	Self Practice	Peer Practice	Peer Testing	Final Testing	Total Earned
18. Calculate correct amount to be aspirated and injected using newly reconstituted mixture.	7					
19. Always use new syringe and needle to aspirate reconstituted medication before administering medication to client.	5					
20. Discard used vials in proper waste containers.	7					
TOTAL POSSIBLE POINTS	100					

Comments: _____

_____

_____

_____

_____

_____

_____

_____

_____

_____

_____

Signatures: _____ Date: _____

SCORING See Preface for scoring instructions.

The Physician's Office

PROCEDURE LM15-7:
Performing Injections

PROCEDURE ASSESSMENT

Procedure Steps	Suggested Points	Self Practice	Peer Practice	Peer Testing	Final Testing	Total Earned
PREPROCEDURE						
1. Check physician's order and get correct medication.	3					
2. Refer to drug reference book to note:	3					
• Correct dosages.	1					
• Route of administration.	1					
• Contraindications.	1					
• Special administration instructions.	1					
3. Compare medication label on vial or ampule with physician's order.	3					
4. Wash hands and gather needed supplies.	3					
5. Calculate dosage according to amount ordered by physician and how medication is supplied.	3					
• Reconstitute powder medications if necessary.	1					
6. Always check medication label 3 times for accuracy:	3					
• First, when you get medication from storage area.	1					
• Second, before you withdraw medication from ampule or vial.	1					
• Third, after you aspirate medication.	1					
PROCEDURE						
7. Assemble syringe and needle.	2					
Intramuscular injection:						
• Assemble a 3-milliliter syringe and a needle size from 18 to 23 gauge, with shaft of 1 to 3 inches in length.	2					
• To determine needle length: Deltoid muscle—1-inch needle. Dorsogluteal muscle—$1\frac{1}{2}$-inch needle. Vastus lateralis muscle—$1\frac{1}{2}$-inch needle.	1					
Subcutaneous injection:						
• Assemble a 3-milliliter syringe and a needle size from 23 to 27 gauge, with shaft of $\frac{1}{2}$ to $\frac{3}{4}$ inches in length.	2					
Intradermal injection:						
• Assemble a 1-milliliter syringe and a needle size from 25 to 26 gauge, with shaft of $\frac{3}{8}$ to $\frac{1}{2}$ inch in length.	2					

PROCEDURE LM15-7: Performing Injections *(continued)*

Procedure Steps	Suggested Points	Self Practice	Peer Practice	Peer Testing	Final Testing	Total Earned
8. Aspirate correct amount of medication from vial or ampule.	2					
9. Place the following on tray to carry to exam room:						
• Syringe and needle filled with correct amount of medication.	1					
• Antiseptic wipe.	1					
• Small gauze pad.	1					
• Clean gloves.	1					
• Adhesive bandages.	1					
• Also, biohazard sharps container should be in room.	1					
10. Identify client by asking his/her full name.	1					
11. Check client's medical record for documentation of any allergy.	3					
• Also, ask client about medication allergies.	1					
12. Instruct client on clothing removal and positioning.	1					
13. Put on clean gloves.	3					
14. Find correct site:						
• Intramuscular—Use proper landmarks on body.	1					
• Subcutaneous.	1					
• Intradermal—Usually, anterior forearm is used for tuberculin screening tests.	1					
15. Clean chosen site with antiseptic wipe.	2					
• Start in center and move in a circular and outward motion.	1					
16. Remove needle cap.	2					
• Ensure sharps container is within easy reach.	1					
Intramuscular Injection:						
a. Hold muscle firmly between thumb and index finger of your nondominant hand.	1					
b. With needle at 90° angle to muscle, insert needle quickly and smoothly with your dominant hand.	1					
c. Release muscle and aspirate by pulling back on plunger to ensure needle isn't in a blood vessel. If blood appears in hub of needle, don't proceed with injection. Withdraw needle, Begin procedure over after getting new syringe and needle. If no blood appears, continue injection.	3					
d. Slowly inject medication into muscle by pressing on plunger.	1					

Procedure Steps	Suggested Points	Self Practice	Peer Practice	Peer Testing	Final Testing	Total Earned
e. Use dominant hand to keep syringe and needle steady during aspiration and injection of medication.	1					
f. When all medication has been injected, put gauze pad above injection site with nondominant hand and quickly remove needle.	1					
g. Gently massage injection site, unless contraindicated, with gauze pad and apply adhesive bandage, if necessary.	1					
Subcutaneous Injection:						
a. Pinch and lift subcutaneous tissue between thumb and index finger of nondominant hand.	1					
b. With needle at 45° angle to skin, insert needle quickly and smoothly with dominant hand with bevel of needle up. Use 90° angle for abdominal SC injections for heavier clients.	2					
c. Release tissue and aspirate to check for blood appearance, do not aspirate when administering certain medications such as insulin and heparin.	1					
d. Slowly inject medication into muscle by pressing on plunger.	1					
e. Use dominant hand to keep syringe and needle steady during aspiration and injection of medication.	1					
f. When all medication has been injected, put gauze pad above injection site with nondominant hand and quickly remove needle.	2					
g. Gently massage injection site with gauze pad. Never massage when giving a heparin injection. Apply adhesive bandage if necessary.	1					
Intradermal Injection:						
a. Tightly stretch skin between thumb and index finger of nondominant hand.	1					
b. With needle at a 10° to 15° angle to skin, insert needle smoothly, with bevel of needle up. Insert needle only until bevel is completely under skin. Don't aspirate for this injection.	3					
c. Release skin and slowly inject medication by pressing on plunger. A small bubble on skin will appear.	1					
d. Use dominant hand to keep syringe and needle steady during aspiration and injection of medication.	1					
e. When all medication has been injected, gently remove needle. Don't apply bandage or massage injection site.	3					

PROCEDURE LM15-7: Performing Injections *(continued)*

Procedure Steps	Suggested Points	Self Practice	Peer Practice	Peer Testing	Final Testing	Total Earned
17. Remove gloves and wash hands.	3					
18. Tell client how to report results, if necessary.	3					
POSTPROCEDURE						
19. Document injection by recording in client's record:	1					
• Date, time, and name.	1					
• Dose of medication.	1					
• Route and site of administration.	1					
• Your name.	1					
20. Observe and report to physician immediately any reactions to medication.	1					
TOTAL POSSIBLE POINTS	**100**					

Comments:

_____

_____

_____

_____

_____

_____

_____

_____

Signatures: _____   Date: _____

SCORING   *See Preface for scoring instructions.*

Mental Health

PROCEDURE LM16-1:
Administering Chemical Restraints

PROCEDURE ASSESSMENT

Procedure Steps	Suggested Points	Self Practice	Peer Practice	Peer Testing	Final Testing	Total Earned
PREPROCEDURE						
1. Check to ensure there's a written order for restraints.	4					
• The order should be in plan of care of supervising nurse or licensed practitioner.						
2. Nurse or licensed practitioner must have instructed you on medication to be given.	5					
3. Wash your hands.	5					
4. Identify client.	5					
5. Introduce yourself to client, if necessary.	4					
6. Provide for privacy of client.	4					
7. Explain procedure to client.	4					
8. Ensure client is in comfortable position.	4					
9. Have glass of water close by.	3					
PROCEDURE						
10. Help client sit up.	3					
11. Hand medication to client.	4					
12. Help client put medication in mouth, if necessary.	4					
13. Hand glass of water to client.	4					
• If client has trouble swallowing medication, suggest he/she take a drink of water before trying again.	3					
14. Ensure client has put medication in mouth and swallowed it.	5					
15. Ensure client can reach signal bell.	5					
16. Ensure client is comfortable.	5					
17. Wash your hands.	5					
18. Record procedure in client's record.	3					
19. Report to supervisor that you have done procedure.	4					
• Report any abnormal occurrence.						
POSTPROCEDURE						
20. Check on client frequently to ensure his/her safety.	5					
• Offer fluids, as necessary.	4					
• Check to see if client needs to use bathroom.	4					
21. Report any adverse findings to supervisor immediately.	4					
TOTAL POSSIBLE POINTS	**100**					

PROCEDURE LM16-1: Administering Chemical Restraints *(continued)*

Comments: _____
_____
_____
_____
_____
_____
_____
_____
_____

Signatures: _____ **Date:** _____

SCORING *See Preface for scoring instructions.*

Rehabilitation

PROCEDURE LM19-1:
Assisting with an Examination of the Ear

PROCEDURE ASSESSMENT

Procedure Steps	Suggested Points	Self Practice	Peer Practice	Peer Testing	Final Testing	Total Earned
PREPROCEDURE						
1. Gather needed equipment.	5					
2. Identify client and introduce yourself.	7					
3. Explain procedure.	7					
4. Ask client to remove glasses and hearing aid(s) if client is wearing these items.	5					
PROCEDURE						
5. Pass lighted otoscope to doctor or nurse.	5					
6. Help client sit in correct position for exam.	7					
• Client should tip head slightly toward shoulder.	6					
• Ear to be examined should be pointing up.	6					
• Doctor may hold earlobe as he/she inserts speculum into ear.						
• Client may need to adjust position so doctor can get a better look.						
• Both ears are usually examined, even if there is a problem with just one.	6					
POSTPROCEDURE						
7. When exam is done, help client put on glasses and hearing aid(s).	6					
8. Provide for client's safety and comfort.	9					
• If you're in an in-patient facility, put call signal within easy reach of client.						
9. Clean and replace all equipment.	8					
• Dispose of cone-shaped plastic tip.	7					
10. Wash your hands.	9					
11. Record all required information.	7					
TOTAL POSSIBLE POINTS	**100**					

Comments: _____

_____

_____

_____

_____

_____

_____

_____

Signatures: _____ Date: _____

SCORING   See Preface for scoring instructions.

CHAPTER 20

Name _____ Date _____

Sports Medicine

PROCEDURE LM20-1:
Using a Cool Whirlpool

-------- PROCEDURE ASSESSMENT --------

Procedure Steps	Suggested Points	Self Practice	Peer Practice	Peer Testing	Final Testing	Total Earned
PREPROCEDURE						
1. Gather needed equipment.	4					
2. Test client's sensation to touch by lightly running fingers across area.	7					
• If client reports decreased sensation or hypersensitivity in area, tell physical therapist immediately.	5					
3. If sensation is normal, fill whirlpool:	5					
• Close drain to whirlpool.	4					
• Turn on faucet to facilitate filling.	4					
• Use scoops or buckets of ice to regulate temperature of water, which should be between 50° and 60°F.	4					
• Add proper amount of disinfectant to water, and turn on turbine to mix it.	4					
• Ensure water is deep enough to cover lower 2/3 of turbine.	7					
• Run turbine for 5 minutes to ensure proper disinfecting.	4					
PROCEDURE						
4. Help client put affected extremity in whirlpool.	3					
5. Turn turbine on.	3					
6. Aim jet of turbine at affected limb.	5					
7. Adjust force of output of turbine by opening or closing outflow valve.	4					
8. Set timer for time specified by therapist.	3					
9. Periodically check client's condition.	7					
• If client reports feeling dizzy or lightheaded or looks pale, immediately assist client out of whirlpool.	5					
• Stop treatment and tell therapist.	5					
POSTPROCEDURE						
10. When timer rings, help client out of whirlpool.	3					
11. Examine skin for adverse effects.	7					
12. Help client dry extremities with towel.	3					
13. You may need to help client put on clothes or walk initially.	4					
• Altered sensation may result in decreased balance or hazardous condition.						
TOTAL POSSIBLE POINTS	**100**					

PROCEDURE LM20-1: Using a Cool Whirlpool *(continued)*

Comments: _____
_____
_____
_____
_____
_____
_____
_____
_____

Signatures: _____   Date: _____

SCORING   *See Preface for scoring instructions.*

Sports Medicine

PROCEDURE LM20-2:
Calculating Body Fat

PROCEDURE ASSESSMENT

Procedure Steps	Suggested Points	Self Practice	Peer Practice	Peer Testing	Final Testing	Total Earned
PREPROCEDURE						
1. Gather needed equipment.	6					
2. If client is male, have him take off shirt and put on short pants.	5					
• If client is female, have her put on short pants and a short-sleeved shirt.	5					
3. Adjust age and sex settings on caliper to match client.	7					
4. Have client stand for the measurements.	6					
5. Take measurements on right side of body.	7					
6. Don't take measurements immediately after exercise or if skin is wet.	6					
• This can lead to inaccurate readings.						
PROCEDURE						
Male						
7. Hold body fat caliper in one hand.	5					
8. With other hand, pinch chest with thumb and forefinger vertically 2 inches above and lateral to nipple.	7					
• Try to pinch only skin and fat, not underlying muscle.	5					
• It may help to lift skin away from muscle.	5					
9. Open caliper by squeezing trigger and allow it to close over skin held in your opposite hand.	6					
10. Click switch on side of caliper to lock in measurement.	6					
11. Repeat steps 7 to 10 for abdominal region just lateral to umbilicus and mid-thigh.	7					
12. Caliper will calculate percent body fat for client and show it on display.	6					
Female						
Repeat steps 7 to 12, but take measurements on back of arm (mid-tricep with arm relaxed by side), on abdominal region just above iliac crest, and at mid-thigh.						
• Note: Some calipers use measurements taken just inferior to scapula. Check directions before using.						

PROCEDURE LM20-2: Calculating Body Fat (continued)

Procedure Steps POSTPROCEDURE	Suggested Points	Self Practice	Peer Practice	Peer Testing	Final Testing	Total Earned
13. Tell client to put his/her clothes back on.	4					
14. Provide results to therapist. Discuss findings with client if appropriate.	7					
TOTAL POSSIBLE POINTS	100					

Comments:

_____

_____

_____

_____

_____

_____

_____

_____

_____

Signatures: _____   Date: _____

SCORING   *See Preface for scoring instructions.*

Alternative Medicine

PROCEDURE LM21-1:
Performing a Foot Massage

-------------------- **PROCEDURE ASSESSMENT** --------------------

Procedure Steps	Suggested Points	Self Practice	Peer Practice	Peer Testing	Final Testing	Total Earned
PREPROCEDURE						
1. Prepare table or bed.	2					
• Cover it with sheet and put large towel or blanket to side.	1					
• Place rolled towel or small blanket under feet.	1					
2. Explain procedure and what client is to do.	2					
3. Adjust table or bed to correct position.	3					
4. Leave room while client removes shoes, socks, and any clothing on lower leg.	2					
• Tell client to lie on table or bed in prone position.	1					
• Help client, if necessary.						
5. Warm the oil, if needed.	2					
6. Wash your hands.	3					
PROCEDURE						
7. If possible, dim room lights and turn on relaxing music.	1					
8. Arrange blanket or towel so only client's lower leg and foot are exposed.	2					
• Ensure any clothing is covered by blanket.	1					
9. Put a quarter-sized amount of oil in your hand.	2					
• Spread oil over your hands and forearms.	1					
• If you notice friction while performing massage, use more oil.						
• Always apply oil to your hands and arms, not client.	1					
10. Don't massage over open sores or rashes.	3					
• Don't massage calf if there is a warm, red, tender area, which could be a blood clot.						
11. Stand on left side of table or bed with feet 18 to 24 inches apart.	3					
• Point your left foot toward client's head.	1					
• Point your right foot toward bed or table.	1					
• Bend slightly at knees and rock from front to back as you do strokes.	1					
12. Spread oil on client's left foot and lower leg, using flat part of fingers.	2					
• Stroke from foot toward knee and back down to foot.	1					

PROCEDURE LM21-1: Performing a Foot Massage *(continued)*

Procedure Steps	Suggested Points	Self Practice	Peer Practice	Peer Testing	Final Testing	Total Earned
13. Shift your weight and turn your body so you face foot of bed or table.	3					
• Point your right foot straight.	1					
• Point your left foot toward bed or table.	1					
• Bend slightly at knees.	1					
14. Gently lift client's leg, bending it at knee.	2					
• Support leg in this position during massage.	1					
15. Use palm of left hand to cup client's heel.	2					
• Rotate your palm over heel, massaging it firmly.	1					
16. Use sides of thumbs to gently but firmly massage sole and ball of foot and lower side of each toe.	2					
17. Shift your weight and turn your body so you face the head of table or bed again.	3					
• Point your left foot straight.	1					
• Point your right foot toward table or bed.	1					
• Bend slightly at knees.	1					
18. Massage client's arch by firmly stroking it with lateral portion of your left forearm.	2					
• Rotate your arm, using lateral side on upstroke, and medial side on down stroke.	1					
• Repeat 3 to 5 times.	1					
19. Use sides of thumbs to gently but firmly massage top of foot.	2					
• Cover all areas with thumb strokes.	1					
20. Massage tops of toes using thumb strokes.	2					
• Pull gently on each toe.	1					
21. Massage around inner and outer ankle bones using thumb strokes.	1					
22. Gently lower leg and foot to table or bed.	1					
23. Using thumb strokes, massage from ankle up calf to back of knee.	1					
• Don't massage popliteal area (behind knee).						
24. Massage entire calf with thumb strokes.	2					
• Work from ankle toward back of knee.	1					
• Use sides, not tips, of thumbs.	1					
• If massage hurts client, use lighter pressure.						
• Don't massage calves of clients who have history of blood clots.						

Procedure Steps	Suggested Points	Self Practice	Peer Practice	Peer Testing	Final Testing	Total Earned
25. Massage calf from ankle to knee and back to ankle.	2					
• Use flat part of your fingers.	1					
• Lighten your touch as you do this stroke.	1					
26. Stroke from client's leg to knee again.	2					
• Use very tips of your fingers with extremely light pressure.	1					
27. Cover client's leg and foot with blanket or towel.	1					
28. Move to right side of table.	2					
• Repeat steps 11 to 27 on client's right leg.	1					
• Reverse your foot position in steps 11, 13, and 17.	1					
POSTPROCEDURE						
29. Tell client you will leave room while he/she dresses.	2					
• Tell client to use towel or blanket to wipe off excess oil before dressing.	1					
• Help client, if necessary.						
30. Leave room and provide privacy for client.	2					
31. Wash your hands thoroughly to remove oil.	3					
32. Remove used linens from table or bed.	2					
• Put them in dirty linen bin.	1					
33. Clean table using a 1:5 solution of bleach and water.	3					
TOTAL POSSIBLE POINTS	**100**					

Comments:

_____

_____

_____

_____

_____

_____

_____

Signatures: _____ **Date:** _____

SCORING   *See Preface for scoring instructions.*

Dental Care

PROCEDURE LM22-1:
One-Handed Instrument Transfer

PROCEDURE ASSESSMENT

Procedure Steps	Suggested Points	Self Practice	Peer Practice	Peer Testing	Final Testing	Total Earned
PREPROCEDURE						
1. Gather needed equipment.	3					
2. Prepare the treatment area.	3					
3. Assemble dental tray with basic setup and additional pen grasp instruments.	3					
4. Seat client and yourself.	3					
5. Wash hands and put on:	5					
• Protective glasses.	1					
• Mask.	1					
• Gloves.	1					
PROCEDURE						
6. Using two-handed transfer, simultaneously pass the mirror and explorer, in their position of use, to the operator.	4					
7. From dental tray, pick up pen grasp instrument on handle away from working end.	4					
8. Grasp between thumb and index and middle fingers of left hand.	3					
9. Move instrument to transfer zone.	3					
10. Receive explorer with little finger of left hand.	3					
11. Place pen grasp instrument in operator's hand in position of use then return explorer to tray or rotate back into passing position.	3					
12. Repeat process with other pen grasp instruments.	3					
13. From dental tray, pick up palm grasp instrument near working end.	4					
14. Grasp between your thumb and index and middle finger.	3					
15. Receive used instrument with little finger of left hand.	4					
16. Place palm instrument in operator's hand in position of use.	4					
17. Return used instrument to tray.	3					

PROCEDURE LM22-1: One-Handed Instrument Transfer *(continued)*

Procedure Steps	Suggested Points	Self Practice	Peer Practice	Peer Testing	Final Testing	Total Earned
18. During procedure:	4					
• Operator is able to maintain a fulcrum.	3					
• Instrument is placed in operator's hand firmly and distinctly.	3					
• Instrument is removed from operator's hand distinctly and without hesitation.	3					
• Instruments are kept parallel to one another during transfer.	3					
• When receiving instrument that will be needed immediately, rotate instrument into passing position using the one-handed technique.	3					
POSTPROCEDURE						
19. Wash your hands. Remove:	5					
• Glasses.	2					
• Mask.	2					
• Gloves.	2					
20. Dismiss client.	4					
21. Return to treatment room and put on utility gloves, complete posttreatment aseptic procedures.	5					
TOTAL POSSIBLE POINTS	**100**					

Comments: _____
_____
_____
_____
_____
_____
_____
_____
_____

Signatures: _____   Date: _____

SCORING   *See Preface for scoring instructions.*

Dental Care

PROCEDURE LM22-2:
Using the Oral Evacuator

········· P R O C E D U R E   A S S E S S M E N T ·········

Procedure Steps	Suggested Points	Self Practice	Peer Practice	Peer Testing	Final Testing	Total Earned
PREPROCEDURE						
1. Gather needed equipment.	3					
2. Prepare treatment area.	4					
3. Assemble dental tray with basic setup.	4					
4. Seat client.	4					
5. Wash hands and put on:	6					
• Protective glasses.	2					
• Mask.	2					
• Gloves.	2					
PROCEDURE						
6. Place high-volume evacuator (HVE) in right hand using thumb-to-nose grasp. See textbook Figure 22-68.	4					
7. Position HVE appropriately.	4					
• For procedure on maxillary right posterior, with tip slightly distal and opening parallel to lingual surface of tooth being treated. See textbook Figure 22-70.	3					
• For procedure on maxillary left posterior, position tip slightly distal, with opening parallel to buccal surface of tooth being treated.	3					
• For procedure on facial surface of maxillary or mandibular anterior area, position tip parallel to lingual surface of tooth being treated, with tip slightly beyond incisal edge. See textbook Figure 22-69.	3					
• For procedure on lingual surface of maxillary or mandibular anterior area, position tip parallel to facial of tooth being treated, with tip slightly beyond incisal edge.	3					
• For procedure on mandibular right position, position tip slightly distal, with opening parallel to lingual surface of tooth being treated.	3					
• For procedure on mandibular left posterior, position tip slightly distal, with opening parallel to buccal surface of tooth being treated.	3					

Procedure Steps	Suggested Points	Self Practice	Peer Practice	Peer Testing	Final Testing	Total Earned
8. Retract cheek and tongue from preparation area.	3					
9. Remove all fluid and debris from oral cavity.	3					
10. When dentist pauses, rotate evacuator opening toward maxillary occlusal surface and clear excess fluid.	4					
11. Maintain client comfort.	3					
12. Use air-water syringe to clear mirror.	3					
POSTPROCEDURE						
13. Wash hands. Remove:	6					
• Glasses.	3					
• Mask.	3					
• Gloves.	3					
14. Dismiss the client.	4					
15. Return to treatment room.	6					
• Put on utility gloves.	3					
• Complete posttreatment aseptic procedures.	3					
TOTAL POSSIBLE POINTS	**100**					

Comments:

Signatures: Date:

SCORING   *See Preface for scoring instructions.*

Dental Care

PROCEDURE LM22-3:
Preparing the Anesthetic Syringe and Assisting with the Administration

PROCEDURE ASSESSMENT

Procedure Steps	Suggested Points	Self Practice	Peer Practice	Peer Testing	Final Testing	Total Earned
PREPROCEDURE						
1. Gather needed equipment.	3					
2. Prepare treatment area.	3					
3. Assemble instruments and materials for procedure.	3					
4. Seat client.	3					
5. Wash your hands. Put on:	5					
• Protective glasses.	2					
• Mask.	2					
• Gloves.	2					
PROCEDURE						
6. Prepare anesthetic syringe out of client's vision.	4					
• Insert cartridge into syringe by pulling down on thumb ring of syringe, inserting rubber stopper end into barrel of syringe and releasing pressure on thumb ring.	3					
• Place needle on syringe by removing shorter, clear protective cap, then pushing exposed end of needle through opening in hub of anesthetic syringe. Ensure needle is straight to pierce rubber diaphragm in aluminum cap of carpule. Screw needle onto hub.	3					
• Gently tap bottom of thumb ring to engage harpoon in rubber stopper.	3					
• Loosen and remove colored needle cap.	3					
• Express a few drops of solution to ensure syringe is functioning properly.	3					
• Recap needle using one-handed scoop technique or a recapping device.	3					
7. Moisten cotton swab with small amount of topical anesthetic.	3					
8. After dentist has explained procedure to client, pass 2 x 2 gauze pad to the dentist to dry injection site.	3					
9. Receive gauze pad and pass topical anesthetic on moistened cotton swab.	3					
10. After 1 to 2 minutes, dentist will remove cotton swab.	3					
11. Pass anesthetic syringe under client's chin and place thumb ring over dentist's thumb.	3					

Procedure Steps	Suggested Points	Self Practice	Peer Practice	Peer Testing	Final Testing	Total Earned
12. Remove needle guard while stabilizing syringe in dentist's hand.	3					
13. Watch client for adverse reactions as dentist administers anesthetic.	3					
14. Rinse and evacuate to remove any excess anesthetic solution.	3					
POSTPROCEDURE						
15. Wash your hands. Remove:	5					
• Glasses.	2					
• Mask.	2					
• Gloves.	2					
16. Dismiss client.	2					
17. Return to treatment room and don utility gloves.	5					
• Disassemble syringe.	2					
• Unscrew needle.	2					
• Pull back thumb ring, pull down on cartridge and remove from syringe.	2					
• Place used needle and cartridge in biohazardous sharps container.	2					
18. Complete other posttreatment aseptic procedures.	5					
TOTAL POSSIBLE POINTS	**100**					

Comments:

_____

_____

_____

_____

_____

_____

_____

_____

Signatures: _____ Date: _____

SCORING *See Preface for scoring instructions.*

Dental Care

PROCEDURE LM22-4A:
Preparing Alginate and Assisting with an Alginate Impression

···· P R O C E D U R E   A S S E S S M E N T ····

Procedure Steps	Suggested Points	Self Practice	Peer Practice	Peer Testing	Final Testing	Total Earned
PREPROCEDURE						
1. Gather needed equipment.	2					
2. Prepare treatment area.	3					
3. Assemble instruments and materials for procedure.	3					
4. Seat client in upright position.	2					
5. Wash hands. Put on:	4					
• Protective glasses.	1					
• Mask.	1					
• Gloves.	1					
6. Gently turn canister over several times to fluff alginate.	2					
7. Measure alginate powder for mandibular impression.	3					
• Place it on paper towel next to bowl.	1					
• Scoop powder from canister, gently tap and level powder with alginate spatula.	1					
• Follow manufacturers' directions and use their measuring scoop.						
8. Repeat procedure for maxillary impression.	3					
9. Measure water for mandibular impression and pour into bowl next to 2 scoops.	2					
10. Measure water for maxillary impression and pour into bowl next to 3 scoops.	2					
11. Check temperature of water. Best to use room-temperature water as warmer water will speed up setting time and cooler will slow down.	3					
PROCEDURE						
12. Explain procedure to client.	2					
13. Add two scoops of powder to water in bowl after dentist determines correct size of tray.	2					
14. With tip of spatula toward bottom of bowl, use circular motion and quickly incorporate all powder into water.	2					
15. Tilt bowl toward you while in palm of hand.	3					
• Beat and press alginate against side of bowl using figure 8 motion.	1					
• Turn bowl while you mix.	1					
• Mix should be creamy and smooth in 1 minute.						

PROCEDURE LM22-4A: Preparing Alginate and Assisting with an Alginate Impression (continued)

Procedure Steps	Suggested Points	Self Practice	Peer Practice	Peer Testing	Final Testing	Total Earned
16. Gather material into single mass.	3					
17. Place one-half of material on each side of impression tray and press down and spread material over entire surface of tray.	2					
18. Wet fingers and smooth alginate.	2					
19. With tray handle directed toward dentist, transfer the tray.	2					
20. Clean spatula while impression is setting.	2					
• In 2 to 3 minutes material will be firm.						
• It will not lose its form with finger pressure.						
21. Receive impression from dentist when material is set.	2					
22. Repeat process for maxillary impression.	3					
• Load maxillary tray from posterior.	1					
• Load all alginate at once.	1					
POSTPROCEDURE						
23. Wash your hands. Remove:	4					
• Glasses.	1					
• Mask.	1					
• Gloves.	1					
24. Dismiss client.	2					
25. Return to treatment room and put on utility gloves.	4					
26. Gently rinse impressions under running water to remove any blood, saliva, or debris.	4					
27. Spray impressions with approved surface disinfectant.	4					
28. Unless models will be poured immediately, wrap impressions in moistened paper towel and place in sealed plastic bag labeled with client's name.	4					
• Impression can be safely transported or poured in office later when proposed this way.						
• Not all offices pour models.						
29. Place any excess alginate in trash container. Clean and disinfect alginate bowls.	4					
30. Clean and sterilize alginate spatula.	4					
31. Complete all other posttreatment aseptic procedures.	4					
TOTAL POSSIBLE POINTS	100					

Comments: _____
_____
_____
_____
_____
_____
_____
_____

Signatures: _____ **Date:** _____

SCORING   *See Preface for scoring instructions.*

Name _____   Date _____

Dental Care

PROCEDURE LM22-4B:
Mixing and Assisting with an Elastomeric Impression

PROCEDURE ASSESSMENT

Procedure Steps	Suggested Points	Self Practice	Peer Practice	Peer Testing	Final Testing	Total Earned
PREPROCEDURE						
1. Gather needed equipment.	3					
2. Prepare treatment area.	4					
3. Assemble instruments and materials.						
4. Seat client.	3					
5. Wash hands. Put on:	6					
• Protective glasses.	3					
• Mask.	3					
• Gloves.	3					
6. Coat inside of tray with adhesive.	4					
7. Extrude equal lengths of base and accelerator onto paper mixing pad.	3					
• Strips should be close together without touching.	2					
• Accelerator strip is thinner than base strip.	2					
• Equal lengths of material, not equal amounts, are needed. Refer to Figure LM 22-6a.	2					
8. Place syringe tip on impression paste syringe.	3					
PROCEDURE						
9. Mix material when dentist is ready to take impression.	4					
• With tip of spatula, use a spiral motion working from top to bottom of strips to mix accelerator into the base very quickly.	3					
• Use flat side of spatula to thoroughly mix the material.	3					
• Should take 30 to 45 seconds. Refer to Figure LM 22-6b and c.						
10. Load syringe by using back end of syringe barrel and in short sweeping motions scoop material into syringe.	3					
11. Place plunger in syringe barrel and extrude material into tip.	4					
12. Load tray with remainder of material.	3					
13. Pass syringe to dentist.	4					
14. Receive syringe and pass filled tray to dentist.	3					
15. Impression material will set in 6 to 10 minutes depending upon type of material used.	4					

PROCEDURE LM22-4B: Mixing and Assisting with an Elastomeric Impression (continued)

Procedure Steps POSTPROCEDURE	Suggested Points	Self Practice	Peer Practice	Peer Testing	Final Testing	Total Earned
16. Disassemble syringe.	3					
17. Remove excess material from spatula and syringe.	4					
• Material will be rubbery and peel off spatula and syringe when set.						
• Brush may be used to clean inside barrel of syringe.						
18. Tear off and dispose top sheet of mixing pad.	3					
19. Clean and sterilize syringe spatula.	6					
20. Rinse, dry and disinfect impression.	6					
21. Place impression in labeled bag for transfer to laboratory.	6					
TOTAL POSSIBLE POINTS	100					

Comments: _____
_____
_____
_____
_____
_____
_____
_____
_____
_____

Signatures: _____ Date: _____

SCORING *See Preface for scoring instructions.*

Name _____ Date _____

Dental Care

PROCEDURE LM22-4C:
Mixing Dental Plaster and Stone and Fabricating a Model

PROCEDURE ASSESSMENT

Procedure Steps	Suggested Points	Self Practice	Peer Practice	Peer Testing	Final Testing	Total Earned
PREPROCEDURE						
1. Gather needed equipment.	2					
2. Place plastic cover over top of vibrator.	3					
PROCEDURE						
3. Wash hands. Put on:	4					
• Masks.	1					
• Gloves.	1					
4. Gently dry air-impression with air-water syringe.	3					
5. Measure 30 mL of water for stone or 50 mL of paste for plaster.	2					
6. Pour water into rubber mixing bowl.	2					
7. Place towel on scale and weigh out 100 g of stone or plaster.	2					
8. Pick up towel and gradually slide stone or plaster into water.	2					
9. Mix water and powder together but DO NOT whip. Whipping causes air bubbles to form.	3					
10. Turn vibrator to low or medium speed.	2					
11. Press mixing bowl on vibrator.	3					
• Press down.	2					
• Rotate bowl to bring bubbles to surface.	2					
• Mixing and vibrating should be completed in less than 2 minutes.						
12. Pick up impression and place tray edge near handle on vibrator.	2					
13. With spatula, place a small amount of plaster or stone in posterior area on one side of dental arch.	3					
14. Tilt tray to allow plaster or stone to flow into teeth around arch.	3					
15. Continue adding small increments until all tooth areas of impression are covered.	3					
16. Add larger increments until entire impression is filled.	3					
17. Place remaining plaster or stone on a plastic or glass slab or tile and shape base approximately same size as impression tray and ½ to 1 inch thick.	2					
18. Invert filled impression onto base without pushing into base.	3					

PROCEDURE LM22-4C: Mixing Dental Plaster and Stone and Fabricating a Model (continued)

Procedure Steps	Suggested Points	Self Practice	Peer Practice	Peer Testing	Final Testing	Total Earned
19. Hold impression by handle to keep it level while smoothing base mix up into inverted material.	3					
• Do not cover edges of impression tray.	1					
• If edges of impression tray are covered, tray will be locked in place when the plaster hardens.						
20. Allow model to set for 1 hour before separating.	2					
POSTPROCEDURE						
21. Place any excess plaster in trash container.	2					
22. Clean and disinfect the plaster bowl and spatula.	2					
23. Rinse all plaster from sink.	4					
24. Remove and discard vibrator cover.	2					
25. Remove gloves and mask.	2					
26. Wash your hands.	4					
27. Separating models:	4					
• When models are set, put gloves on again and use lab knife to remove any excess plaster from around margins on impression tray.	4					
• Pull straight up on tray handle to remove impression from model.	3					
28. If reusable trays were used:	4					
• Remove impression material from tray.	3					
• Clean and sterilize tray.	3					
29. Remove gloves and wash hands.	4					
TOTAL POSSIBLE POINTS	100					

Comments:

_____

_____

_____

_____

_____

_____

Signatures: _____   Date: _____

SCORING   *See Preface for scoring instructions.*

Dental Care

PROCEDURE LM22-5A:
Preparing Amalgam and Assisting with an Amalgam Restoration

PROCEDURE ASSESSMENT

Procedure Steps	Suggested Points	Self Practice	Peer Practice	Peer Testing	Final Testing	Total Earned
PREPROCEDURE						
1. Gather needed equipment.	2					
2. Prepare treatment area.	3					
3. Prepare amalgam tray setup. Refer to textbook Procedure 22D.	2					
4. Prepare anesthetic syringe.	2					
5. Read amalgam manufacturer's direction for mixing time and speed and adjust settings on amalgamator.	3					
6. Seat client.	2					
7. Wash hands and put on:	4					
• Protective glasses.	1					
• Mask.	1					
• Gloves.	1					
PROCEDURE						
8. Transfer mouth mirror and explorer to dentist.	2					
9. Transfer 2 x 2 gauze pad to dentist for use in drying injection site.	3					
10. Receive gauze pad and pass a cotton swab moistened with topical anesthetic.	2					
11. Pass anesthetic syringe.	2					
12. Rinse and evacuate to remove any excess anesthetic solution.	2					
13. A dental dam may be placed to isolate treatment area.	2					
14. Dentist uses handpiece and burs to remove decay and prepare cavity.	2					
15. During cavity preparation:	3					
• Use oral evacuation and air-water syringe.	1					
• Retract oral tissues.	1					
• Adjust light as needed to maintain a clear operating field.	1					
16. Pass explorer and hand cutting instruments as required.	2					
17. When cavity preparation is complete, cavity is thoroughly rinsed and dried.	2					
18. If required, mix bases or liners and transfer them to dentist.	2					
19. Assemble and transfer matrix band if cavity involves a proximal surface.	2					

Procedure Steps	Suggested Points	Self Practice	Peer Practice	Peer Testing	Final Testing	Total Earned
20. Activate premeasured amalgam capsule by pressing ends of capsule together to break membrane in capsule that separates mercury and silver alloy.	3					
21. Place amalgam capsule in amalgamator and mix.	2					
22. Open capsule and drop mix onto a squeeze cloth or amalgam well.	3					
23. Fill amalgam carrier and transfer to dentist.	2					
24. Transfer amalgam condenser and refill carrier.	3					
• Repeat until cavity is overfilled.						
• It may be necessary to use more than one capsule depending on size of cavity.						
25. Transfer carving instrument to shape amalgam to proper contour and to make contact with adjacent and opposing teeth.	2					
26. Use oral evacuator to remove excess amalgam as dentist is carving.	2					
27. Remove rubber dam.	2					
28. Transfer articulating paper to check occlusion.	2					
29. Rinse and evacuate.	2					
30. Advise client to avoid chewing on area for several hours and hot drinks and food until numbness is gone.	2					
POSTPROCEDURE						
31. Wash hands. Remove:	4					
• Gloves.	1					
• Mask.	1					
• Protective glasses.	1					
32. Dismiss the client.	2					
33. Return to treatment room and put on utility gloves.	4					
34. Disassemble syringe and place used needle and cartridge in biohazardous sharps container.	4					
35. Put scrap amalgam in container reserved for this purpose.	4					
• Since mercury is hazardous material, excess amalgam should not be thrown into trash.						
• It could contaminate groundwater. If incinerated, it could release hazardous materials.						
36. Complete all other posttreatment aseptic procedures.	4					
TOTAL POSSIBLE POINTS	**100**					

PROCEDURE LM22-5A: Preparing Amalgam and Assisting with an Amalgam Restoration (continued)

Comments: _____
_____
_____
_____
_____
_____
_____
_____
_____

Signatures: _____   Date: _____

SCORING   *See Preface for scoring instructions.*

Name _____   Date _____

Dental Care

PROCEDURE LM22-5B:
Preparing Composite and Assisting with a Composite Restoration

PROCEDURE ASSESSMENT

Procedure Steps	Suggested Points	Self Practice	Peer Practice	Peer Testing	Final Testing	Total Earned
PREPROCEDURE						
1. Gather needed equipment.	2					
2. Prepare treatment area.	3					
3. Prepare composite resin tray setup. Refer to textbook Procedure 22D.	2					
4. Prepare anesthetic syringe.	2					
5. Read composite manufacturer's directions.	3					
6. Seat client.	2					
7. Wash your hands and put on:	4					
• Protective glasses.	1					
• Mask.	1					
• Gloves.	1					
PROCEDURE						
8. Transfer mouth mirror and explorer to dentist.	2					
9. Transfer 2 x 2 gauze pad to dentist for use in drying injection site.	2					
10. Receive gauze pad and pass topical anesthetic moistened cotton swab.	2					
11. Pass the anesthetic syringe.	3					
12. Rinse and evacuate to remove any excess anesthetic solution.	2					
13. A dental dam may be placed to isolate treatment area.	2					
14. Dentist uses handpiece and burs to remove decay and prepare cavity.	2					
15. During cavity preparation:	2					
• Use oral evacuator and air-water syringe.	1					
• Retract oral tissues.	1					
• Adjust light as needed to maintain a clear operating field.	1					
16. Pass explorer and hand cutting instruments as required.	2					
17. When cavity preparation is complete, thoroughly rinse and dry cavity.	2					
18. If required, mix bases or liners and transfer them to dentist.	2					
19. Transfer acid etch syringe to dentist.	2					
20. Rinse and dry tooth after approximately 15 to 30 seconds.	3					
21. Plastic matrix strip is placed interproximally (between two teeth).	2					

Procedure Steps	Suggested Points	Self Practice	Peer Practice	Peer Testing	Final Testing	Total Earned
22. Place bonding agent on applicator tip and transfer to dentist.	2					
23. Transfer curing light to harden bonding material.	3					
• Curing light is very high-intensity light.	4					
• Do not look directly at light.						
• Clients and dental staff can wear special glasses for protection.						
24. Transfer composite material.	3					
• This is supplied in compules or unit doses and can be expressed directly into the cavity.						
• Or, a small amount from a larger syringe can be placed on small mixing pad and placed with a plastic instrument.						
25. Dentist places material.	3					
• Matrix is pulled tightly around tooth.						
• Material is light-cured.						
26. Transfer sandpaper strips and discs, finishing burs, diamonds, and polishing points as needed for smoothing restoration.	2					
27. Remove rubber dam.	2					
28. Transfer articulating paper to check occlusion.	2					
29. Rinse and evacuate.	2					
30. Advise client to avoid chewing on area for several hours and to avoid hot drinks and food until numbness is gone.	2					
POSTPROCEDURE						
31. Wash your hands. Remove:	4					
• Gloves.	1					
• Mask.	1					
• Protective glasses.	1					
32. Dismiss the client.	2					
33. Return to treatment room and put on utility gloves.	4					
34. Disassemble syringe and place used needle and cartridge in sharps container.	4					
35. Complete all other posttreatment aseptic procedures.	4					
TOTAL POSSIBLE POINTS	100					

PROCEDURE LM22-5B: Preparing Composite and Assisting with a Composite Restoration *(continued)*

Comments: _____

_____

_____

_____

_____

_____

_____

_____

Signatures: _____   **Date:** _____

SCORING   *See Preface for scoring instructions.*

Dental Care

PROCEDURE LM22-6A:
Mixing Zinc Oxide Eugenol Cement

PROCEDURE ASSESSMENT

Procedure Steps	Suggested Points	Self Practice	Peer Practice	Peer Testing	Final Testing	Total Earned
PREPROCEDURE						
1. Gather needed equipment.	4					
2. Assemble instruments and materials needed for procedure.	6					
3. Read cement manufacturer's instructions.	6					
• Some zinc oxide eugenol cements are two-paste systems.						
• They are mixed in same manner as calcium hydroxide.						
PROCEDURE						
4. Fluff powder in closed bottle.	4					
5. Measure powder.	6					
• Use scoop and level it with cement spatula.	4					
• Amount of powder needed is determined by amount of cement needed for procedure.						
6. Place powder on right side of pad.	4					
7. Replace cap on powder bottle.	3					
8. Draw up liquid into dropper and replace bottle cap.	4					
9. Hold dropper perpendicular to pad.	6					
• Dispense drops close to powder without touching powder.	4					
• Use one drop of liquid for each scoop of powder.	4					
10. Divide powder into two sections and then divide one section into two or three smaller sections.	4					
11. Draw larger section into liquid and incorporate powder using a figure 8 rotary motion.	4					
12. Continue mixing in small increments of powder until desired consistency is reached.	6					
• For temporary luting, mix should be creamy.						
• As spatula is lifted off pad, cement should follow spatula for about 1 inch before breaking into a thin thread.						
• For a base or temporary restoration, cement should be puttylike and capable of being rolled into a ball.						

Procedure Steps	Suggested Points	Self Practice	Peer Practice	Peer Testing	Final Testing	Total Earned
• Dentist's preferences also dictate consistency required.						
• Mixing time is 1 to 1½ minutes.						
13. Once mixing is completed, gather all material into one area.	6					
14. Remove excess cement from the spatula with a 2 x 2 gauze pad.	4					
15. Hold pad and a clean 2 x 2 gauze pad at the client's chin and pass the plastic instrument to dentist.	4					
POSTPROCEDURE						
16. Remove excess cement from plastic instrument.	5					
17. Tear off top sheet from paper pad and throw away.	4					
18. Disinfect all surfaces touched during procedure including exterior of bottles and dropper.	4					
19. Sterilize instruments.	4					
TOTAL POSSIBLE POINTS	**100**					

Comments:

_____
_____
_____
_____
_____
_____
_____
_____
_____

Signatures: _____ **Date:** _____

SCORING   *See Preface for scoring instructions.*

Dental Care

PROCEDURE LM22-6B:
Mixing Calcium Hydroxide Cement

PROCEDURE ASSESSMENT

Procedure Steps	Suggested Points	Self Practice	Peer Practice	Peer Testing	Final Testing	Total Earned
PREPROCEDURE						
1. Gather needed equipment.	8					
2. Read cement manufacturer's instructions.	10					
PROCEDURE						
3. Express very small, equal amounts of both catalyst and base in close proximity on mixing pad.	10					
4. Replace caps on both tubes.	9					
5. Using a circular motion, quickly (10 to 15 seconds) mix two pastes together until color is uniform.	10					
6. Remove excess cement from mixing instrument with a 2 x 2 gauze pad.	9					
7. Hold mixing pad and clean 2 x 2 gauze pad at client's chin and pass ball-ended instrument or an explorer to dentist.	8					
POSTPROCEDURE						
8. Remove excess cement from placement instrument.	8					
9. Tear off top sheet from paper pad and throw away.	9					
10. Disinfect all surfaces touched during the procedure including exteriors of paste tubes.	9					
11. Sterilize instruments.	10					
TOTAL POSSIBLE POINTS	100					

Comments: _____
_____
_____
_____
_____
_____
_____
_____

Signatures: _____ Date: _____

SCORING
See Preface for scoring instructions.

Dental Care

PROCEDURE LM22-6C:
Mixing Polycarboxylate Cement

PROCEDURE ASSESSMENT

Procedure Steps	Suggested Points	Self Practice	Peer Practice	Peer Testing	Final Testing	Total Earned
PREPROCEDURE						
1. Gather needed equipment.	4					
2. Read current manufacturer's instructions.	7					
PROCEDURE						
3. Fluff powder in closed bottle.	4					
4. Measure powder using dispenser supplied by manufacturer.	6					
5. Place powder on right side of pad.	5					
6. Replace cap on powder bottle.	5					
7. Hold bottle or syringe perpendicular to pad.	7					
• Dispense drops close to powder without touching powder.	5					
• Follow manufacturer's directions for appropriate number of drops or calibrations per scoop of powder.	5					
8. Incorporate all powder into liquid at once.	5					
9. Mix quickly using a folding motion and some pressure, finishing mix within 45 seconds.	6					
10. For luting, mix should be creamy.	5					
• As spatula is lifted off pad, cement should follow spatula for about 1 inch before breaking into a thin thread.						
• For a base, the liquid is decreased and mix will be glossy but consistency will be tacky and stiff.						
11. Once mixing is completed, gather all material into one area then use material immediately before mix becomes dull and stringy.	5					
12. Remove excess cement from spatula with a moist 2 x 2 gauze pad.	6					
13. For luting, use a plastic instrument to coat internal surfaces of crown or bridge then transfer crown or bridge to dentist occlusal side up.	5					
14. If you use polycarboxylate as a base, hold slab and a clean 2 x 2 gauze pad at the client's chin and pass plastic instrument to dentist.	4					

PROCEDURE LM22-6C: Mixing Polycarboxylate Cement (continued)

Procedure Steps POSTPROCEDURE	Suggested Points	Self Practice	Peer Practice	Peer Testing	Final Testing	Total Earned
15. Remove excess cement from plastic instrument.	5					
16. Tear off top sheet from paper pad and throw it away.	5					
17. Disinfect all surfaces touched during procedure including exteriors of bottles and dropper.	6					
18. Sterilize instruments.						
TOTAL POSSIBLE POINTS	100					

Comments:

_____

_____

_____

_____

_____

_____

_____

_____

Signatures: _____ Date: _____

SCORING   See Preface for scoring instructions.

Name _____ Date _____

Dental Care

PROCEDURE LM22-6D:
Mixing Glass Ionomer Cement

P R O C E D U R E   A S S E S S M E N T

Procedure Steps	Suggested Points	Self Practice	Peer Practice	Peer Testing	Final Testing	Total Earned
PREPROCEDURE						
1. Gather needed equipment.	5					
2. Read cement manufacturer's instructions.	6					
PROCEDURE						
3. Fluff powder in closed bottle.	4					
4. Measure powder with scoop.	6					
• Level with cement spatula.	5					
• Amount of powder needed is determined by amount needed and manufacturer's recommendations.						
5. Place powder on right side of pad.	5					
6. Replace cap on powder bottle.	5					
7. Hold dropper or liquid bottle perpendicular to pad and dispense recommended amount of liquid close to powder without touching powder.	6					
8. Replace cap on liquid immediately to prevent evaporation.	6					
9. With spatula, add powder to liquid in small, even increments.	5					
10. Incorporate powder using a figure 8 rotary motion and complete mixing in 60 seconds.	6					
11. Once mixing is complete, gather all material into one area.	6					
• Manipulation time is an additional 2 minutes.						
• Surface of cement remains glossy.						
12. Remove excess cement from spatula with a moist 2 x 2 gauze pad.	5					
13. For luting, use a plastic instrument to thinly coat internal surfaces of crown or bridge; then transfer crown or bridge to dentist occlusal side up.	4					
14. If using glass ionomer as a base or restorative material, hold slab and a clean 2 x 2 gauze pad at client's chin; then pass plastic instrument to dentist.	5					

PROCEDURE LM22-6D: Mixing Glass Ionomer Cement *(continued)*

Procedure Steps POSTPROCEDURE	Suggested Points	Self Practice	Peer Practice	Peer Testing	Final Testing	Total Earned
15. Remove excess cement from plastic instrument.	4					
16. Tear off top sheet from paper pad and throw it away.	5					
17. Disinfect all surfaces touched during procedure, including exterior of bottles.	6					
18. Sterilize instruments.	6					
TOTAL POSSIBLE POINTS	100					

Comments: _____

_____

_____

_____

_____

_____

_____

_____

Signatures: _____ Date: _____

SCORING *See Preface for scoring instructions.*

Dental Care

PROCEDURE LM22-7A:
Manual Processing of Dental Radiographs

PROCEDURE ASSESSMENT

Procedure Steps	Suggested Points	Self Practice	Peer Practice	Peer Testing	Final Testing	Total Earned
PREPROCEDURE						
1. Gather needed equipment.	2					
2. Put on safety glasses and gloves.	5					
3. Fill water tank.	2					
4. Stir developer.	3					
• Rinse stirring rod thoroughly.	1					
• Stir fixer.	1					
5. Check temperature of developer and adjust water temperature until developer is 68°F.	3					
6. Cover work surface with paper towel.	2					
7. Label film rack with client's name and date.	3					
8. Turn on safelights and turn off overhead lights.	2					
PROCEDURE						
9. Open outer film packet.	3					
• Remove inner paper packet.	1					
• Without touching film inside, pull back paper wrapping and drop film onto towel.						
• Continue with all film packets.						
10. Dispose of all contaminated film packets.	5					
11. Remove gloves and wash hands.	5					
12. Attach each film to film rack keeping films parallel to avoid contact.	3					
13. Smoothly immerse film rack into left side of developer tank.	2					
14. Slowly agitate, or raise the rack up and down, several times.	3					
15. Hook rack on edge of developer tank and place cover on processing tank.	2					
16. Set timer for $4\frac{1}{2}$ minutes.	2					
17. When timer rings, remove rack from developer.	3					
• Place film in rinsing area, middle portion of processing tank.	1					
• Agitate slowly for 30 seconds.	1					

PROCEDURE LM22-7A: Manual Processing of Dental Radiographs *(continued)*

Procedure Steps	Suggested Points	Self Practice	Peer Practice	Peer Testing	Final Testing	Total Earned
18. Smoothly immerse film rack in fixer tank, or right side of tank.	4					
• Agitate it carefully.	2					
• Hook rack over edge of tank.	2					
• Replace cover.	2					
19. Set timer for 10 minutes.	3					
20. When timer rings, remove rack from fixer.	4					
• Place rack in rinsing section.	2					
• Hook rack over edge of tank.	2					
• Replace cover.	2					
21. Set timer for 20 minutes.	3					
22. When timer rings, remove rack and hang to dry and do not handle rack until thoroughly dry.	5					
23. When films are dry, place them in a labeled mount.	5					
POSTPROCEDURE						
24. Dry off all work surfaces.	3					
25. When finished processing for day, turn off water and drain rinsing tank.	2					
26. Replace tank cover.	2					
27. Turn off safelights.	2					
TOTAL POSSIBLE POINTS	**100**					

Comments:

_____

_____

_____

_____

_____

_____

_____

_____

Signatures: _____ Date: _____

SCORING *See Preface for scoring instructions.*

Dental Care

PROCEDURE LM22-7B:
Mounting Dental Radiographs

P R O C E D U R E   A S S E S S M E N T

Procedure Steps	Suggested Points	Self Practice	Peer Practice	Peer Testing	Final Testing	Total Earned
PREPROCEDURE						
1. Wash your hands.	9					
2. Gather needed equipment.	6					
3. Turn on view box.	5					
PROCEDURE						
4. Label film mount with client's name, dentist's name and date.	7					
5. Place all films on work surface with dot rounding up.	7					
6. Locate four bitewings. Both maxillary and mandibular crowns will be on film.	6					
7. Mount bitewings:	7					
• Bitewing closest to center of mount has both premolars.						
• Bitewing toward outside of mouth has second and third molars.						
• Occlusal plane is curved as if "smiling."						
8. Locate six anterior films with length of teeth in same direction as length of film.	6					
9. Mount anterior films:	7					
• Maxillary teeth are larger.						
• Maxillary cuspid is longest tooth in mouth.						
• Place incisal edge of films toward middle of mouth.	6					
• Place roots of maxillary teeth toward top and roots of mandibular teeth toward bottom edges of mount.	6					
10. Locate eight posterior films and mount them:	7					
• Maxillary molars have three roots that are not clearly distinct.						
• Mandibular molars have two roots, a distinct mesial and a distinct distal root.						
• Roots generally curve toward distal.						
• Occlusal plane is curved as if "smiling."						
• Film closest to center of mount shows both premolars.						
• Film toward outside of mount shows second and third molars.						
• Teeth on film are oriented as in mouth, with roots of maxillary teeth at top and roots of mandibular teeth at bottom.						

Procedure Steps	Suggested Points	Self Practice	Peer Practice	Peer Testing	Final Testing	Total Earned
11. Review entire mount for accuracy.	8					
POSTPROCEDURE						
12. Place radiographs in client's chart.	7					
13. Turn off view box.	6					
TOTAL POSSIBLE POINTS	**100**					

Comments:

_____
_____
_____
_____
_____
_____
_____
_____
_____

Signatures: _____   **Date:** _____

SCORING   *See Preface for scoring instructions.*

CHAPTER 23

Name _____   Date _____

Animal Health Care

PROCEDURE LM23-1:
Performing a Fecal Exam

PROCEDURE ASSESSMENT

Procedure Steps	Suggested Points	Self Practice	Peer Practice	Peer Testing	Final Testing	Total Earned
PREPROCEDURE						
1. Identify the animal.	4					
2. Gather needed equipment.	2					
3. Put on gloves.	5					
4. Collect fresh fecal sample from animal.	4					
• If sample is in refrigerator, ensure it's properly identified.	3					
• Evaluate only samples that are properly labeled.	5					
• Using wrong sample will cause reporting errors.						
PROCEDURE						
5. Examine feces for color, texture, form, and presence of mucus, blood, or tapeworms.	4					
• Normal dog stool is cylindrical, solid, and brown.						
• Normal dog stool has no blood, mucus, or parasites.						
• Undigested food items sometimes appear in normal dog stool.						
• It's normal for clothing to pass through dog's digestive tract.						
6. Note any abnormalities in animal's record.	3					
7. Use applicator stick to put fecal matter on slide; add drop of saline.	2					
8. Mix feces with saline using application stick.	3					
9. Examine slide under low power on microscope. Look for protozoan organisms.	4					
10. Look for presence of any parasite larvae or eggs.	4					
11. Put gumball-sized fecal mass in cup and add 20 mL of flotation solution; mix until liquid turns brown.	3					
12. Pour liquefied feces through strainer into a 15-mL test tube. Fill tube.	3					
13. Put tube in centrifuge. Balance centrifuge with another tube filled with water directly across from it.	5					
14. Operate centrifuge for 3 to 5 minutes at 1,500 rpm.	4					
15. Remove tube from centrifuge and put in test tube rack.	3					

PROCEDURE LM23-1: Performing a Fecal Examination (continued)

Procedure Steps	Suggested Points	Self Practice	Peer Practice	Peer Testing	Final Testing	Total Earned
16. Add flotation solution to fill tube so fluid is just over top.	3					
17. Put 22mm-square cover slip over top of tube and leave in place for 5 minutes.	4					
18. Put cover slip in center of clean, dry microscope slide.	2					
19. Put slide on microscope stage. Examine under low power for presence of larva or eggs.	3					
20. Reexamine entire slide under high power.	4					
21. Note any positive findings in animal's medical record.	3					
POSTPROCEDURE						
22. Put microscope slide in glass waste receptacle.	3					
23. Thoroughly wash out test tube and put in drying rack.	5					
24. Thoroughly rinse strainer.	5					
25. Turn off microscope light.	2					
26. Remove gloves and wash hands.	5					
TOTAL POSSIBLE POINTS	**100**					

Comments: _____
_____
_____
_____
_____
_____
_____
_____
_____

Signatures: _____ Date: _____

SCORING *See Preface for scoring instructions.*

Animal Health Care

PROCEDURE LM23-2:
Performing a Urinalysis on a Dog

PROCEDURE ASSESSMENT

Procedure Steps	Suggested Points	Self Practice	Peer Practice	Peer Testing	Final Testing	Total Earned
PREPROCEDURE						
1. Gather needed equipment.	2					
2. Take dog for a walk on a leash.	1					
3. Take clean, dry container for urine collection. You can attach container to stick that is 2 to 3 feet long.	1					
4. Let dog urinate for a few seconds, then put container under urine stream. You need $\frac{1}{4}$ to $\frac{1}{2}$ ounce or 7 to 15cc or mL of urine.	2					
5. Return dog to enclosure.	2					
6. Wash your hands.	4					
7. Label urine container with name of animal and date.	4					
8. Take sample to lab for analysis. Put sample in refrigerator if analysis won't be done for several hours.	2					
PROCEDURE						
9. Examine urine for color, transparency, and odor.	4					
• Normal dog urine is clear yellow to almost colorless.						
• Darkest urine is seen in morning.						
• As dog drinks water during day, urine becomes diluted and colorless.						
• Medications can turn urine green or blue.						
• Red color indicates bleeding, common in urinary tract diseases.						
10. Note any abnormalities on animal's medical record.	2					
11. If you are using sample from refrigerator, let it come to room temperature before testing.	1					
12. Using dropper, put drop of urine on prism cover glass of refractometer (TS meter).	2					
13. Close cover plate over urine, hold refractometer up to light, and look in eyepiece.	1					
14. You will see light-dark interface.	4					
• Read value for specific gravity that is intersected by light-dark interface.	2					
• Value should be between 1.000 and 1.055.	2					
15. Record value in animal's record.	2					

PROCEDURE LM23-2: Performing a Urinalysis on a Dog *(continued)*

Procedure Steps	Suggested Points	Self Practice	Peer Practice	Peer Testing	Final Testing	Total Earned
16. Clean refractometer according to manufacturer's recommendations.	2					
17. Open bottle of urine reagent strips, remove one strip, and close jar immediately. Read directions on bottle.	3					
18. Insert strip into urine so all colored squares are covered.	1					
19. Remove strip and hold it in horizontal position, tapping it slightly on edge of jar.	3					
20. Compare colors of squares with colors on chart on bottle, which correspond to certain values.	4					
21. Record values in animal's record.	2					
22. Dispose of reagent strip.	2					
23. Remove gloves, if worn, and wash hands thoroughly.	4					
24. Put 5 to 7 mL of urine in centrifuge tube and put in centrifuge.	2					
• Fill similar-sized tube to same level with water.	4					
• Put tube directly across from urine tube to balance centrifuge.	2					
25. Centrifuge urine for 2 to 5 minutes at 1,000 to 2,000 rpm.	3					
26. Once centrifuge stops, remove urine-filled tube and pour off supernatant, leaving a drop or two in tube.	2					
27. Gently flick bottom of tube with finger, to suspend urine sediment in remaining few drops.	1					
28. Use dropper to put drop of sediment suspension on clean, dry microscope slide.	3					
29. You may choose to add a stain or put cover slip on top of slide.	2					
30. Examine slide under low power on microscope.	2					
• Note cells and other structures.	1					
• You may want to use higher power for smaller objects.	1					
• Compare objects to photographic chart, if available, or ask instructor or professional for assistance.	1					
• Record results in animal's record.	1					

PROCEDURE LM23-2: Performing a Urinalysis on a Dog *(continued)*

Procedure Steps POSTPROCEDURE	Suggested Points	Self Practice	Peer Practice	Peer Testing	Final Testing	Total Earned
31. Clean lab area.	4					
32. Ensure top is securely on reagent strip bottle.	4					
33. Ensure you have turned off microscope light.	2					
34. Put dust cover over microscope.	2					
35. Remove gloves and wash hands.	4					
TOTAL POSSIBLE POINTS	**100**					

Comments: _____

_____

_____

_____

_____

_____

_____

_____

_____

Signatures: _____   **Date:** _____

SCORING   *See Preface for scoring instructions.*

Animal Health Care

PROCEDURE LM23-3:
Administering a Medication by Subcutaneous Injection

PROCEDURE ASSESSMENT

Procedure Steps	Suggested Points	Self Practice	Peer Practice	Peer Testing	Final Testing	Total Earned
PREPROCEDURE						
1. Gather needed equipment.	2					
2. Identify animal and verify medication needed and amount to be given.	3					
3. Locate drug.	4					
• Determine how many ccs or mLs are required.	3					
• Double-check name of dog.	3					
• Double-check amount of medication to be given.	3					
4. Get correct size syringe (usually 3-cc) and correct size hypodermic needle (usually 22-gauge, 1-inch).	3					
5. Wipe rubber area on top of vial with cotton moistened with alcohol.	2					
6. Remove needle guard and attach it firmly to hub of syringe.	3					
• Draw plunger back.	2					
• Fill syringe with volume of air equal to volume of drug to be given.	2					
7. Insert needle through rubber area and inject air.	2					
8. Turn needle and bottle upside down.	3					
• Keep tip of needle below level of medication.	2					
• Pull plunger back until correct volume of medication enters syringe.	2					
9. Remove needle from vial.	3					
• Hold syringe with needle upright.	2					
• Flick it with your finger to move any air to top.	3					
• Keeping syringe upright, push plunger to expel any excess air.	4					
10. Check medication amount again before giving injection.	4					
PROCEDURE						
11. Have someone restrain the animal.	4					
12. Wipe an area of skin between animal's shoulder blades with alcohol-moistened cotton.	4					
13. Gently tent skin by pulling it away from animal.	2					

PROCEDURE LM23-3: Administering a Medication by Subcutaneous Injection (continued)

Procedure Steps	Suggested Points	Self Practice	Peer Practice	Peer Testing	Final Testing	Total Earned
14. Quickly insert needle through skin at 45° angle.	3					
15. Pull slightly back on plunger and ensure no blood appears in needle hub.	4					
• Blood means needle tip is in blood vessel.						
• If you see blood, don't inject medication, because it could cause serious damage or death. (Move needle forward into another location.)						
16. If you don't see any blood, completely depress plunger.	3					
17. Remove needle from animal.	2					
18. Put needle in biohazard waste container.	4					
19. Put syringe in trashcan, or follow procedures of facility.	2					
POSTPROCEDURE						
20. Return animal to its cage.	2					
21. Return drug to its proper storage place.	2					
22. Clean up work area.	4					
23. Wash your hands.	4					
24. Record medication and dose administered.	2					
25. Mark procedure as completed on treatment sheet.	3					
TOTAL POSSIBLE POINTS	100					

Comments:

_____
_____
_____
_____
_____
_____
_____
_____
_____

Signatures: _____   Date: _____

SCORING   *See Preface for scoring instructions.*

Medical Laboratory

PROCEDURE LM24-1:
Performing the Test for Infectious Mononucleosis

PROCEDURE ASSESSMENT

Procedure Steps	Suggested Points	Self Practice	Peer Practice	Peer Testing	Final Testing	Total Earned
PREPROCEDURE						
1. Gather needed equipment.	4					
2. Wash hands and put on gloves and face shield.	6					
3. Review client's request form.	4					
4. Label tubes with client's name.	5					
5. Verify that controls for test have been run for the day.	5					
• Verify that controls are within normal range.	4					
• Controls should be run daily.						
6. If controls haven't been run, review manufacturer's directions and run controls. Your supervisor may have to check results.	5					
7. Confirm that test kit has been brought to room temperature.	5					
8. Check expiration date of kit.	4					
PROCEDURE						
9. Fill disposable capillary tube to calibration mark with serum or plasma.	5					
10. Drop specimen (serum or plasma) onto test slide.	5					
11. Immediately dispose of capillary tube in biohazard waste container.	6					
12. Mix reagents by rolling bottle gently between palms of hands.	5					
13. Hold dropper in vertical position. Don't touch dropper to slide.	5					
14. Follow manufacturer's directions for adding reagents.	5					
15. Use clean stirrer for each area to avoid cross-contamination.	5					
16. Follow manufacturer's directions for timing and observation of agglutination.	5					
POSTPROCEDURE						
17. Disinfect work area.	6					
18. Remove gloves and face shield and wash hands.	6					
19. Record test results in client's record or on lab form.	5					
TOTAL POSSIBLE POINTS	100					

PROCEDURE LM24-1: Performing the Test for Infectious Mononucleosis *(continued)*

Comments: _____
_____
_____
_____
_____
_____
_____
_____
_____

Signatures: _____ Date: _____

SCORING *See Preface for scoring instructions.*

Name _____ Date _____

Medical Laboratory

PROCEDURE LM24-2A:
Testing Urine for Glucose Using Copper Reduction

PROCEDURE ASSESSMENT

Procedure Steps	Suggested Points	Self Practice	Peer Practice	Peer Testing	Final Testing	Total Earned
PREPROCEDURE						
1. Gather needed equipment.	3					
2. Check expiration date of tablets.	4					
3. Wash hands and put on gloves.	6					
4. Put on a face shield.	6					
PROCEDURE						
5. Gently swirl container to mix specimen.	4					
• Aspirate urine into disposable dropper.	3					
• Squeeze dropper bulb before placing it in urine.	3					
• When you release bulb, urine will be drawn into dropper tip.						
6. Put tube in rack.	5					
• Hold dropper vertically.	4					
• Add amount of urine and water specified by manufacturer's directions.	4					
7. With dry hands, pour tablet from bottle into bottle cap.	4					
8. Tap tablet into test tube and recap container tightly. Don't touch tablet.	6					
9. Observe entire reaction to avoid missing a rapid pass-through phase.	4					
• This phase happens when glucose level is so high, it goes beyond orange color that indicates highest level of glucose.						
• If you miss this phase, you may obtain result that indicates a trace of glucose instead of a high level.						
10. When bubbling stops, follow timing precisely.	4					
• Use manufacturer's directions.	3					
• Gently shake tube to mix entire contents.	3					
11. Immediately compare color of specimen with five-drop color chart. Results are recorded as trace, 1+, 2+, 3+, or 4+.	5					
12. If orange color appears briefly during reaction, rapid pass-through has occurred. Repeat test using alternate color procedure and chart.	5					

PROCEDURE LM24-2A: Testing Urine for Glucose Using Copper Reduction *(continued)*

Procedure Steps	Suggested Points	Self Practice	Peer Practice	Peer Testing	Final Testing	Total Earned
POSTPROCEDURE						
13. Disinfect work area.	6					
14. Return items to their proper storage location.	3					
15. Remove face shield and gloves.	4					
16. Wash hands.	6					
17. Record results in client's chart or on lab form.	5					
TOTAL POSSIBLE POINTS	100					

Comments: _____
_____
_____
_____
_____
_____
_____
_____
_____

Signatures: _____ Date: _____

SCORING *See Preface for scoring instructions.*

Medical Laboratory

PROCEDURE LM24-2B:
Testing Urine for Protein Using the Sulfosalicylic Acid Precipitation Test

PROCEDURE ASSESSMENT

Procedure Steps	Suggested Points	Self Practice	Peer Practice	Peer Testing	Final Testing	Total Earned
PREPROCEDURE						
1. Gather needed materials.	6					
2. Wash hands and put on gloves.	10					
3. Put on face shield.	10					
4. If urine is cloudy, filter specimen or use a centrifuged specimen.	7					
PROCEDURE						
5. Using a clear test tube in a rack and a dropper, mix equal amounts of urine and 3% sulfosalicylic acid.	7					
6. Observe for cloudiness, which indicates presence of protein.	10					
7. Record results. Test is reported according to degree of cloudiness as negative, trace, 1+, 2+, 3+, or 4+.	8					
POSTPROCEDURE						
8. Disinfect work area.	10					
9. Return items to their proper storage location.	7					
10. Remove face shield and gloves.	7					
11. Wash hands.	10					
12. Record results in client's chart or on lab form.	8					
TOTAL POSSIBLE POINTS	100					

Comments: _____
_____
_____
_____
_____
_____
_____
_____
_____

Signatures: _____ Date: _____

SCORING *See Preface for scoring instructions.*

Medical Laboratory

PROCEDURE LM24-2C:
Performing a Pregnancy Test

PROCEDURE ASSESSMENT

Procedure Steps	Suggested Points	Self Practice	Peer Practice	Peer Testing	Final Testing	Total Earned
PREPROCEDURE						
1. Gather needed equipment.	7					
2. Check expiration date of kit.	8					
3. Let pregnancy test kit come to room temperature, if so directed by manufacturer's instructions.	9					
4. Wash hands and put on gloves and face shield.	10					
PROCEDURE						
5. Label test tube with client's name and label control tubes.	7					
6. Follow manufacturer's guidelines exactly regarding timing and methods.	8					
7. Read results using color comparison charts or examples in directions.	7					
POSTPROCEDURE						
8. Disinfect work area.	10					
9. Return items to proper storage location.	8					
10. Remove face shield and gloves.	7					
11. Wash hands.	10					
12. Record results on client's chart or on lab form.	9					
TOTAL POSSIBLE POINTS	100					

Comments: _____

_____

_____

_____

_____

_____

_____

_____

Signatures: _____   **Date:** _____

SCORING   *See Preface for scoring instructions.*

Medical Laboratory

PROCEDURE LM24-3:
Collecting a Capillary Blood Sample

PROCEDURE ASSESSMENT

Procedure Steps	Suggested Points	Self Practice	Peer Practice	Peer Testing	Final Testing	Total Earned
PREPROCEDURE						
1. Gather needed equipment.	3					
2. Review requisition and calculate amount of sample needed.	3					
3. If you need more than one tube of blood, arrange microtubes in order of draw.	3					
4. Introduce yourself to client.	3					
5. Identify client, verify client information, and explain procedure to client.	4					
6. Seat client in collection chair or have client lie in bed with hand and arm resting on bed.	2					
7. Wash hands and put on gloves and face shield.	5					
PROCEDURE						
8. Load lancet device with sterile lancet.	3					
9. Select puncture site on side of middle finger of nondominant hand or on heel for an infant.	2					
10. Rub area to promote circulation.	2					
• If client's fingers are very cold, warm them first.						
• Apply a warm, moist washcloth or paper towel to area.						
11. Clean site with alcohol and let it air-dry.	2					
• Or, dry site with sterile gauze.						
• Don't blow on skin to accelerate drying.						
12. Remove sterile lancet from package or remove plastic tip.	3					
• Don't touch point of lancet, and don't lay it on work surface.						
• If lancet or plastic tip becomes contaminated, discard it and obtain a new one.						
13. With nondominant forefinger and thumb, grasp client's finger on sides near puncture site.	3					
14. Hold lancet at right angle to client's finger.	4					
• Make a rapid, deep puncture across fingerprint on side of fingertip.	2					
• Puncture should not be parallel to fingerprint.	2					

PROCEDURE LM24-3: Collecting a Capillary Blood Sample (continued)

Procedure Steps	Suggested Points	Self Practice	Peer Practice	Peer Testing	Final Testing	Total Earned
15. Dispose of lancet and tip cover immediately in a sharps container.	5					
16. Wipe away first drop of blood using sterile gauze.	2					
17. Use gentle pressure to start blood flow.	2					
• Don't apply too much pressure, which could cause tissue fluid to mix with blood.						
• If that happened, sample would be diluted, and test results would be incorrect.						
18. Collect samples in capillary tubes or micro blood collection tubes.	4					
• Hold tube horizontally by colored end to drop of blood.	2					
• Let tube fill.	2					
• Don't let air bubbles enter tube or touch tube to skin.						
• If either happens, discard tube and start with new tube.						
19. Seal tubes with clay and put them in test tube.	3					
20. Mix by gently rotating any microtubes that contain an anticoagulant.	3					
21. Apply pressure to puncture site and apply nonallergenic adhesive strip, if needed.	3					
22. Label all tubes with client's name, date, and other information required.	3					
23. Thank and dismiss client.	2					
POSTPROCEDURE						
24. Disinfect work area.	5					
25. Return items to proper storage location.	4					
26. Remove face shield and gloves.	5					
27. Wash hands.	5					
28. Record procedure on client's chart or on lab form.	4					
TOTAL POSSIBLE POINTS	100					

Comments: _____

_____

_____

Signatures: _____ Date: _____

SCORING *See Preface for scoring instructions.*

Medical Laboratory

PROCEDURE LM24-4:
Performing a Hematocrit

PROCEDURE ASSESSMENT

Procedure Steps	Suggested Points	Self Practice	Peer Practice	Peer Testing	Final Testing	Total Earned
PREPROCEDURE						
1. Gather needed equipment. Be sure microhematocrit centrifuge has been tested for accurate speed.	3					
2. Obtain EDTA anticoagulated blood specimen tube or draw capillary blood using 2 capillary tubes with anticoagulant, capillary tubes, and sealing clay.	4					
3. Wash hands and put on face shield and gloves.	6					
PROCEDURE						
4. Gently mix EDTA anticoagulated blood. For capillary specimen, go to step 7.	5					
5. Fill 2 plain capillary tubes 3/4 full with anticoagulated blood or blood from a capillary puncture site.	3					
6. Seal dry end of each tube with sealing clay.	4					
7. Put tubes opposite each other to balance microcentrifuge.	5					
• Ensure sealed ends are secure against rubber tubing.	3					
8. Note and record numbers on centrifuge slots, plus client's name.	6					
9. Secure locking top, fasten lid down, and lock.	5					
10. Set timer and adjust speed as needed. Follow manufacturer's guidelines for time and speed.	5					
11. Let centrifuge come to complete stop and unlock lids.	6					
12. Read tubes immediately.	5					
13. Read microhematocrit values.	5					
• Centrifuge may have built-in reader.						
• You will locate the bottom line of packed red blood cells.						
14. Average results of 2 capillary tube readings.	4					
15. Dispose of capillary tubes in a biohazard sharps container.	5					

PROCEDURE LM24-4: Performing a Hematocrit *(continued)*

Procedure Steps	Suggested Points	Self Practice	Peer Practice	Peer Testing	Final Testing	Total Earned
POSTPROCEDURE						
16. If any tubes have broken during procedure, clean and decontaminate centrifuge.	6					
17. Return items to proper storage location.	4					
18. Disinfect work area.	6					
19. Remove face shield and gloves and wash hands.	6					
20. Record results on client's record or on lab record.	4					
TOTAL POSSIBLE POINTS	**100**					

Comments: _____
_____
_____
_____
_____
_____
_____
_____
_____
_____

Signatures: _____   **Date:** _____

SCORING *See Preface for scoring instructions.*

Medical Laboratory

PROCEDURE LM24-5:
Performing a Hemoglobin Test

······· P R O C E D U R E   A S S E S S M E N T ·······

Procedure Steps	Suggested Points	Self Practice	Peer Practice	Peer Testing	Final Testing	Total Earned
PREPROCEDURE						
1. Gather needed equipment.	4					
2. Introduce yourself to client.	5					
3. Identify client, verify information, and explain procedure.	6					
4. Seat client in collection chair or have client lie in bed with hand and arm resting on bed.	5					
5. Wash hands and put on face shield and gloves.	6					
PROCEDURE						
6. Prepare hemoglobinometer following manufacturer's instructions.	5					
7. Clean site with alcohol.	5					
8. Follow procedure for a capillary puncture.	5					
9. Wipe away first drop of blood.	5					
10. Put a drop of blood on the chamber slide or hemoglobin instrument.	5					
11. Follow guidelines for proper calculation of client's hemoglobin, including:	5					
• Rotate hemolysis applicator on slide until specimen turns from red and cloudy to clear, which usually takes 30 seconds.	4					
• Cover chamber with cover glass.	4					
• Insert chamber into hemoglobinometer, turn on light, and view specimen.	4					
12. Dispose of waste in biohazard waste container, and dispose of sharps in proper container.	6					
13. Thank and dismiss client.	4					
POSTPROCEDURE						
14. Disinfect work area.	6					
15. Return items to proper storage location.	5					
16. Remove gloves and face shield and wash hands.	6					
17. Record test results in client's medical record or on lab form.	5					
TOTAL POSSIBLE POINTS	100					

Comments:

_____

_____

_____

_____

_____

_____

_____

Signatures: _____ Date: _____

SCORING   *See Preface for scoring instructions.*

Name _____   Date _____

Medical Laboratory

PROCEDURE LM24-6:
Making a Blood Smear

PROCEDURE ASSESSMENT

Procedure Steps	Suggested Points	Self Practice	Peer Practice	Peer Testing	Final Testing	Total Earned
PREPROCEDURE						
1. Gather needed equipment.	3					
2. Label frosted end of 2 slides with client's name and date.	4					
3. Review request form to verify test ordered.	4					
4. Introduce yourself to client.	4					
5. Identify client, verify information, and explain procedure.	6					
6. Have client sit in collection chair or lie in bed with hand and arm resting on bed.	3					
7. Wash hands and put on gloves and face shield.	6					
PROCEDURE						
8. Obtain blood specimen using facility's preferred method: venipuncture, butterfly puncture, or capillary puncture.	3					
9. Put small drop of blood 1/4 inch from frosted end of each glass slide.	4					
• Place labeled side of slide up.	3					
• If you do a capillary puncture, don't let client's finger touch slide.	3					
10. Hold corners of frosted end of 1 slide on flat surface. With other hand, hold second slide at 45° angle.	4					
11. Put upright (spreader) slide against first one.	4					
• Draw spreader slide against drop of blood.	3					
• Blood should spread across edge of spreader slide in straight line.	3					
12. Move angled slide toward frosted end and gently spread out blood.	4					
13. Let blood smear air-dry.	3					
14. Put blood smear in proper container, along with completed lab form.	4					
15. If a CBC has been ordered, the EDTA tube should accompany blood slide.	3					
16. Recheck puncture site for bleeding, bruising, or swelling.	3					
17. Thank and dismiss client.	3					

PROCEDURE LM24-6: Making a Blood Smear *(continued)*

Procedure Steps	Suggested Points	Self Practice	Peer Practice	Peer Testing	Final Testing	Total Earned
POSTPROCEDURE						
18. Immediately dispose of all biohazardous materials in waste container and all lancets in sharps container.	6					
19. Disinfect work area.	6					
20. Remove gloves and face shield and wash hands.	6					
21. Record test results in client's record or on lab form.	5					
TOTAL POSSIBLE POINTS	100					

Comments:

_____

_____

_____

_____

_____

_____

_____

_____

_____

Signatures: _____   **Date:** _____

SCORING   *See Preface for scoring instructions.*

Name _____ Date _____

Medical Laboratory

PROCEDURE LM24-7:
Manual Method for Counting Blood Cells

PROCEDURE ASSESSMENT

Procedure Steps	Suggested Points	Self Practice	Peer Practice	Peer Testing	Final Testing	Total Earned
PREPROCEDURE						
1. Gather needed equipment.	4					
2. Wash and dry hands.	8					
3. Put on gloves and face shield.	8					
PROCEDURE						
4. Put hemocytometer on lowered microscope stage under low-power magnification.	5					
5. Center ruled area over opening in stage.	4					
6. Adjust light so you can see cells to be counted.	5					
7. Follow correct path sequence for counting cells to avoid counting cells twice or missing them.	6					
8. When you have finished one area, record number.	5					
9. Return tally to zero, move to next square, and count cells using same sequence.	5					
10. Counts from each square shouldn't vary by more than:	6					
• 10 cells, for white blood cells.	5					
• 20 cells, for red blood cells.	5					
• If this happens, wash chamber, refill it, and count again.						
11. Total cells counted and average counts from both sides of chamber.	6					
12. Calculate results following instructions for your counting instrument.	6					
POSTPROCEDURE						
13. Record results in client's record or on lab form.	6					
14. Disinfect work area.	8					
15. Remove gloves and face shield and wash hands.	8					
TOTAL POSSIBLE POINTS	**100**					

Procedure LM24-7: Manual Method for Counting Blood Cells (continued)

Comments: _____

_____

_____

_____

_____

_____

_____

_____

_____

Signatures: _____ **Date:** _____

SCORING   *See Preface for scoring instructions.*

Name _____   Date _____

Medical Laboratory

PROCEDURE LM24-8:
Collecting a Venous Blood Sample

PROCEDURE ASSESSMENT

Procedure Steps	Suggested Points	Self Practice	Peer Practice	Peer Testing	Final Testing	Total Earned
PREPROCEDURE						
1. Check requisition form to determine test ordered.	2					
• Calculate amount of specimen needed.	1					
• Select correct tubes for tests ordered.	1					
2. Gather needed equipment.	1					
3. Check all tubes for expiration dates. Arrange tubes in order of draw according to method to be used.	2					
4. Wash and dry hands. Put on gloves and face shield.	4					
5. Introduce yourself to client.	2					
6. Identify client, verify information, and explain procedure to client.	4					
7. Have client sit in collection chair or lie on bed.	1					
8. Ensure arm will be well supported in slightly downward position.	2					
9. Select venipuncture site by palpating antecubital space.	1					
10. Ask client to open and close hand to make veins prominent. You may tie tourniquet to help locate vein.	1					
11. Use index finger to locate median vein and trace path of vein.	2					
• Judge depth of vein.	1					
• Don't use thumb to palpate; if you do this, you will feel your own pulse.						
• Remove tourniquet.	1					
12. Determine if you will use vacutainer or syringe for venipuncture. Ensure all equipment is available.	2					
13. Don't remove shield from needle at this time.	4					
PROCEDURE						
14. Clean venipuncture site.	4					
• Start in center and work in circular pattern using alcohol prep pads.	1					
• Don't recontaminate area.						
15. Tie tourniquet 3 to 4 inches above client's elbow. Don't recontaminate area with tourniquet.	1					

PROCEDURE LM24-8: Collecting a Venous Blood Sample (continued)

Procedure Steps	Suggested Points	Self Practice	Peer Practice	Peer Testing	Final Testing	Total Earned
16. Remove needle sheath.	1					
17. Hold evacuated system adapter in your dominant hand.	2					
• Or, hold syringe in your dominant hand.						
• Keep thumb on top and fingers underneath.	1					
18. Grasp client's arm with your nondominant hand.	2					
• Use your thumb and forefinger to draw skin tightly over site.	1					
• This will help to anchor the vein.						
19. Insert needle quickly and smoothly through skin and into vein.	2					
• Bevel of needle should be up at 15° angle, aligned parallel to vein.	1					
• If you use evacuated system, push tube onto needle inside adapter holder. Don't move needle after it enters vein. Let tube fill completely.	1					
• If you use syringe, slowly pull back plunger with nondominant hand. Don't move needle after it enters vein. Let syringe fill completely, or to amount needed.	1					
20. Remove evacuated tube from adapter smoothly.	2					
• Insert next tube.	1					
• Or, remove needle from vein.	1					
21. Release tourniquet when venipuncture is complete, BEFORE you remove needle from arm.	4					
22. Put sterile gauze over site as you withdraw needle.	4					
23. Tell client to apply direct pressure on puncture site with sterile gauze pad. Client may elevate arm.	2					
24. Put evacuated needle immediately in sharps container. Don't recap used needles.	4					
25. If you use evacuated system, gently invert tubes with anticoagulants to mix thoroughly with blood.	2					
• If you use syringe, transfer blood to tubes that are in rack.	1					
• Gently invert any tubes containing anticoagulants.	1					
26. Dispose of syringe and needle in sharps container. Don't recap used needles.	4					

Procedure Steps	Suggested Points	Self Practice	Peer Practice	Peer Testing	Final Testing	Total Earned
27. Label tubes with:	2					
• Client's name, date, and time.	1					
• Any other information needed (your initials, tests requested, whether client was fasting, etc.)	1					
28. Check puncture site for bleeding.	4					
29. Apply a hypoallergenic bandage.	1					
30. Thank and dismiss client.	1					
POSTPROCEDURE						
31. Disinfect area.	4					
32. Return items to proper storage location.	2					
33. Remove gloves and face shield and wash hands.	4					
34. Complete lab requisition and label specimen.	2					
35. Record procedure in client's chart or on lab form.	2					
TOTAL POSSIBLE POINTS	**100**					

Comments:

Signatures: Date:

SCORING *See Preface for scoring instructions.*

Medical Laboratory

PROCEDURE LM24-9:
Performing a Butterfly Blood Collection

PROCEDURE ASSESSMENT

Procedure Steps	Suggested Points	Self Practice	Peer Practice	Peer Testing	Final Testing	Total Earned
PREPROCEDURE						
1. Gather needed equipment.	2					
2. Check requisition and calculate amount of sample needed.	3					
3. Select and arrange tubes in order of the draw.	2					
4. Introduce yourself to client.	3					
5. Identify client, verify information, and explain procedure.	4					
6. Wash hands and put on gloves and face shield.	5					
7. Seat client in collection chair.	2					
8. Ensure both arms will be well supported in slightly downward position.	2					
9. Select a vein at the bifurcation (site where a vein divides).	2					
10. Use alcohol gauze and clean venipuncture site by starting in center.	5					
• Work in circular pattern.	2					
• Don't recontaminate site.	2					
PROCEDURE						
11. Remove butterfly device from package.	2					
12. Attach butterfly device to syringe or evacuated tube holder.	2					
13. Insert first tube into evacuated tube holder.	2					
14. Apply tourniquet to client's wrist, just proximal to wrist bone.	3					
15. Hold client's hand in your nondominant hand, with fingers lower than wrist.	2					
16. Using thumb, pull client's skin tightly.	2					
17. With needle at 10° to 15° angle and bevel up, align needle with vein.	3					
18. Gently thread needle up lumen, or center of vein.	2					
19. Push blood collection tube onto end of adapter or draw blood into syringe.	3					
20. Release tourniquet when blood appears in tube or syringe. Keep needle in place.	3					
21. Keep tube and holder in downward position so tube will fill from bottom up.	2					
22. Put gauze pad over puncture site and remove needle.	2					

PROCEDURE LM24-9: Performing a Butterfly Blood Collection *(continued)*

Procedure Steps	Suggested Points	Self Practice	Peer Practice	Peer Testing	Final Testing	Total Earned
23. Immediately put needle and tubing in sharps container.	5					
24. Label tubes with:	4					
• Client's name, date, and time.	2					
• Any other information needed (your initials, tests requested, whether client was fasting, etc).	2					
25. Check puncture site for bleeding.	2					
26. Apply hypoallergenic bandage.	2					
27. Thank and dismiss client.	2					
POSTPROCEDURE						
28. Disinfect area.	5					
29. Return items to proper storage location.	3					
30. Remove gloves and face shield and wash hands.	5					
31. Complete lab requisition.	3					
32. Record procedure in client's chart or on lab form.	3					
TOTAL POSSIBLE POINTS	100					

Comments: _____

_____

_____

_____

_____

_____

_____

_____

Signatures: _____   Date: _____

SCORING   *See Preface for scoring instructions.*

Medical Laboratory

PROCEDURE LM24-10:
Performing an Erythrocyte Sedimentation Rate Test

P R O C E D U R E   A S S E S S M E N T

Procedure Steps	Suggested Points	Self Practice	Peer Practice	Peer Testing	Final Testing	Total Earned
PREPROCEDURE						
1. Gather needed equipment.	5					
2. Check expiration date of reagents.	7					
3. Wash hands and put on gloves and face shield.	8					
4. Check sedimentation rack for levelness.	7					
PROCEDURE						
5. Mix blood sample.	6					
6. Fill pipette with blood and insert tip of pipette in bottom of tube.	6					
7. Slowly fill tube while moving pipette to top of tube. Avoid air bubbles.	6					
8. Put tube in rack without jarring rack.	7					
9. Set timer as instructed by manufacturer.	6					
10. Record number of client's tube for identification.	7					
11. Measure distance the erythrocytes have fallen after specified time.	7					
• The ESR scale measures from 0 at top to 100 at bottom.						
• Each line is 1 mm.						
POSTPROCEDURE						
12. Disinfect work area.	8					
13. Remove face shield and gloves.	5					
14. Wash hands.	8					
15. Record ESR result in client's record or on lab form.	7					
TOTAL POSSIBLE POINTS	100					

Comments: _____

_____

_____

_____

Signatures: _____   **Date:** _____

SCORING   *See Preface for scoring instructions.*

Medical Laboratory

PROCEDURE LM24-11:
Performing a Cholesterol Test

PROCEDURE ASSESSMENT

Procedure Steps	Suggested Points	Self Practice	Peer Practice	Peer Testing	Final Testing	Total Earned
PREPROCEDURE						
1. Gather needed equipment.	4					
2. Label test tubes or slides with client's name and the controls.	4					
3. Review request form to verify test ordered.	5					
4. Introduce yourself to client.	5					
5. Identify client, verify information, and explain procedure.	6					
6. Have client sit in collection chair or lie in bed with arm supported.	4					
7. Wash hands and put on gloves and face shield.	7					
PROCEDURE						
8. Obtain blood specimen required for test procedure.	5					
9. Follow manufacturer's directions for proper testing method.	4					
10. Neither you nor client should touch a reagent pad with fingers.	6					
11. Give client clean gauze square to hold over puncture site.	6					
12. Read result.	4					
13. Recheck puncture site.	5					
14. Thank and dismiss client.	4					
POSTPROCEDURE						
15. Immediately put all biohazardous materials and lancets in proper containers.	7					
16. Return items to proper storage location.	5					
17. Disinfect work area.	6					
18. Remove gloves and face shield and wash hands.	7					
19. Record test results in client's record or on lab form.	6					
TOTAL POSSIBLE POINTS	**100**					

PROCEDURE LM24-11: Performing a Cholesterol Test *(continued)*

Comments: _____

_____

_____

_____

_____

_____

_____

_____

Signatures: _____ **Date:** _____

SCORING   *See Preface for scoring instructions.*

Name _____ Date _____

Medical Laboratory

PROCEDURE LM24-12:
Determining ABO Group

PROCEDURE ASSESSMENT

Procedure Steps	Suggested Points	Self Practice	Peer Practice	Peer Testing	Final Testing	Total Earned
PREPROCEDURE						
1. Gather needed equipment.	3					
2. Review request form to verify test ordered.	4					
3. Check expiration date of reagents.	4					
4. Introduce yourself to client.	5					
5. Identify client, verify information, and explain procedure.	6					
6. Have client sit in collection chair or lie in bed with arm supported.	3					
7. Wash hands and put on gloves and face shield.	6					
8. Label slides in frosted area with client's name.	5					
9. Verify that controls have been run for day and are within correct range.	4					
PROCEDURE						
10. Put 1 drop of anti-A serum on slide 1.	4					
• Put 1 drop of anti-B serum on slide 2.	3					
• Put 1 drop of anti-A serum and anti-B serum on slide 3.	3					
11. Follow procedure for capillary puncture. Let site air-dry.	4					
12. Wipe away first drop of blood with sterile gauze square.	4					
13. Put 1 large drop of blood on each of the 3 prepared slides.	3					
14. Cover puncture site with sterile gauze square and tell client to apply gentle pressure to site.	4					
15. Mix antiserum and blood thoroughly, using a clean applicator stick for each slide.	3					
16. Read and interpret results of reaction of each slide. Agglutination indicates positive reaction.	3					
17. Recheck puncture site.	4					
18. Thank and dismiss client.	3					

PROCEDURE LM24-12: Determining ABO Group *(continued)*

Procedure Steps POSTPROCEDURE	Suggested Points	Self Practice	Peer Practice	Peer Testing	Final Testing	Total Earned
19. Immediately put all biohazardous materials and lancets in proper containers.	6					
20. Disinfect work area.	6					
21. Remove gloves and face shield and wash hands.	6					
22. Record test results in client's record or on lab form.	4					
TOTAL POSSIBLE POINTS	100					

Comments: _____
_____
_____
_____
_____
_____
_____
_____

Signatures: _____ **Date:** _____

SCORING   *See Preface for scoring instructions.*

Medical Laboratory

PROCEDURE LM24-13:
Determining Rh Blood Factor

P R O C E D U R E   A S S E S S M E N T

Procedure Steps	Suggested Points	Self Practice	Peer Practice	Peer Testing	Final Testing	Total Earned
PREPROCEDURE						
1. Gather needed equipment.	3					
2. Review requisition to verify test ordered.	4					
3. Check expiration date of reagents.	4					
4. Introduce yourself to client.	5					
5. Identify client, verify information, and explain procedure.	5					
6. Have client sit in collection chair or lie in bed with arm supported.	4					
7. Wash hands and put on gloves and face shield.	6					
8. Label slides in frosted area with client's name.	5					
9. Verify that controls have been run for day and are within correct range.	5					
10. Label 1 slide D and 1 slide C.	4					
11. Put 1 drop of anti-D serum on the D slide.	3					
12. Put 1 drop of control reagent on the C slide.	3					
PROCEDURE						
13. Wipe away first drop of blood with sterile gauze square.	3					
14. Add 2 drops of client's blood to each slide.	4					
15. Thoroughly mix blood on both slides. Use clean applicator stick for each slide.	5					
16. Read results immediately. Agglutination on slide indicates position reaction.	5					
17. Recheck puncture site.	5					
18. Thank and dismiss client.	4					
POSTPROCEDURE						
19. Immediately put all biohazardous materials and lancets in proper containers.	6					
20. Disinfect work area.	6					
21. Remove gloves and face shield and wash hands.	6					
22. Record test results in client's record or on lab form.	5					
TOTAL POSSIBLE POINTS	**100**					

PROCEDURE LM24-13: Determining Rh Blood Factor (continued)

Comments:
_____
_____
_____
_____
_____
_____
_____
_____

Signatures: _____ Date: _____

SCORING   *See Preface for scoring instructions.*

Radiology

PROCEDURE LM26-1:
Adult PA Chest Radiographic Film Evaluation Procedure

PROCEDURE ASSESSMENT

Procedure Steps	Suggested Points	Self Practice	Peer Practice	Peer Testing	Final Testing	Total Earned
PREPROCEDURE						
1. Gather needed equipment and obtain the completed film to be evaluated.	4					
PROCEDURE						
2. Put developed PA chest radiograph on view box.	6					
• Ensure radiograph is placed correctly for viewing.	5					
• Normal heart shadow should fall on right side of lung field as you look directly at radiograph.						
3. Ensure there are no visible radiopaque items (artifacts) within chest area of consideration.	4					
4. Evaluate contrast of film.	6					
• Contrast should be adequate to demonstrate anatomy.	5					
• If film is high contrast (starkly black-and-white), it may be hard to see through thick anatomical parts.						
• If film is low contrast (gray or washed out), it may be hard to see details inside thinner anatomical parts.						
5. Ensure density is adequate to demonstrate anatomy.	4					
• Radiographs with too much density are dark and overexposed.						
• Radiographs with too little density are light and underexposed.						
• In both cases, it may be hard to see chest anatomy.						
6. Ensure film size and placement is correct (14 by 17 inches, placed lengthwise).	4					
7. Ensure essential anatomical structures are on film.	6					
• Entire lung field should be present.	5					
• Ensure top (apices) and bottom (bases) areas of both lungs are displayed, without edges cut off.	5					
• Ensure that both right and left lateral sides of lungs are displayed, without edges cut off.	5					

Procedure Steps	Suggested Points	Self Practice	Peer Practice	Peer Testing	Final Testing	Total Earned
8. Ensure that correct letter marker is displayed in correct location.	6					
• If right "R" letter marker is in upper right hand corner of cassette, it will correspond with client's right side.	5					
• If radiograph were placed correctly on view box, then the "R" would face opposite your left side.	5					
9. Ensure there is appropriate collimation (a thin white border of $^1/_4$ inch or more around edge of chest radiograph is right).	4					
• This may be hard to achieve with larger patients without cutting off edge of lung fields.						
10. Ensure that motion (blurred areas) isn't visible on radiograph.	4					
11. Ensure chest is not rotated.	4					
12. Ensure chest is centered on film.	4					
13. Ensure client's correct ID data has been stamped on film ID corner.	5					
• If radiographic film evaluation of PA chest is OK, then radiographer will take the PA chest radiograph to radiologist for diagnostic reading.						
• If film evaluation is not OK, then another film has to be taken.						
POSTPROCEDURE						
14. Once a correct film has been completed, put it in proper area for radiologist to review and create a diagnostic report.	4					
TOTAL POSSIBLE POINTS	100					

Comments:

_____

_____

_____

_____

_____

_____

_____

Signatures: _____   Date: _____

SCORING   *See Preface for scoring instructions.*

Ophthalmic Care

PROCEDURE LM27-1:
Instilling Eye Drops

PROCEDURE ASSESSMENT

Procedure Steps	Suggested Points	Self Practice	Peer Practice	Peer Testing	Final Testing	Total Earned
PREPROCEDURE						
1. Gather equipment.	3					
2. Check expiration date on medication bottle.	4					
• Date bottle the first time it's used.						
• After bottle is open, medication is used for only two weeks.						
• Check appearance of medication; don't use any that looks abnormal.						
3. Verify medication order from bottle and client's chart. Ensure you know how many drops to put in each eye.	4					
4. Wash hands and put on gloves.	5					
PROCEDURE						
5. Identify client and explain procedure.	5					
6. Have client sit or lie on back with head tilted back and towards affected eye.	4					
7. Remove dropper from bottle.	3					
• If necessary, draw medication into it.	5					
• Don't contaminate tip of dropper by touching it to anything.						
8. Hold dropper in your dominant hand	3					
9. With tissue in other hand, pull down lower lid until you see the conjunctival sac.	4					
10. Have client look up and away.	5					
11. Put drops in eye:	4					
• Rest palm of dominant hand on client's forehead.	3					
• Hold tip of dropper 1/2 inch from eye.	3					
• Do not touch eye.	3					
• Do not put drops directly on colored portion of eye.	3					
• Do not touch eye, eyelid or eye lashes with dropper tip.	3					
12. Release lower eyelid and tell client to blink.	4					
13. If medication went outside eye, use tissue to pat away excess medication from inside to outside of eye. Do not rub eye	7					

PROCEDURE LM27-1: Instilling Eye Drops *(continued)*

Procedure Steps POSTPROCEDURE	Suggested Points	Self Practice	Peer Practice	Peer Testing	Final Testing	Total Earned
14. Discard medication in dropper before reinserting in bottle. Discard dropper if contaminated and get a new one.	9					
15. Recap bottle.	3					
16. Record procedure.	4					
17. Remove gloves and wash hands.	5					
18. Clean area and put away equipment.	4					
TOTAL POSSIBLE POINTS	**100**					

Comments:

Signatures: Date:

SCORING *See Preface for scoring instructions.*

Medical Office

PROCEDURE LM28-1:
Evaluating Client Charts

PROCEDURE ASSESSMENT

Procedure Steps	Suggested Points	Self Practice	Peer Practice	Peer Testing	Final Testing	Total Earned
PREPROCEDURE						
1. Gather needed supplies.	10					
PROCEDURE						
2. Obtain medical record to be evaluated and determine whether it is active, inactive, or closed according to office policy.	12					
3. Check all pages in record to confirm that client's name is on each page and that record is in reverse chronological order.	12					
4. Securely add any loose pages and ensure client's name is on each page.	11					
5. If record is active, add new or blank pages, if necessary.	10					
6. If record is inactive, mark front of record according to office policy and file it.	11					
7. If record is closed, mark or stamp front of record as closed and file it with other closed files.	12					
• Usually, closed files are kept in storage facilities off-site.						
• Patient charts are required to be kept for 7 years.						
POSTPROCEDURE						
8. Record inactive and closed files in a medical record logbook or cross-reference file.	11					
9. After evaluating medical record, return chart to filing cabinet.	11					
TOTAL POSSIBLE POINTS	100					

Comments: _____

_____

_____

_____

_____

Signatures: _____   **Date:** _____

SCORING   *See Preface for scoring instructions.*

Name _____   Date _____

Medical Office

PROCEDURE LM28-2:
Completing Insurance Forms

PROCEDURE ASSESSMENT

Procedure Steps	Suggested Points	Self Practice	Peer Practice	Peer Testing	Final Testing	Total Earned
PREPROCEDURE						
1. Gather needed supplies.	2					
2. Check encounter form or superbill for accuracy and completeness.	2					
• Check medical record to determine physician diagnosis and treatments given if information isn't clearly indicated on encounter form.						
3. Refer to ICD and CPT coding books:	3					
• To determine accuracy of assigned codes according to superbill.						
• To determine most appropriate codes if no codes were assigned.						
4. Check client medical record for:	4					
• Insurance information, including copy of client's insurance card, front and back.	1					
• Form signed by client giving permission to release confidential information to insurance provider.	1					
• Form signed by client giving permission to have payment from insurance provider sent to medical office and not to client.	1					
• If client is under age 18, parents must sign all forms giving permission to release information.	1					
PROCEDURE						
5. Using black or blue pen, typewriter, or computer with insurance software, fill in name and address of insurance company in top right-hand corner.	3					
6. Continue filling out the CMS-1500 as follows:	4					
a. Box 1: Put a check mark in appropriate box.	1					
b. Box 2: Insert client's last name, first name, and middle initial.	1					
c. Box 5: Insert client's address, street address, city, state and ZIP code.	1					
d. Box 3: Fill in client's date of birth.	1					
e. Box 6: Indicate relationship of client to insured or policyholder.	1					
f. Box 8: Indicate status of client as appropriate.	1					

PROCEDURE LM28-2: Completing Insurance Forms *(continued)*

Procedure Steps	Suggested Points	Self Practice	Peer Practice	Peer Testing	Final Testing	Total Earned
• Box 10: Always check No for each of 3 questions related to reason for office visit, unless questions are applicable. Don't leave this box blank.	1					
• Box 1a: Fill in insured or policyholder identification number as indicated on insurance card; include any extra letters or numbers.	1					
• Box 4: Fill in policyholder's last name, first name, and middle initial.	1					
• Box 7: Complete policyholder's address, including street address, city, state, and ZIP code. Insert word "Same" if client and policyholder live at same location.	1					
• Box. 11: If group number is noted on insurance card, fill it in. If no group number is given, leave this blank.	1					
• Box 11a: If insured or policyholder isn't client, fill in policyholder's date of birth.	1					
• Box 11b: Give name of employer or school, if policyholder is full-time student.	1					
• Box 11c: Leave this blank. Name of insurance company will be printed in top right-hand corner of form.	1					
• Box 11d: If client is covered by another insurance plan, check Yes box and go to the 9 form locators. If another insurance company doesn't cover client, check No box and leave 9 form locators blank.	1					
• Box 12: If medical record contains form signed by client giving permission to release information to insurance company, write words "Signature on file." If record doesn't contain that form, client must sign on this line before insurance claim form can be processed.	1					
• Box 13 (Assignment of benefits): If client has signed a form giving permission to do so, write "Signature on file," indicating that reimbursement from insurance company should be sent to medical office instead of client.	1					
• Boxes 14 through 20: Leave these blank unless insurance company has told you to complete them.	1					
• Box 21: Indicate numerical diagnosis code. The CMS form allows for total of 4 diagnosis codes to be entered.	1					
• Boxes 22 and 23: Leave blank unless insurance company has told you to complete them.	1					

Procedure Steps	Suggested Points	Self Practice	Peer Practice	Peer Testing	Final Testing	Total Earned
• Box 24:	1					
a. Column A: For each line used for procedural codes, write in date when service was provided, even if all procedures were administered on same day. Leave "To" columns blank.	1					
b. Column B: Using place of service codes, fill in code determined by location where service was provided. Use POS code of 11 for services provided in office.	1					
c. Column C: Leave blank unless insurance company has told you to complete it.	1					
d. Column D: Using CPT book if needed, fill in correct procedural codes and modifiers, if appropriate.	1					
e. Column E: For each procedural code listed, indicate most appropriately linked diagnostic code by writing in number 1, 2, 3, or 4 located beside diagnostic codes in Box 21. Don't repeat diagnostic codes in these boxes.	1					
f. Column F: Use office fee schedule to fill in appropriate charges for corresponding procedural codes in Column D.	1					
g. Column G: Indicate number of days or units by writing in correct number (usually, 1). Don't leave this blank.	1					
h. Columns H, I, J, and K: Leave blank unless insurance company has told you to complete them.	1					
i. Box 25: Write in physician or practice employee identification number (EIN) or federal tax ID number or physician's social security number. Depending on number used, put check mark in appropriate box indicating SSN or EIN.	1					
j. Box 26: Leave this blank.	1					
k. Box 27: If form is being completed for a government-sponsored insurance plan, indicate Yes or No according to whether physician has agreed to accept assignment, or payment, in full. Other insurance plans permit this box to be left blank.	1					
l. Box 28: Total charges in Column F and put total amount due in this box.	1					
m. Box 29: If client made a payment, such as a co-payment, co-insurance, or deductible, indicate amount paid. If no payment was received, write in zeros.	1					
n. Box 30: Subtract Box 29 from Box 28 and place balance on this line.	1					

PROCEDURE LM28-2: Completing Insurance Forms *(continued)*

Procedure Steps	Suggested Points	Self Practice	Peer Practice	Peer Testing	Final Testing	Total Earned
o. Box 31: Physician must sign the CMS before it leaves the office.	1					
p. Box 32: Leave this blank.	1					
q. Box 33: Indicate physician's name and full address. In bottom of box, write in physician's identification number and group number, if appropriate.	1					
7. Check completed form for accuracy. Have another employee check form, if dictated by office policy.	2					
POSTPROCEDURE						
8. Verify that CMS-1500 form is accurately and completely filled out and make a copy.	4					
• Put original into envelope and mail it.	2					
• If you completed form electronically, save document in separate file and either print it out to mail or submit it electronically.	2					
9. Note claim information in claims register and put copy of CMS in separate file (claims pending file).	2					
10. Make a note on client's ledger card or electronic financial record, indicating that an insurance form was sent, date, and amount billed.	2					
11. In 6 to 8 weeks, an EOB should arrive with a reimbursement check.	2					
• If claim has been denied or if form is incomplete, this will be indicated on EOB.						
• Correct problem or begin appeals process as soon as possible.	2					
• Resubmit claim form.	2					
12. If EOB hasn't been received in a timely manner, follow up with insurance provider to determine cause for delay.	3					
13. When payment has been made and received by medical office, remove copy of claim form from claims pending file.	4					
• Attach EOB to copy of claim form.	2					
• Place them in a separate file for inactive insurance claims.	2					
• Don't discard these forms.						
14. Indicate payment on office day sheet and individual client account ledger.	3					
15. Process check received from insurance provider for deposit into medical practice bank account.	3					

Procedure Steps	Suggested Points	Self Practice	Peer Practice	Peer Testing	Final Testing	Total Earned
16. Bill client for any balance due or notify billing and collections specialist of a balance due.	3					
TOTAL POSSIBLE POINTS	100					

Comments: _____

_____

_____

_____

_____

_____

_____

_____

_____

_____

Signatures: _____   **Date:** _____

SCORING *See Preface for scoring instructions.*

Health Information

PROCEDURE LM29-1:
Documenting Health Care

PROCEDURE ASSESSMENT

Procedure Steps	Suggested Points	Self Practice	Peer Practice	Peer Testing	Final Testing	Total Earned
PREPROCEDURE						
1. Obtain a sample client chart from your supervisor for evaluation.	10					
PROCEDURE						
2. Complete and date records.	15					
3. Ensure records are legible.	15					
4. Entries must be signed.	15					
5. Clearly make changes.	15					
POSTPROCEDURE						
6. List four standards cited under Procedure and for each write how you evaluated the standard when you examined the discharge summary.	30					
TOTAL POSSIBLE POINTS	100					

Comments: _____

_____

_____

_____

_____

_____

_____

_____

Signatures: _____   **Date:** _____

SCORING   *See Preface for scoring instructions.*

Name _____   Date _____

Health Information

PROCEDURE LM29-2:
Billing Review

PROCEDURE ASSESSMENT

Procedure Steps	Suggested Points	Self Practice	Peer Practice	Peer Testing	Final Testing	Total Earned
PREPROCEDURE						
1. Study encounter form and UB-92 form.	8					
PROCEDURE						
2. Compare data in Patient Identification Information section of encounter form with corresponding data on UB-92.	10					
• Verify all data is correctly reported on claim form.	8					
• Write down any incorrect items.	8					
3. Compare data in Insurance Information section of encounter form with corresponding data on UB-92.	10					
• Verify all data is correctly reported on claim form.	8					
• Write down any incorrect items.	8					
4. Compare data in Procedures and Services section on encounter form with corresponding data on UB-92.	10					
• Verify all data is correctly reported on claim form.	8					
• Write down any missing or incorrect items.	8					
5. Calculate total charge amount based on review.	7					
POSTPROCEDURE						
6. Compare findings with instructor's answers.	7					
TOTAL POSSIBLE POINTS	100					

Comments: _____
_____
_____
_____
_____

Signatures: _____   Date: _____

SCORING   *See Preface for scoring instructions.*

Central Supply/ Processing

PROCEDURE LM31-1:
Donning Sterile Gloves

PROCEDURE ASSESSMENT

Procedure Steps	Suggested Points	Self Practice	Peer Practice	Peer Testing	Final Testing	Total Earned
PREPROCEDURE						
1. Gather needed equipment.	6					
• Gloves come in various sizes (S, M, L, and XL).						
• Check package for tears.						
• Ensure expiration date hasn't passed.						
2. Perform a surgical scrub.	5					
PROCEDURE						
3. Peel outer wrap from gloves and place inner wrapper on a clean surface above waist level.	5					
4. Position gloves so cuff end is closest to your body.	5					
5. Touch only the flaps as you open the package.	5					
• Use instructions provided on inner package, if available.						
• Avoid reaching over sterile inside of inner package.	4					
• Follow these steps if there are no instructions:						
a. Open package so first flap is opened away from you.	4					
b. Pinch corner and pull to one side.	4					
c. Put fingertips under side flaps and gently pull until package is completely open.	4					
6. Use non-dominant hand to grasp inside cuff of opposite glove (folded edge).	7					
• Don't touch outside of glove.						
• If you're right-handed, use left hand to put on right glove first, and vice versa.						
7. Holding glove at arm's length and waist level.						
• Insert dominant hand into glove with palm facing up.	4					
• Don't let outside of glove touch any other surface.						
8. With sterile gloved hand, slip gloved fingers into cuff of other glove.	7					
• Pick up other glove, touching only outside.	4					
• Don't touch any other surfaces.						

PROCEDURE LM31-1: Donning Sterile Gloves (continued)

Procedure Steps PROCEDURE	Suggested Points	Self Practice	Peer Practice	Peer Testing	Final Testing	Total Earned
9. Pull glove up and onto your hand.	4					
• Ensure sterile gloved hand doesn't touch skin.						
• Adjust fingers as necessary, touching only glove to glove.						
• Don't adjust cuffs, as your forearms may contaminate the gloves.						
POSTPROCEDURE						
10. Keep hands in front of you, between shoulders and waist. If you move hands out of this area, they are considered contaminated.	7					
11. If contamination or possibility of contamination occurs, change gloves.	5					
12. Remove gloves the same way you remove clean gloves, by touching only the inside.	7					
13. Clean area and put equipment away.	6					
14. Wash hands.	7					
TOTAL POSSIBLE POINTS	**100**					

Comments:

_____

_____

_____

_____

_____

_____

_____

_____

Signatures: _____ Date: _____

SCORING *See Preface for scoring instructions.*

Name _____   Date _____

Central Supply/ Processing

PROCEDURE LM31-2:
Preparing a Sterile Field and Opening Sterile Packages

PROCEDURE ASSESSMENT

Procedure Steps	Suggested Points	Self Practice	Peer Practice	Peer Testing	Final Testing	Total Earned
PREPROCEDURE						
1. Gather needed equipment.	6					
2. Check expiration date and sterilization indicator on packages.	6					
3. Clean and disinfect tray or counter to be used.	8					
4. Wash hands.	8					
PROCEDURE						
5. Create sterile field using a commercially prepared sterile field or a sterile instrument pack. Follow these steps:	6					
• Place sterile package on tray or counter, with first flap pointing away from you.	5					
• Unfold outmost fold away from yourself.	5					
• Unfold sides of package one at a time. Touch only outside of sterile package.	5					
• Open last flap towards yourself.	5					
6. Open packaged sterile packages to place on sterile field.	6					
• Ensure you have the correct item or instrument.	5					
• Stand away from sterile field.	5					
• Grasp package flaps and pull apart about halfway.	5					
• Hold package over sterile field with opening down; with quick movement, pull flap completely open and drop sterile item onto field.	5					
POSTPROCEDURE						
7. Apply sterile gloves after sterile field is completed.	6					
8. Assist or perform sterile procedure as required.	6					
9. Clean area and wash hands.	8					
TOTAL POSSIBLE POINTS	**100**					

Comments: _____

_____

_____

_____

_____

_____

_____

_____

Signatures: _____ Date: _____

SCORING   *See Preface for scoring instructions.*

CHAPTER 32

Name _____ Date _____

Dietetics

PROCEDURE LM32-1:
Taking a Diet History

PROCEDURE ASSESSMENT

Procedure Steps	Suggested Points	Self Practice	Peer Practice	Peer Testing	Final Testing	Total Earned
PREPROCEDURE						
1. Have pen or pencil and blank paper or blank diet history form and 24-hour dietary recall form on hand.	4					
• Use these items to record client's answers to your diet history questions and to record usual food intake.	3					
• Bring food models and measuring cups and spoons to interview with client, if possible.						
2. Review client's medical history. Get this information from client's medical chart, a nurse, or the client.	5					
3. Introduce yourself to client and explain why you'll be asking diet questions and how you'll use this information.	5					
PROCEDURE						
Ask the following questions when you take the diet history.						
4. How many meals and snacks does client eat in average day?	4					
5. How many servings does client eat from 4 food groups on most days?	5					
• Grains—breads, cereals, rice, pasta, etc.						
• Fruits—fresh, canned, dried, juices.						
• Vegetables—fresh, canned, frozen, or juice.						
• Dairy products—milk, yogurt, and cheese.						
• Protein foods—meat, poultry, fish, eggs, dried beans and peas, nuts, and seeds.						
6. Does client have any food intolerances or allergies?	4					
7. Does client avoid any specific foods or food groups?	5					
8. Does client have any problems with eating (i.e. chewing, dry mouth).	4					
9. Does client follow special diet prescribed by doctor or dietitian (i.e., low fat or low sodium)?	5					
10. Does client take any medications or vitamins, minerals, or herbal supplements?	5					

Procedure Steps PROCEDURE	Suggested Points	Self Practice	Peer Practice	Peer Testing	Final Testing	Total Earned
11. Where does client obtain food (i.e. home, restaurants)?	4					
12. Does client ever skip meals? If client says yes, ask whether client skips meals for any of these reasons:	4					
• Not enough food or money to buy food.	3					
• No transportation to grocery stores.	3					
• No working appliances (stove or kitchen utensils) to prepare foods.	3					
• No place to store perishable foods (refrigerator or freezer).	3					
• No access to food shelters or congregate meal programs.	3					
13. What is client's level of physical activity?	4					
14. What foods and beverages does client consume, and in what amounts, in a 24-hour period?	5					
POSTPROCEDURE						
15. Review client's answers to diet history questions and clarify answers you don't understand.	5					
16. Review 24-hour dietary recall form if appropriate.	4					
• Count number of servings from each food group.	3					
• Compare results with recommended number of servings from each food group for client's age, gender, and activity level.	3					
• Refer to Chapter 8, "Nutrition," if necessary.						
17. Give information you obtained from diet history and food group evaluation to client's registered dietitian for further evaluation.	4					
TOTAL POSSIBLE POINTS	100					

Comments:

_____

_____

_____

_____

_____

Signatures: _____   Date: _____

SCORING *See Preface for scoring instructions.*

Photo
Credits